Pediatric Medicine: A Clinical Guide

Pediatric Medicine: A Clinical Guide

Editor: Iris Murdock

AMERICAN
MEDICAL PUBLISHERS
www.americanmedicalpublishers.com

AMERICAN
MEDICAL PUBLISHERS
www.americanmedicalpublishers.com

Cataloging-in-Publication Data

Pediatric medicine : a clinical guide / edited by Iris Murdock.
p. cm.
Includes bibliographical references and index.
ISBN 978-1-63927-427-7
1. Pediatrics. 2. Children--Diseases. 3. Children--Diseases--Treatment. I. Murdock, Iris.
RJ45 .P43 2022
618.92--dc23

American Medical Publishers,
41 Flatbush Avenue,
1st Floor, New York,
NY 11217, USA

ISBN 978-1-63927-427-7 (Hardback)

Contents

Preface

Pediatrics is the branch of medicine that is related to the medical care of infants, children and adolescents. Pediatric medicine treats the congenital defects, genetic variance and developmental issues. Pediatric physiology affects the pharmacokinetic properties of drugs entering the body. The absorption, distribution, metabolism and elimination properties of pediatric medicine are different than the medications used by adults. Some of its subspecialties are child neurology, adolescent medicine, neonatology, pediatric radiology, neurocritical care, pediatric dermatology, pediatric surgery, etc. This book presents the complex subject of pediatric medicine in the most comprehensible and easy to understand language. It explores all the important aspects of pediatric medicine in the present day scenario. The book will serve as a valuable source of reference for graduate and postgraduate students.

This book is a comprehensive compilation of works of different researchers from varied parts of the world. It includes valuable experiences of the researchers with the sole objective of providing the readers (learners) with a proper knowledge of the concerned field. This book will be beneficial in evoking inspiration and enhancing the knowledge of the interested readers.

In the end, I would like to extend my heartiest thanks to the authors who worked with great determination on their chapters. I also appreciate the publisher's support in the course of the book. I would also like to deeply acknowledge my family who stood by me as a source of inspiration during the project.

Editor

1

A novel fibrillin-1 gene missense mutation associated with neonatal Marfan syndrome

Qian Peng[1,2,3], Yan Deng[4], Yuan Yang[5] and Hanmin Liu[1,2*]

Abstract

Background: Marfan syndrome (MFS) is a heritable disorder of connective tissue resulting from pathogenic variants of the fibrillin-1 gene (*FBN1*). Neonatal Marfan syndrome (nMFS) is rare and the most severe form of MFS, involving rapidly progressive cardiovascular dysfunction leading to death during early childhood. The constant enrichment of the nMFS mutation spectrum is helpful to improve our understanding of genotype–phenotype correlations in the disease. Herein, we report a novel dominant mutation in exon 26 of *FBN1* (c.3331 T > C) in a sporadic case with nMFS.

Case presentation: An 8-month-old Han Chinese girl presented with the classic nMFS phenotype, including prominent manifestations of bone overgrowth, aortic root dilatation, and multiple cardiac valve dysfunctions. Genetic analysis revealed that she was heterozygous for a *de novo FBN1* missense mutation (c.3331 T > C). The mutation leads to the substitution of a highly conserved FBN1 cysteine residue (p.Cys1111Arg), which is likely to severely perturb the FBN1 structure because of an alteration of the disulfide bond pattern in the calcium-binding epidermal growth factor-like (cbEGF) 12 domain. This variant was absent in 208 ethnically matched controls, providing further evidence that it may be causative of nMFS. An analysis of nMFS-associated mutations from the UMD-FBN1 database indicates that those *de novo* mutations altering disulfide bonds or Ca^{2+} binding sites of the cbEGF domains encoded by exons 25–33, and a lack of phenotypic heterogeneity may be associated with an increased risk for nMFS.

Conclusion: We diagnosed an infant with rare nMFS showing rapidly progressive cardiovascular dysfunction and widely systemic features. As the only causal *FBN1* mutation identified in the patient, the missense mutation c.3331 T > C (p.Cys1111Arg) was associated with the severe phenotype of MFS. However, the pathogenicity of the novel mutation needs further confirmation in other patients with nMFS. Our review of the prominent characteristics of nMFS mutations relative to classic or incomplete MFS-related mutations will be helpful for the recognition of novel nMFS-associated variants.

Keywords: Calcium-binding EGF-like domain, Cysteine substitution, Disulfide bond, *FBN1*, Neonatal Marfan syndrome

* Correspondence: liuhscu@163.com
[1]Department of Pediatric Cardiology, West China Second University Hospital/West China Women's and Children's Hospital, West China School of Medicine, Sichuan University, Chengdu 610041, China
[2]Key Laboratory of Birth Defects and Related Diseases of Women and Children (Sichuan University), Ministry of Education, Chengdu 610041, China

Background

Marfan syndrome (MFS) (OMIM 154700) is an autosomal dominant disorder of fibrous connective tissue involving the ocular, skeletal, and cardiovascular systems. MFS patients present with clinical variability, in which the rare neonatal Marfan syndrome (nMFS) has the most severe presentation in early childhood [1]. The prognosis of nMFS is very poor, with a mean survival age of only 16.3 months [2]. Valvular insufficiencies and diaphragmatic hernias have been associated with shorter survival in patients diagnosed before the age of 1 year [3].

nMFS has been correlated with a limited number of mutations in the neonatal region of the fibrillin-1 gene (*FBN1*) (OMIM 134797) [4–6]. In the UMD-FBN1 mutations database (http://www.umd.be/), a total of 1,318 different *FBN1* mutations for MFS have been included to date, of which only 59 (4.8 %) including 37 missense mutations (2.8 %) are associated with nMFS. Here, we present a novel missense mutation associated with nMFS, which leads to a cysteine substitution in the calcium-binding epidermal growth factor-like (cbEGF) 12 domain of FBN1.

Case presentation

An 8-month-old Han Chinese girl, the only child of her parents, was born full-term weighing 2.60 kg by vaginal delivery. Her father was 32 years old and her mother 26 years old. She was diagnosed with suspected MFS at birth caused by the presence of finger and toe arachnodactyly, elbow and knee flexion contractures, a characteristic 'senile' facial appearance, and loose skin, so was referred to the pediatrician. At the age of 8 days, an x-ray of the bilateral knee and elbow joints showed bone overgrowth with no apparent abnormalities of the joints or bone substance. After that, she received continuous follow-up at the Division of Children's Healthcare, West China Second University Hospital, Chengdu, China. During this period, she was shown to have pectus excavatum, malnutrition, growth retardation, and feeding difficulties, with vitamin D levels at the lower end of normal limits; she was therefore administered vitamin D3 and calcium, although she failed to respond to treatment.

At the age of 6 months, she was admitted to hospital with bronchial pneumonia and then transferred to a pediatric cardiovascular ward because of a newly found grade 2–3 precordium murmur. On physical examination, in addition to malnutrition, she was observed to have a 'senile' facial appearance, loose skin, downslanting palpebral fissures, frontal bossing, downturned corners of the mouth, and skeletal abnormalities including big ears, micrognathia, arachnodactyly, a pectus deformity, pes planus, and dolichocephaly (Additional file 1). X-ray analysis of her bilateral calves showed that the margins of the distal tibial and fibular metaphysis were not smooth, and that the gap around the ankle was blurred. Cardiac enlargement and pectus excavatum were confirmed by computed tomography. Electrocardiography (ECG) suggested a sinus rhythm with abnormal Q waves in I and aVL leads. Echocardiography indicated mitral valve prolapse and regurgitation with a grade 3 insufficiency, tricuspid valve hypertrophy and regurgitation with a grade 1 insufficiency, left atrial chamber enlargement, and aortic root dilatation at the sinuses of Valsalva (23 mm, $Z > 2$) (Fig. 1). Ectopia lentis could not be determined because of the failure of pupils to dilate during several ophthalmologic examinations.

Neither parent had experienced any symptoms similar to those of their daughter, and their ECG examination and echocardiography were normal. According to the revised Ghent criteria for the diagnosis of MFS [7], the detected systemic features (scores) of the present patient included the wrist and thumb sign (3), pectus excavatum (1), pes planus (1), facial features (1), skin striae (1), and mitral valve prolapse (1). These systemic features (score >7) combined with the presentation of severe aortic root dilation ($Z > 2$) resulted in a diagnosis of MFS. After 5 days of antibiotic therapy administered intravenously for bronchial pneumonia, the patient recovered and was discharged. She was advised continuous follow-up at the Pediatric Cardiovascular Division to monitor cardiac function.

At the age of 8 months, the patient presented to the Department of Medical Genetics, West China Hospital, Chengdu, China. Her mother stated that no disease or condition had potentially affected the pregnancy, including hypertension, diabetes, thyroid disease, infection, medication, or toxic exposure. Moreover, the parents are not consanguineous and there is no family history of unexplained disorders or hereditary disease. After informed consent had been obtained, peripheral blood samples of the patient and her parents were collected for genetic testing to identify the causal *FBN1* mutation. All 65 exons of *FBN1* and their splice sites in the patient were sequenced by Sanger sequencing. This identified four variants, including a homozygous synonymous variant in exon 15 (c.1875 T > C, p.Asn625Asn) (rs25458), two heterozygous missense variants in exon 26 (c.3331 T > C, p.Cys1111Arg) (Fig. 1) and exon 27 (c.3442C > G, p.Pro1148Ala) (rs140598), and a heterozygous intronic variant (c.3464-5G > A) (rs11853943).

Total RNA was extracted from buccal epithelial cells and Sanger sequencing of the reverse transcriptase (RT)-PCR product further confirmed the presence of the variant c.3331 T > C. Direct sequencing of parental PCR products showed that substitution c.3331 T > C was absent in both parents, and also from 208 ethnically matched controls without the MFS phenotype. There was no evidence of parental mosaicism of the missense mutation. The patient's mother was found to be homozygous for the c.3442C > G substitution. At this time, an echocardiogram of the patient showed a progression of

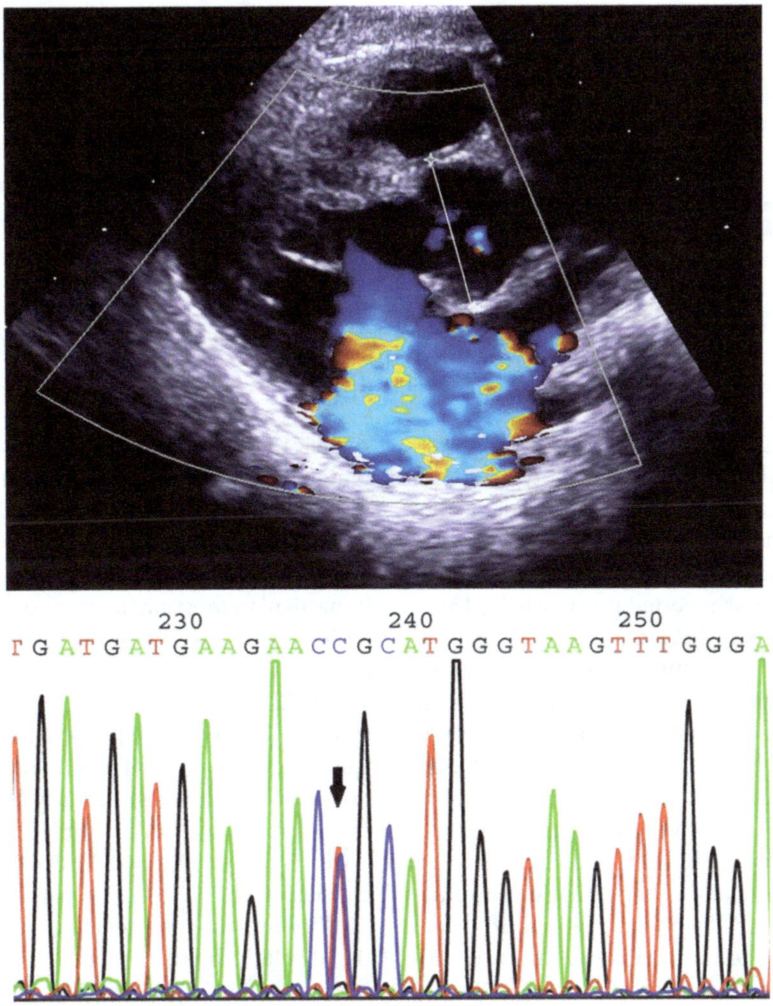

Fig. 1 Echocardiograph showing aortic root dilatation at the sinuses of Valsalva (line in-between two asterisks) and the sequencing result showing the heterozygous missense mutation c.3331 T > C in the patient (arrow)

mitral valve regurgitation with a grade 3–4 insufficiency. She was advised of the possibility of cardiovascular surgery if the severe mitral valve insufficiency led to further ventricular dysfunction. The CARE Checklist of information of the case report is available as Additional file 2.

Discussion

The term neonatal Marfan syndrome was first used in 1991 to describe the most severe phenotype of MFS similar to cases previously known as infantile Marfan syndrome, congenital Marfan syndrome, and severe perinatal Marfan syndrome [1, 8–10]. Recently, it has been suggested that the term neonatal MFS should be replaced by early onset and rapidly progressive MFS to represent the most severe features of MFS in early childhood [11]. Of the 2,088 MFS patients on the UMD-FBN1 mutations database (last update, 28/08/14), only 80 (3.8 %) were recorded as suffering from nMFS, indicating that nMFS is a rare condition relative to classic and incomplete MFS. Its incidence rate is therefore far lower than that estimated for MFS, at 1/5,000–1/10,000 [11]. Although the characteristics of nMFS have been previously discussed [6, 12], there are currently no diagnostic criteria. In combination with systemic manifestations, the identification of *FBN1* mutations responsible for nMFS is helpful for disease diagnosis in the absence of any family history [7].

Our patient carries a *de novo* variant of *FBN1*, c.3331 T > C, which has not been reported previously. This missense substitution affects a cysteine residue in the cbEGF 12 domain (p.Cys1111Arg) of FBN1. Moreover, its absence in more than 200 ethnically matched controls suggested that it is a causative mutation [7]. It is of note that there is another missense mutation in the same codon (c.3332G > A, p.Cys1111Tyr) in the UMD-FBN1 mutations database leading to incomplete MFS. Although phenotypic variation of different mutations in the same codon has been observed

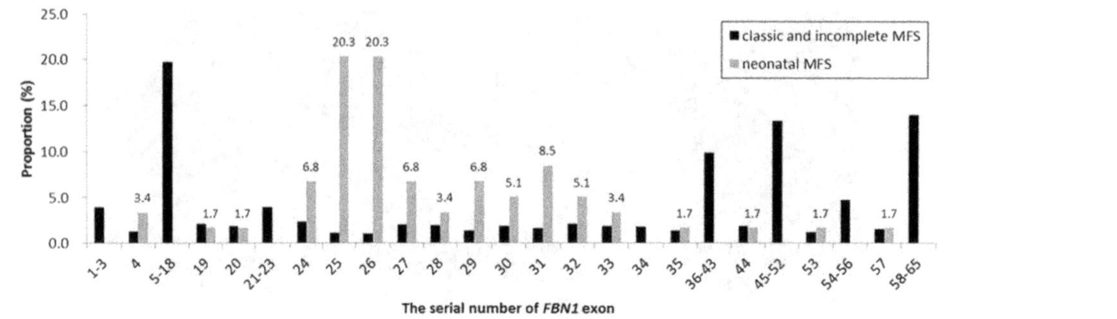

Fig. 2 Different distributions of neonatal and classic or incomplete Marfan syndrome-associated mutations among *FBN1* exons based on the UMD-FBN1 mutations database

in other codons encoding the disulfide bond-related cysteine residue of the cbEGF domain, the phenotypic consequence of the novel mutation in our patient needs further confirmation in other patients with nMFS. The nMFS diagnosis of our patient is supported by the high-degree similarity of clinical features to those reported previously [5, 13].

Most previously identified nMFS-associated *FBN1* mutations are known to cluster between exons 24 and 32, which is the neonatal region of *FBN1* [3, 4, 11, 12]. A recent hypothesis to explain this is that some mutations in the region may cause enhanced proteolytic susceptibility of FBN1 and loss of function for heparin binding, leading to a more severe phenotype relative to other mutations responsible for milder forms of MFS [14]. However, it is still difficult to predict the correlations between a given mutation in the region and the nMFS phenotype [11]. In recent years, more nMFS-causative mutations have been identified which may offer clues for the recognition of others.

Based on information from the UMD-FBN1 mutations database, we have determined a number of characteristics of nMFS-associated mutations compared with those of classic and incomplete MFS. First, 92.3 % (60/65) of nMFS mutations were *de novo*, which is significantly higher than the number of *de novo* classic and incomplete MFS mutations (35.3 %, 417/1,181) (Fisher's exact test, $\alpha = 0.05$; $P < 0.001$). Second, at the genome level, the distribution of the two types of mutations differs among *FBN1* exons (Pearson's χ test, $\alpha = 0.05$; $P < 0.001$); in particular, most nMFS mutations (86.4 %, 51/59) cluster within exons 24–33 while the distribution of mutations for classic and incomplete MFS is more even with only 17.4 % (221/1274) in the exon 24–33 region (Fisher's exact test, $\alpha = 0.05$; $P < 0.001$) (Fig. 2). Third, at the protein level, 91.5 % (54/59) of nMFS mutations are located in cbEGF domains, which is significantly higher than that of mutations for classic and incomplete MFS (71.7 %, 914/1,274) (Fisher's exact test, $\alpha = 0.05$; $P < 0.001$). Within the domain cluster of cbEGFs 11–19 encoded by exons 25–33, 47 nMFS mutations are located, of which 43 (91.5 %) affect the disulfide bond or Ca^{2+} binding site. This compares with only 58.2 % (111/191) of classic and incomplete MFS mutations (Fisher's exact test, $\alpha = 0.05$; $P < 0.001$). An nMFS genotype–phenotype analysis showed that most of the mutations (88.4 %, 52/59) present exclusively in patients with nMFS. Further, of all missense mutations associated with nMFS, only 8.1 % (3/37) also

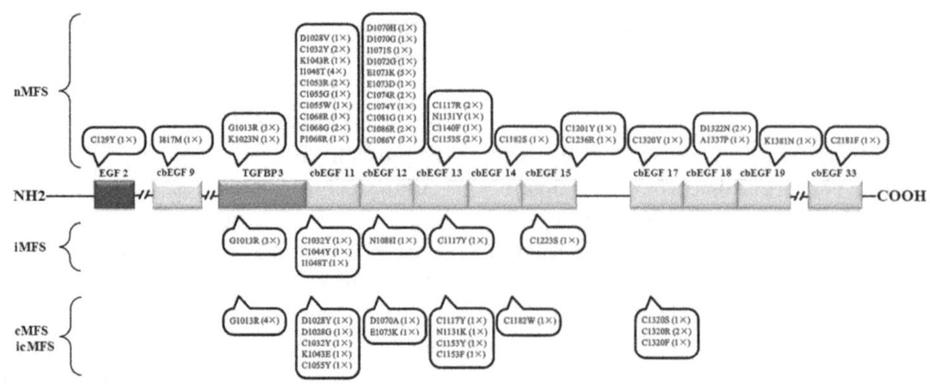

Fig. 3 The location and phenotypic heterogeneity of amino acid substitutions in the FBN1 protein associated with neonatal Marfan syndrome, and the number of such substitutions in patients with MFS based on the UMD-FBN1 mutations database. nMFS, neonatal Marfan syndrome; iMFS, infantile Marfan syndrome; cMFS, classic Marfan syndrome; icMFS, incomplete Marfan syndrome

present in patients with classic or incomplete MFS (Fig. 3). These observations strongly suggest that limited phenotypic heterogeneity of nMFS-associated mutations is evident, although it should not be ignored that some mutations can also result in a later onset or classic presentation of MFS.

A bicuspid aortic valve (BAV) is a common congenital heart abnormality [15] that appears to be associated with mutations in *FBN1* because of the significantly higher frequency of these mutations in affected patients relative to the general population [16, 17]. One of the *FBN1* variants in the current patient, c.3442C > G, has previously been reported to be a pathogenic mutation for BAV [18]. In the present study, the patient was a heterozygote and her mother a homozygote of the variant. However, echocardiography did not reveal BAV in either individual, which does not support causality of this variant for BAV.

Conclusions

The diagnosis of the severe disease nMFS can be aided by identifying known nMFS-causing variants through continuous enrichment of the nMFS mutation spectrum. In the present study, we identified a novel dominant *FBN1* mutation, c.3331 T > C (p.Cys1111Arg), which was associated with the most severe phenotype of MFS. This finding will be helpful for the clinical diagnosis, prenatal diagnosis, and genetic counseling in patients with the same mutation. Our brief review, based on the latest database information, summarized the distinctive features of nMFS-associated mutations relative to mutations for classic and incomplete MFS, which will be valuable for evaluating the pathogenicity of novel *FBN1* variants for nMFS.

Abbreviations

BAV: bicuspid aortic valve; cbEGF: calcium-binding epidermal growth factor-like; ECG: electrocardiograph; *FBN1*: fibrillin-1; nMFS: neonatal marfan syndrome.

Competing interests

The authors declare that they have no competing interests.

Authors' contributions

QP and HL cared for the patient. YD and QP performed echocardiography of the patient and her parents. YY and QP were responsible for genetic testing and counselling. QP drafted the manuscript. HL and YY made critical revisions. All of the authors discussed the content of the manuscript and approved the final version of the manuscript.

Acknowledgments

We are grateful to all study participants including the patient, her parents, and the physicians who provided clinical data. This study was funded by the Science & Technology Department of Sichuan Province (Grand number: 2013sz0040). We thank Edanz (http://www.liwenbianji.cn/) for English editing assistance.

Author details

[1]Department of Pediatric Cardiology, West China Second University Hospital/ West China Women's and Children's Hospital, West China School of Medicine, Sichuan University, Chengdu 610041, China. [2]Key Laboratory of Birth Defects and Related Diseases of Women and Children (Sichuan University), Ministry of Education, Chengdu 610041, China. [3]Department of Pediatrics, Sichuan Academy of Medical Sciences & Sichuan Provincial People's Hospital, Chengdu 610072, China. [4]Department of Cardiovascular Ultrasound and Non-invasive Cardiology, Sichuan Academy of Medical Sciences & Sichuan Provincial People's Hospital, Chengdu 610072, China. [5]Department of Medical Genetics, West China Hospital, West China School of Medicine, Sichuan University, Chengdu 610041, China.

References

1. Buntinx IM, Willems PJ, Spitaels SE, Van Reempst PJ, De Paepe AM, Dumon JE. Neonatal Marfan syndrome with congenital arachnodactyly, flexion contractures, and severe cardiac valve insufficiency. J Med Genet. 1991;28:267–3.
2. Strigl S, Quagebeur JM, Gersony WM. Quadrivalvar replacement in infantile Marfan syndrome. Pediatr Cardiol. 2007;28:403–5.
3. Stheneur C, Faivre L, Collod-Béroud G, Gautier E, Binquet C, Bonithon-Kopp C, et al. Prognosis factors in probands with an FBN1 mutation diagnosed before the age of 1 year. Pediatr Res. 2011;69:265–70.
4. Kainulainen K, Karttunen L, Puhakka L, Sakai L, Peltonen L. Mutations in the fibrillin gene responsible for dominant ectopia lentis and neonatal Marfan syndrome. Nat Genet. 1994;6:64–9.
5. Booms P, Cisler J, Mathews KR. Novel exon skipping mutation in the fibrillin-1 gene: two 'hot spots' for the neonatal Marfan syndrome. Clin Genet. 1999;55:110–7.
6. Dietz HC, Cutting GR, Pyeritz RE, Maslen CL, Sakai LY, Corson GM, et al. Marfan syndrome caused by a recurrent de novo missense mutation in the fibrillin gene. Nature. 1991;352:337–9.
7. Loeys BL, Dietz HC, Braverman AC, Callewaert BL, De Backer J, Devereux RB, et al. The revised Ghent nosology for the Marfan syndrome. J Med Genet. 2010;47:476–85.
8. Morse RP, Rockenmacher S, Pyeritz RE, Sanders SP, Bieber FR, Lin A, et al. Diagnosis and management of infantile marfan syndrome. Pediatrics. 1990;86:888–95.
9. Edwards RH. Congenital Marfan syndrome. Birth Defects Orig Artic Ser. 1975;11:329–31.
10. Gross DM, Robinson LK, Smith LT, Glass N, Rosenberg H, Duvic M. Severe perinatal Marfan syndrome. Pediatrics. 1989;84:83–9.
11. Dietz HC. Marfan Syndrome. 2001 Apr 18 [updated 2014 Jun 12]. In: Pagon RA, Adam MP, Ardinger HH, Wallace SE, Amemiya A, Bean LJH, et al. GeneReviews® [Internet]. Seattle (WA): University of Washington, Seattle; 1993–2015. Available from http://www.ncbi.nlm.nih.gov/books/NBK1335/. Accessed 25 April 2015.
12. Faivre L, Collod-Beroud G, Loeys BL, Child A, Binquet C, Gautier E, et al. Effect of mutation type and location on clinical outcome in 1,013 probands with Marfan syndrome or related phenotypes and FBN1 mutations: an international study. Am J Hum Genet. 2007;81:454–66.
13. Faivre L, Masurel-Paulet A, Collod-Béroud G, Callewaert BL, Child AH, Stheneur C, et al. Clinical and molecular study of 320 children with Marfan syndrome and related type I fibrillinopathies in a series of 1009 probands with pathogenic FBN1 mutations. Pediatrics. 2009;123:391–8.
14. Kirschner R, Hubmacher D, Iyengar G, Kaur J, Fagotto-Kaufmann C, Brömme D, et al. Classical and neonatal Marfan syndrome mutations in fibrillin-1 cause differential protease susceptibilities and protein function. J Biol Chem. 2011; 286:32810–23.
15. Siu SC, Silversides CK. Bicuspid aortic valve disease. J Am Coll Cardiol. 2010; 55:2789–800.
16. Nistri S, Porciani MC, Attanasio M, Abbate R, Gensini GF, Pepe G. Association of Marfan syndrome and bicuspid aortic valve: frequency and outcome. Int J Cardiol. 2012;155:324–5.
17. Pepe G, Nistri S, Giusti B, Sticchi E, Attanasio M, Porciani C, et al. Identification of fibrillin 1 gene mutations in patients with bicuspid aortic valve (BAV) without Marfan syndrome. BMC Med Genet. 2014;15:23.
18. Balakrishnan P, Ganesan K, Bhima Shankar PR, Kabra M. Gene symbol: FBN1. Hum Genet. 2007;120:917.

2

Predicting the severity of dengue fever in children on admission based on clinical features and laboratory indicators

Khansoudaphone Phakhounthong[1], Pimwadee Chaovalit[2], Podjanee Jittamala[1,3], Stuart D. Blacksell[3,4], Michael J. Carter[5], Paul Turner[4,6], Kheng Chheng[6], Soeung Sona[6], Varun Kumar[6], Nicholas P. J. Day[3,4], Lisa J. White[3,4] and Wirichada Pan-ngum[1,3*]

Abstract

Background: Dengue fever is a re-emerging viral disease commonly occurring in tropical and subtropical areas. The clinical features and abnormal laboratory test results of dengue infection are similar to those of other febrile illnesses; hence, its accurate and timely diagnosis for providing appropriate treatment is difficult. Delayed diagnosis may be associated with inappropriate treatment and higher risk of death. Early and correct diagnosis can help improve case management and optimise the use of resources such as hospital staff, beds, and intensive care equipment. The goal of this study was to develop a predictive model to characterise dengue severity based on early clinical and laboratory indicators using data mining and statistical tools.

Methods: We retrieved data from a study of febrile illness in children at Angkor Hospital for Children, Cambodia. Of 1225 febrile episodes recorded, 198 patients were confirmed to have dengue. A classification and regression tree (CART) was used to construct a predictive decision tree for severe dengue, while logistic regression analysis was used to independently quantify the significance of each parameter in the decision tree.

Results: A decision tree algorithm using haematocrit, Glasgow Coma Score, urine protein, creatinine, and platelet count predicted severe dengue with a sensitivity, specificity, and accuracy of 60.5%, 65% and 64.1%, respectively.

Conclusions: The decision tree we describe, using five simple clinical and laboratory indicators, can be used to predict severe cases of dengue among paediatric patients on admission. This algorithm is potentially useful for guiding a patient-monitoring plan and outpatient management of fever in resource-poor settings.

Keywords: Classification tree, Dengue, Severity, Cambodia, Data mining, Children

Background

Dengue fever causes a high burden of disease and mortality across tropical and subtropical regions in Southeast Asia, Africa, the Western Pacific, and the Americas [1]. Dengue virus comprises five serotypes, DENV-1, DENV-2, DENV-3, DENV-4 and DENV-5, which are transmitted by *Aedes aegypti* mosquitoes [2–4]. An estimated 2.5 billion people worldwide are at risk of dengue. More than 50 million dengue infections are estimated to occur annually, of which approximately 500,000 result in hospital admissions for severe dengue in the form of dengue haemorrhagic fever (DHF) or dengue shock syndrome (DSS), principally among children [5].

Dengue infection is frequently confounded with other febrile illnesses (OFI), presenting with non-specific clinical symptoms and clinical features analogous to OFI. During the early stages of dengue, the presence of non-specific febrile illness makes precise diagnosis strikingly

* Correspondence: pan@tropmedres.ac
[1]Department of Tropical Hygiene (Biomedical and Health Informatics), Faculty of Tropical Medicine, Mahidol University, Bangkok, Thailand
[3]Mahidol-Oxford Tropical Medicine Research Unit, Faculty of Tropical Medicine, Mahidol University, Bangkok, Thailand

difficult, resulting in inefficient treatment and possible increases in morbidity and mortality [2, 6]. Severe dengue fever, if not appropriately managed, may lead to rapid death, particularly in children [7, 8]. In addition, the lack of necessary laboratory facilities, particularly in remote, rural areas, may cause difficultly in discriminating dengue infection from OFI [9]. Dengue is one of the most common vector-borne diseases in Southeast Asia, and one of the most important mosquito-borne viral diseases with an epidemic potential in the world [10].

Dengue was first included in Cambodia's national surveillance programme in 1980. Since 2000, between 10,000 and 40,000 dengue cases have been reported annually by the Dengue National Control Program [11], from a total population of approximately 13.5 million people [12]. The true incidence of the burden of disease in Cambodia remains under-reported due to difficulties in diagnosing dengue infection, especially in hospitals [13]. In this study, data from a cohort of children that were admitted with febrile illness to Angkor Hospital for Children, Siem Reap, Cambodia, during a one-year period were retrospectively analysed using a data mining approach. This approach used a classification and regression tree, or CART, which was first introduced by Breiman et al. [14]. This is a common tool used in data mining, which creates a model or algorithm that predicts the value of a target variable based on several input variables. In our study, CART was constructed to predict the severity of dengue infection based on early clinical and laboratory indicators. The model was then evaluated against the final diagnoses.

Methods

Study design and data

We conducted a retrospective study of data derived from an investigation of febrile illness in children ("the fever study") at Angkor Hospital for Children, Cambodia (AHC) [15]. This is a 70-bed children's hospital in Siem Reap province, Cambodia, which provides free, comprehensive healthcare to children aged less than 16 years of age, and includes specialised medical and surgical in-patient and outpatient care. For the fever study, the inclusion criteria were age < 16 years, documented axillary temperature ≥ 38.0 °C within 48 h of admission, and informed consent by a parent or caregiver. Children who developed fever ≥ 48 h after admission or following surgery were excluded since they could be considered as having acquired a healthcare-associated infection [16, 17]. Integrated Management of Childhood Illness (IMCI) was used for the assessment and decision-making on whether to admit a patient to the hospital [18].

Data were collected on admission by clinicians using a specific case report form. Admission blood samples and, where possible, a convalescent serology sample taken on discharge, or seven days after admission, were taken for IgM antibody and NS1 antigen testing. All admitted patients were reviewed twice daily for eligibility and data collection quality. Data were collected between 12th October 2009 and 12th October 2010 from patients who were admitted to AHC.

Dengue diagnosis was based on the following laboratory diagnostic methods: 1) DENV NS1 antigen ELISA (Standard Diagnostics, Korea) to detect dengue-specific antigen in serum samples, 2) Panbio Japanese encephalitis virus (JEV) and dengue IgM Combo ELISA (Standard Diagnostics, Korea) was used to detect anti-JEV- and anti-DENV-specific IgM antibodies in serum samples, and 3) Dengue IgM capture ELISA (Venture Technologies, Malaysia) was used to detect anti-JEV- and anti-DENV-specific IgM antibodies in cerebrospinal fluid (CSF) specimens [15].

Patients were classified as having dengue virus infection if NS1 antigen was detected in their serum by ELISA, or if paired sera from acute and convalescent time points (≥7 days following the acute sample) showed rising or static anti-dengue IgM (and anti-dengue IgM was greater than anti-Japanese encephalitis IgM) [15]. NS1 antigen and IgM antibody results were combined in a Boolean manner using AND/OR operators to ensure that the entire temporal spectrum of patient presentations during the acute phase of dengue infection were covered, with NS1 antigen present in the serum in the early phase of infection and dengue IgM antibodies usually present after 2–5 days of infection [19]. The ratio of anti-dengue to anti-JEV IgM levels was used to determine if the infection was dengue or Japanese encephalitis virus, whose antibodies often have some cross-reactivity when co-circulating in the same area. Children less than 60 days old were not tested for dengue virus infection.

All confirmed dengue cases were further categorised as either severe or non-severe dengue. From our literature review we noted that, although the revised 2009 WHO classification was said to be an improvement on the 1997 WHO classification, there was still a need for training, dissemination of relevant information, and further research on the warning signs of severe dengue [20]. The classification was also considered by many to be too broad, requiring more specific definitions of the warning signs [21], that it increased the workload for health care personnel, and was not simple or user-friendly enough [22]. In our study we categorised dengue cases as severe based on a two–step process. The first step was to take into account all confirmed dengue cases with intensive care unit (ICU) admission, together with the 2009 WHO dengue classification. Secondly, two independent paediatricians' assessments were considered to a) exclude any ICU-admitted cases that might not have had severe dengue as their primary diagnosis and b) to include any non-ICU-admitted cases which may have actually presented with severe dengue but were not admitted for some reason, usually because of resource limitations. Grading the disease severity in these patients was challenging because only the early clinical presentation of dengue and limited laboratory indicators were available on admission i.e. the first recorded haematocrit, platelet counts, white blood cell (WBC) counts, urea, creatinine, and alanine aminotransferase (ALT) results, and the presence of urinary protein or red blood cells (RBC). The results of chest X-rays were not available to evaluate pleural effusion, nor were results of abdominal ultrasound available for the detection of peritoneal fluid (ascites). The presence of bleeding was not assessed other than by examining stool samples for blood. The case-by-case assessment and verification by the two clinicians was used as the reference for the predictive model.

Data analysis and construction of a predictive model

The demographics and clinical characteristics of severe and non-severe dengue cases were described using the mean ± standard deviation (SD) if the data were normally distributed, or by median and range otherwise. Comparisons between the two groups were performed using the Student's *t*-test for continuous variables if the data were normally distributed, otherwise the Mann–Whitney *U* test was used. A chi-square test was used for categorical data. A p value < 0.05 was considered significant. A classification and regression tree (CART) was constructed for predicting the severity of dengue cases based on their early clinical features and laboratory indicators on admission. The J48 algorithm was used for generating decision trees because it is able to handle nominal, categorical and numerical data, as well as missing values. The loss matrix was specified to differently weight misdiagnoses. In this study we assigned five times greater weight to false negatives when compared with false positives, i.e. the cost of misdiagnosing a patient with severe dengue was five times greater than a non-severe case being misdiagnosed as severe. Pruning and tuning parameters were applied to optimise the predictive model by avoiding an over-complex tree, and thus increasing the model's accuracy. The 10-fold cross-validation function provided by Weka was used to estimate the out-of-sample accuracy, given the constraint on data availability and avoiding the over-fitting issue. Put simply, it split the data set into ten partitions, nine of which were for training, with one partition for testing. The tree model was built on the training set, and applied to the testing set. To reduce variability, multiple rounds of cross-validation were performed using different partitions, and the validation results were combined over the rounds to estimate the model's performance [23].

Once the final tree was obtained, the significance of each predictive factor was then quantified through multiple logistic regression with the 'enter' method of selection (i.e. all variables were included in the model) and reported as an odds ratio (OR) and 95% confidence interval (95% CI). Descriptive analysis and multiple logistic regression were performed using the Statistical Package for the Social Sciences (SPSS) software, version 18.0 (SPSS, Inc., Chicago, IL, USA), and the CART was constructed with Weka, version 3.6.10 (University of Waikato, New Zealand).

Parameterisation

Before data mining algorithms can be used, a target data set must be assembled and pre-processed, which involves cleaning, removing, grouping, and transforming the data. There were 24 variables originally available for the analysis. However, three variables were excluded from the analysis i.e. tourniquet test result was with more than 15% missing data points where as pulse rate and respiratory rate were age-dependent parameters. The latter ones were excluded from the analysis since they would not be practical to refer to if presented in the final model. For other variables with fewer than 15% missing values, the missing values were imputed using a one-by-one single imputation approach. The advantage of the imputation method over the tree-based mining algorithm within CART [24] is that it separates the missing data problem from the prediction problem, allowing different predictive modelling methods to be applied to the imputed data set [25]. In our study, some missing values were imputed with a single value, including the mean value for some variables (number of days of fever, capillary refill time, Glasgow Coma Score, and urea result) and the median value for others (haematocrit, creatinine, ALT, respiratory rate of infant, urinary protein and RBC, and WBC, neutrophil, lymphocyte, and platelet counts).

Results

There were 3225 patient admissions during the study year, of which 1361 (42.2%) met the inclusion criteria. Of these, 136 (10.0%) were not enrolled, leaving 1225 febrile episodes in 1180 children, with 1144 children having a single episode, 31 children having two episodes, one child having three episodes, and four children having four episodes. The patients were mainly diagnosed as having lower respiratory tract infection (38.3%), undifferentiated fever (25.5%), or diarrhoeal disease (19.5%) [15]. Out of 1180 enrolled children, there were 69 deaths, the causes of which were: clinical pneumonia with no organism/virus identified (12 cases, 27.5%), dengue virus infection (eleven cases, including one with co-existent melioidosis, two with co-existent scrub typhus, and four with co-existent clinical pneumonia, 15.9%), and melioidosis (four cases, 5.8%). 941 non-dengue episodes and 86 episodes with no samples available were excluded from this analysis. Further details can be found in the original report [15].

Out of 198 confirmed dengue episodes, 43 episodes required ICU admission, with 29 of those classified as severe dengue based on their clinical signs, supported by two independent clinical opinions. Nine additional severe dengue episodes were included from non-ICU admissions, making a total of 38 episodes of severe dengue. There were eleven in-hospital deaths amongst all ICU-admitted patients with dengue virus infection, however dengue was the primary diagnosis in just five of these. Therefore, only these five cases were included in the severe dengue group. The flowchart of the study is shown in Fig. 1.

Clinical features, including blood in the stool, liver enlargement, ICU admission, number of days in ICU, low or high haematocrit, low or high WBC count, high creatinine, high urea, low platelet count, rapid pulse, rapid respiratory rate, low Glasgow Coma Score (GCS), pleural effusion (only one case), abdominal pain, urinary protein, urinary RBC, and high ALT, were considered on a case-by-case basis when clinicians classified dengue as severe or non-severe. The clinical features and laboratory indicators of the 38 severe dengue cases are shown in Table 1. The three most common features among patients with severe disease were ICU admission (76.3%), rapid respiratory rate (81.5%), and rapid pulse (65.7%). Severe dengue was more prevalent in children aged less than five years old. Vomiting and abdominal pain were significantly more common in the severe dengue group, as were rapid pulse and respiratory rate, increased capillary refill time, and low GCS. A significantly higher proportion of patients with severe dengue presented with a lower haematocrit, higher WBC and lymphocyte count, higher ALT level, together with the presence of urinary RBC (Table 2).

The final decision tree algorithm included five clinical and laboratory parameters: haematocrit, GCS, urinary protein, creatinine, and platelet count. The sensitivity and specificity of the model were 60.5% and 65%, respectively (Fig. 2). The accuracy of the model was 64.1%, where the clinical diagnosis was used as the reference value. The area under the receiver operating characteristic (ROC) curve for logistic regression was 0.616. The final decision tree was then restructured using logistic regression analysis to estimate the impact of each CART-selected variable as represented by the OR and 95% CI.

Table 3 gives the estimated OR for each parameter selected by CART. Low haematocrit, low GCS, low platelet count, presence of urine protein, and high creatinine increased the probability of a diagnosis of severe dengue, with significant OR ranging from 1.47 to 13.73. The parameters that were statistically associated with severe dengue were 1) low haematocrit (OR = 7.114, 95% CI = 3.00–16.87, $p < 0.001$) and 2) low GCS (OR = 13.73, 95% CI = 3.46–54.50, $p < 0.001$). Although low platelet count (OR = 2.33, 95% CI = 0.95–5.76), presence of urine protein (OR = 1.83, 95% CI = 0.78–4.32) and increased

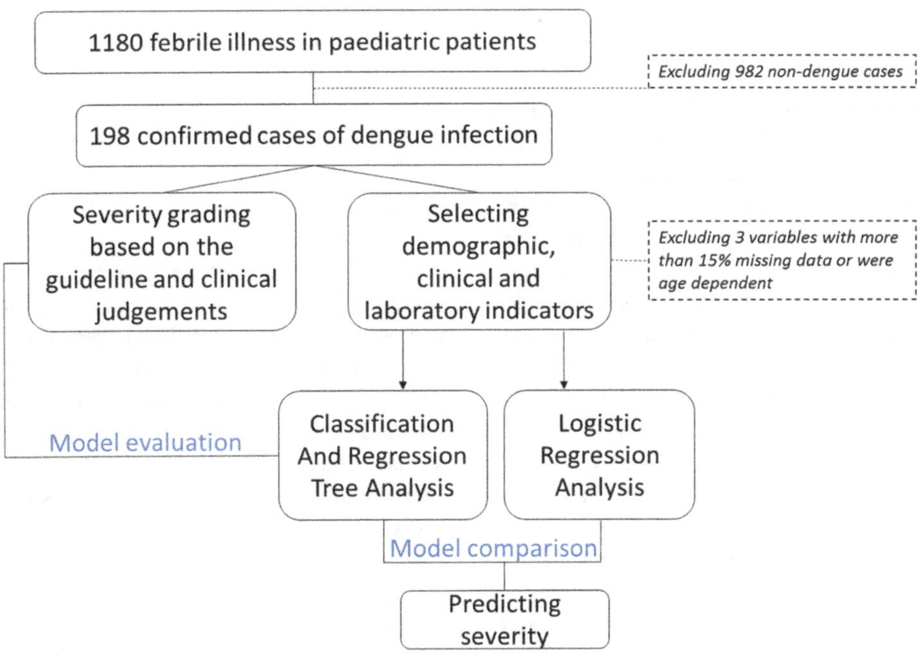

Fig. 1 The flowchart of the study. Boxes show the total number of patients enrolled in the study, reasons for exclusion from the analysis, model construction and evaluation

Table 1 Clinical features and laboratory indicators of 38 severe dengue cases based on the 2009 WHO dengue classification

Factor	N (%)
ICU admission	29 (76.3)
Average number of ICU days	4.6 days
Vomiting	15 (39.4)
Blood in stool	8 (21)
Rapid respiratory rate	31 (81.5)
Rapid pulse	25 (65.7)
Liver enlargement	22 (57.8)
Abdominal pain	9 (23.6)
Low WBC count	10 (26.3)
High WBC count	13 (34.2)
Low haematocrit	22 (57.8)
High haematocrit	3 (7.8)
Low platelet count	12 (31.5)
Low Glasgow Coma Scale	8 (21)
High urea	9 (23.6)
High creatinine	21 (55.2)
ALT > 1000	2 (5.2)
Urine protein > 100	5 (13.1)
Urine red blood cells	12 (31.5)
Death	5 (13)

Table 2 Clinical manifestations of 198 patients with dengue infection, including 38 with severe disease

Variables	Non-severe ($n = 160$)	Severe ($n = 38$)	p value
Demographics			
Male (n, %)	84 (52.5)	23 (60.5)	0.372
Age: 28 days to 1 year (n, %)	40 (25.0)	16 (42.1)	
≥ 1 year to < 5 years	45 (28.1)	14 (36.8)	0.012
≥ 5 years to < 16 years	75 (46.9)	8 (21.1)	
History/symptoms			
Number of days of fever	4.31	4.10	0.683
Vomiting (n, %)	94 (58.7)	15 (39.4)	0.032
Abdominal pain (n, %)	75 (46.8)	9 (23.6)	0.012
Headache or retro-orbital pain (n, %)	63 (39.3)	8 (21)	0.101
Clinical parameters			
Rash (n, %)	18 (11.2)	1 (2.6)	0.153
Temperature (°C)	38.76	38.63	0.234
Pulse/min	131.49	152.26	< 0.001
Capillary refill time	2.03	2.24	0.001
Respiratory rate	38.40	46.42	0.002
Liver enlargement (n, %)	64 (40.0)	22 (57.8)	0.127
Glasgow Coma Score	14.60	13.42	0.003
Laboratory parameters			
Haematocrit (%)	32.56	28.84	0.004
Platelets (per 10^3/μl)	267.87	294.16	0.477
White blood cells (per10^3/μl)	9.46	14.25	0.006
Neutrophils	5.64	8.01	0.46
Lymphocytes	2.76	5.14	< 0.001
Urea (mmol/L)	4.64	4.95	0.712
Creatinine (μmol/l)	68.29	68.71	0.932
Alanine transaminase, IU/l	78.99	177.08	0.002
Urine protein mg/dL	12.34	24.13	0.088
Urine red blood cells	2.84	10.32	0.009

serum creatinine (OR = 1.47, 95% CI = 0.51–4.25) were associated with an increased risk of severity, they were not shown to be statistically significant by regression analysis (Table 3).

Discussion

Using a data mining approach, we have developed an algorithm using both simple clinical manifestations and laboratory indicators to predict the severity of dengue during the early phase of the illness. The final algorithm for predicting severe dengue (Fig. 2) comprised six components in order of their significance. The most significant factor in predicting severe dengue was low haematocrit, followed by a GCS of 11 or below as the second split if haematocrit was greater than 28, the presence of urine protein and creatinine above 84 μmol/l as the third split if GCS was above 11, and finally a platelet count of 146,000 per mm^3 or less as the final split, if the presence of urine protein and creatinine was below 84 μmol/l.

Comparing the algorithm we derived with those reported in previous studies, we found both similarities and differences. Potts et al. constructed decision algorithms for predicting dengue shock syndrome (DSS) or dengue with significant pleural effusion [26]. The algorithm achieved a high sensitivity of 97%. Both low haematocrit and platelet counts were also identified as predictive factors in their work, although the cut-off values used in our algorithm were more extreme, i.e. for haematocrit ≤ 28 vs. ≤ 40, and for platelet count ≤ 146,000 vs. ≤ 160,200. The mechanism by which thrombocytopaenia is caused by dengue virus is complex [27]. Previous studies suggest that the virus probably contributes to bone marrow suppression and platelet destruction [28, 29]. To meet the WHO guidelines for classifying patients with DHF, thrombocytopaenia (platelet count ≤ 100,000) is required. Srikiatkhachorn et al. demonstrated that thrombocytopaenia was related to dengue severity and that not all severe cases would have been classified as DHF according to the WHO criteria [30]. Although thrombocytopaenia suggests that dengue infection is severe, a low platelet

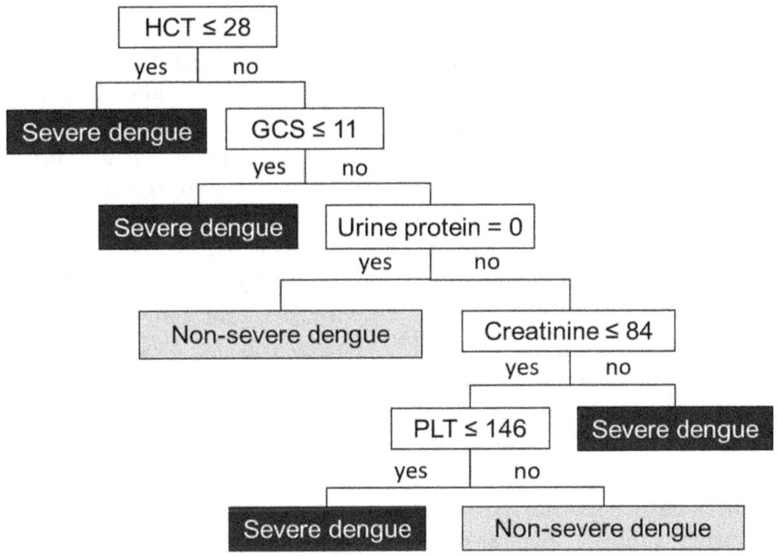

Fig. 2 Clinical decision tree to distinguish severe dengue from all cases of dengue (HCT = haematocrit, GCS = Glasgow Coma Score, PLT = platelets)

count is also common among OFI such as malaria and scrub typhus [31]. The 1997 WHO definition of DHF stated that a low platelet count (≤ 100,000), together with an increased haematocrit of ≥ 20% above the baseline value, is indicative of plasma leakage. In contrast, our results and those of Potts et al. suggested a drop in haematocrit as a sign of severity, especially among patients with internal bleeding in areas such as the gastrointestinal tract [26]. Our results also suggested a more extreme haematocrit value compared with the previous study (28% vs 40%) [27]. Although Potts et al. identified WBC count and monocyte percentage as important, our analysis did not identify monocyte results as significant even when included in the decision tree algorithm. In addition, Potts et al. evaluated predictors for DSS and dengue with significant pleural effusion, whereas in our study severe dengue was differentiated based on clinical features and laboratory indicators.

Table 3 Output from logistic regression using the decision tree algorithm to predict severe dengue infection

Variable	OR	95% CI		*p* value
		Lower	Upper	
Haematocrit (> 28%)	1			
Haematocrit (≤ 28%)	7.114	3.000	16.869	< 0.001
Glasgow Coma Score (> 11)	1			
Glasgow Coma Score (≤ 11)	13.731	3.460	54.501	< 0.001
No urine protein	1			
Urine protein	1.832	0.777	4.319	0.167
Creatinine (≤ 84 μmol/l)	1			
Creatinine (> 84 μmol/l)	1.471	0.509	4.247	0.476
Platelets (> 146 × 10^3/μl)	1			
Platelets (≤ 146 × 10^3/μl)	2.334	0.946	5.763	0.066

Another recent study, by Tamibmaniam et al., used simple logistic regression and identified three parameters, including vomiting, pleural effusion, and low systolic blood pressure, to predict severe dengue based on the 2009 WHO criteria [32]. This study did not specifically focus on children and included only female patients. The sensitivity and specificity achieved in its decision algorithm were 81% and 54%, respectively. Of the three parameters they identified, vomiting was the only parameter available in our study, and although it initially appeared to be significant in the severe group, it was not selected for the final tree.

Despite using a similar approach to predict somewhat similar outcomes to the aforementioned studies, we identified additional parameters that related to the severity of dengue, including GCS, urine protein, and serum creatinine. There are a number of possible explanations for these differences, as outlined below.

GCS is used to measure the level of consciousness (mental status changes) [33]. In our results, the node with GCS ≤ 11 (considered to be moderate) in the model was significant. Rao et al. showed that patients with dengue encephalitis had a GCS of 7–8 and recommended intubation and mechanical ventilator support during their hospitalisation [34].

Previous studies in which urine protein was associated with DHF or DSS used the urine protein-to-creatinine ratio [35, 36], but we used only a urine dipstick for this measure. The presence of urine protein in severe dengue could be due to plasma leakage.

An increased serum creatinine level indicates kidney dysfunction. In patients with DHF, a mild increase in serum creatinine is common, in contrast to the higher levels seen in severe dengue cases. Our model showed that a serum creatinine level > 84 mmol/l (4.6 mg/dl) was associated with severe dengue, a value similar to that found in Thai paediatric patients with DHF, whose mean serum creatinine was 4.9 mg/dl. That analysis also showed that 24 of 25 patients with acute kidney injury (AKI) had DSS as a final diagnosis. Of the 25 patients with DHF-associated AKI, 16 (64%) died as a result of profound shock, together with other conditions such as liver failure, respiratory failure, and severe bleeding [37]. Studies in adults have reported an AKI incidence of 14.2% among dengue patients, and those with AKI saw significant morbidity and mortality, longer hospital stays, and poor renal outcomes [38]. Early diagnosis of dengue infection, known clinical and laboratory characteristics and risk factors together with early detection of AKI using appropriate criteria [39], and monitoring for warning signs of severe dengue, are essential if AKI and other complications are to be avoided [40].

Although the two sets of WHO criteria from 1997 and 2009 are still debatable in terms of their ability to appropriately differentiate dengue from OFI and to classify disease severity [20–22, 41, 42], the problem is compounded by a lack of key data in resource-poor settings, making it difficult to apply the criteria. For instance, we lacked information on clinical bleeding sites, and were only able to detect gastrointestinal bleeding based on stool examinations. In addition, there was a lack of information on blood pressure or narrow pulse pressure to indicate whether a patient was in shock [43], no data on restlessness suggestive of circulatory failure, and no chest X-ray results to evaluate pleural effusion or abdominal ultrasound to detect ascites, both of which are important for identifying plasma leakage. The 1997 and 2009 WHO dengue guidelines also include a tourniquet test as a diagnostic tool for dengue in the early febrile phrase. However, the tourniquet test has been shown to have low sensitivity for dengue diagnosis, such that a negative result does not exclude dengue infection [44–46]. The tourniquet test had not been performed for the majority of patients in our data set and was thus not included in the analysis.

Regarding the two approaches used in this study, CART versus the more conventional approach of logistic regression, some points are worth mentioning here. Firstly, our main focus was on building the decision tree model from CART analysis. CART is non-parametric, and can manipulate numerical data which may be highly skewed, multi-modal, ordinal or non-ordinal in structure. CART is not significantly impacted by outliers in the input variables. The output of CART in the form of a decision tree is easy to follow and gives some visual information on the hierarchical importance of the variables from the top to the bottom of the tree, although calculating the importance matrices of the predictors in CART is not straightforward. In this study, therefore, we quantified the importance of each decision tree predictor via the odds ratio as calculated by logistic regression. Secondly, the ways in which the decision boundaries are generated in the two approaches are different. While the logistic regression generates a single boundary, a decision tree essentially partitions the data space into half-spaces using axis-aligned linear decision boundaries, giving a non-linear decision boundary. Either approach may be more applicable depending on the setting. Finally, the model's accuracy was measured in different ways for each of the two approaches. For the decision tree model, the out-of-sample accuracy was estimated via cross-validation, i.e. the 10-fold cross-validation function in Weka allowed us to conveniently perform the cross-validation and directly report the model's accuracy. For the logistic regression, however, the model's accuracy was estimated from the classification table, which showed the number of observed against predicted outcomes, using a default cut-off value of 0.5 for the predicted probability. For all of the above reasons, it would have been difficult to compare the relative merits of the two methods used in our study.

There were several limitations with regard to the data-set used for this study. Firstly, the data came from just one hospital, a further indicator of the poor resources in the Southeast Asia region where dengue is endemic. Secondly, due to the lack of IgG antibody results it was not possible to interpret whether cases were primary or secondary dengue infections. This information could potentially be a useful early indicator for the severity of a dengue infection. Thirdly, the algorithm was derived from data collected within 48 h of admission among children aged less than 16 years old. If the model were to be used for older patients or in different regions, some adjustments to it may be necessary.

Although the cohort of 198 patients with confirmed dengue was relatively small, with an even smaller subset of just 38 severe dengue cases, the simple model we derived is still likely to be useful because it includes a small number of predictive variables that would probably be available in similar settings. In addition, a previous study by Carter et al. showed that the DENV rapid diagnostic test (RDT) had low sensitivity for the diagnosis of dengue infection [47]. However, the development of diagnostic tests for dengue has advanced rapidly. The NS1 test in particular has become widely available in many resource-limited settings. It is simple to use and has acceptable accuracy. If rapid diagnosis of dengue using

NS1 can be achieved, our algorithm would prove very useful. This also highlights the importance of children attending for testing as soon as dengue is suspected, because NS1 detection is optimal during the first seven days of infection. The algorithm will become more relevant and useful as the rapid diagnosis of dengue becomes more common. By using our simple algorithm to help identify and predict severe dengue, we believe that there would be more room to focus on other, more serious bacterial diseases, which are all-too-common in these types of resource-poor settings.

Conclusions

Our decision tree algorithm using simple clinical and laboratory indicators has a moderate classification accuracy for predicting the development of severe dengue fever among paediatric patients with confirmed DENV infection. The model demonstrates the importance of haematocrit and platelet levels for monitoring the severity of dengue, as indicated by the WHO criteria and previous studies. Our algorithm offers simple indicators for severity, including haematocrit, GCS, urine protein, creatinine, and platelet count, all of which are measured on admission. This model is potentially useful for guiding inpatient monitoring and outpatient management of fever cases. The model does require further validation against other datasets from cohort studies conducted in a variety of settings, with the goal of establishing a universal algorithm for guiding clinical management of severe dengue in resource-limited settings.

Abbreviations

AHC: Angkor Hospital for Children; AKI: Acute kidney injury; ALT: Alanine aminotransferase; CART: Classification and regression tree; CI: Confidence interval; DHF: Dengue haemorrhagic fever; DSS: Dengue shock syndrome; GCS: Glasgow Coma Score; ICU: Intensive care unit; JEV: Japanese encephalitis virus; OFI: Other febrile illnesses; OR: Odds ratio; WBC: White blood cells

Acknowledgements

We wish to thank all staff from the Department of Tropical Hygiene, Faculty of Tropical Medicine, Mahidol University, and Professor Paul Newton from Wellcome Trust - Mahosot Hospital - Oxford Tropical Medicine Research, Lao PDR for their support with this study.

Funding

This study was part of the Wellcome Trust Major Overseas Programme in SE Asia (grant number 106698/Z/14/Z).

Authors' contributions

KP, PC and WP contributed to the conception and design of the study. SB, MC, PT, KC, SS, VK and ND coordinated with Angkor Hospital for Children to obtain data and helped with the pre-processing of data. KP and WP drafted texts of this study. PC, PJ, SB and LW critically revised the manuscript for important intellectual content. All authors have read and approved the final manuscript.

Competing interests

The authors declare that they have no competing interests.

Author details

[1]Department of Tropical Hygiene (Biomedical and Health Informatics), Faculty of Tropical Medicine, Mahidol University, Bangkok, Thailand. [2]National Electronics and Computer Technology Center (NECTEC), Bangkok, Thailand. [3]Mahidol-Oxford Tropical Medicine Research Unit, Faculty of Tropical Medicine, Mahidol University, Bangkok, Thailand. [4]Centre for Tropical Medicine and Global Health, Nuffield Department of Medicine, University of Oxford, Oxford, UK. [5]Institute of Child Health, University College London, London, UK. [6]Angkor Hospital for Children, Siem Reap, Cambodia.

References

1. Tantawichien T. Dengue fever and dengue haemorrhagic fever in adolescents and adults. Paediatrics and international child health. 2012;32(Suppl 1):22–7.
2. Tanner L, Schreiber M, Low JG, Ong A, Tolfvenstam T, Lai YL, Ng LC, Leo YS, Thi Puong L, Vasudevan SG, et al. Decision tree algorithms predict the diagnosis and outcome of dengue fever in the early phase of illness. PLoS Negl Trop Dis. 2008;2(3):e196.
3. Normile D. Tropical medicine. Surprising new dengue virus throws a spanner in disease control efforts. Science (New York, NY). 2013;342(6157):415.
4. Dwivedi VD, Tripathi IP, Tripathi RC, Bharadwaj S, Mishra SK. Genomics, proteomics and evolution of dengue virus. Briefings in functional genomics. 2017;16(4):217–27.
5. Guzman MG, Halstead SB, Artsob H, Buchy P, Farrar J, Gubler DJ, Hunsperger E, Kroeger A, Margolis HS, Martinez E, et al. Dengue: a continuing global threat. Nat Rev Microbiol. 2010;8(12 Suppl):S7–16.
6. Manock SR, Jacobsen KH, de Bravo NB, Russell KL, Negrete M, Olson JG, Sanchez JL, Blair PJ, Smalligan RD, Quist BK, et al. Etiology of acute undifferentiated febrile illness in the Amazon basin of Ecuador. Am J Trop Med Hyg. 2009;81(1):146–51.
7. Huy R, Buchy P, Conan A, Ngan C, Ong S, Ali R, Duong V, Yit S, Ung S, Te V, et al. National dengue surveillance in Cambodia 1980-2008: epidemiological and virological trends and the impact of vector control. Bull World Health Organ. 2010;88(9):650–7.
8. Sam SS, Omar SF, Teoh BT, Abd-Jamil J, AbuBakar S. Review of dengue hemorrhagic fever fatal cases seen among adults: a retrospective study. PLoS Negl Trop Dis. 2013;7(5):e2194.
9. Potts JA, Thomas SJ, Srikiatkhachorn A, Supradish PO, Li W, Nisalak A, Nimmannitya S, Endy TP, Libraty DH, Gibbons RV, et al. Classification of dengue illness based on readily available laboratory data. Am J Trop Med Hyg. 2010;83(4):781–8.
10. WHO. World health organization:a global brief on vector-borne diseases. Geneva: World Health Organization; 2014.
11. Duong V, Henn MR, Simmons C, Ngan C, Y B, Gavotte L, Viari A, Ong S, Huy R, Lennon NJ, et al. Complex dynamic of dengue virus serotypes 2 and 3 in Cambodia following series of climate disasters. Infection, genetics and evolution : journal of molecular epidemiology and evolutionary genetics in infectious diseases 2013, 15:77–86.
12. National Institute of Statistics, Ministry of Planning Phnom Penh, Cambodia. General Population Census of Cambodia 2008. Cambodia: National Institute of Statistics, Ministry of Planning Phnom Penh, Cambodia; 2008.
13. Vong S, Goyet S, Ly S, Ngan C, Huy R, Duong V, Wichmann O, Letson GW, Margolis HS, Buchy P. Under-recognition and reporting of dengue in Cambodia: a capture-recapture analysis of the National Dengue Surveillance System. Epidemiol Infect. 2012;140(3):491–9.
14. L Breiman J Friedman, CJ. Stone, R.A. Olshen: Classification and regression trees, illustrated, reprint, revised edn: Taylor & Francis, 1984; 1984.
15. Chheng K, Carter MJ, Emary K, Chanpheaktra N, Moore CE, Stoesser N, Putchhat H, Sona S, Reaksmey S, Kitsutani P, et al. A prospective study of the causes of febrile illness requiring hospitalization in children in Cambodia. PLoS One. 2013;8(4):e60634.

16. Collins AS. Preventing health care-associated infections. In: Hughes RG, editor. Patient safety and quality: an evidence-based handbook for nurses. Rockville (MD): Agency for Healthcare Research and Quality; 2008.
17. Revelas A. Healthcare - associated infections: a public health problem. Niger Med J. 2012;53(2):59–64.
18. Handbook WHO: Integrated management of childhood illness. World Health Organization: 2005.
19. Blacksell SD. Commercial dengue rapid diagnostic tests for point-of-care application: recent evaluations and future needs? J Biomed Biotechnol. 2012;2012:151967.
20. Barniol J, Gaczkowski R, Barbato EV, da Cunha RV, Salgado D, Martinez E, Segarra CS, Pleites Sandoval EB, Mishra A, Laksono IS, et al. Usefulness and applicability of the revised dengue case classification by disease: multi-centre study in 18 countries. BMC Infect Dis. 2011;11:106.
21. Hadinegoro SR. The revised WHO dengue case classification: does the system need to be modified? Paediatrics and international child health. 2012;32(Suppl 1):33–8.
22. Kalayanarooj S. Dengue classification: current WHO vs. the newly suggested classification for better clinical application? Journal of the Medical Association of Thailand = Chotmaihet thangphaet. 2011;94(Suppl 3):S74–84.
23. Seni G, Elder J. Ensemble Methods in Data Mining: Improving Accuracy Through Combining Predictions. Morgan & Claypool; 2010.
24. Feelders A. Handling missing data in trees: Surrogate splits or statistical imputation? Principles of Data Mining and Knowledge Discovery 1999, 1704. Springer Berlin Heidelberg.
25. Cevallos Valdiviezo H, Van Aelst S: Tree-based prediction on incomplete data using imputation or surrogate decisions. ELSEVIER, Information Sciences 2015, 311:163–181.
26. Potts JA, Gibbons RV, Rothman AL, Srikiatkhachorn A, Thomas SJ, Supradish PO, Lemon SC, Libraty DH, Green S, Kalayanarooj S. Prediction of dengue disease severity among pediatric Thai patients using early clinical laboratory indicators. PLoS Negl Trop Dis. 2010;4(8):e769.
27. Chuansumrit A: Pathophysiology and management of dengue hemorrhagic fever. 2006:3–11. Blackwell Publishing.
28. Lei HY, Yeh TM, Liu HS, Lin YS, Chen SH, Liu CC. Immunopathogenesis of dengue virus infection. J Biomed Sci. 2001;8(5):377–88.
29. Hottz E. Platelets in dengue infection. Drug Discovery Today. 2011;8(No. 1-2):e33-e38. Elsevier.
30. Srikiatkhachorn A, Gibbons RV, Green S, Libraty DH, Thomas SJ, Endy TP, Vaughn DW, Nisalak A, Ennis FA, Rothman AL, et al. Dengue hemorrhagic fever: the sensitivity and specificity of the world health organization definition for identification of severe cases of dengue in Thailand, 1994-2005. Clinical infectious diseases : an official publication of the Infectious Diseases Society of America. 2010;50(8):1135–43.
31. Chadwick D, Arch B, Wilder-Smith A, Paton N. Distinguishing dengue fever from other infections on the basis of simple clinical and laboratory features: application of logistic regression analysis. Journal of clinical virology : the official publication of the Pan American Society for Clinical Virology. 2006;35(2):147–53.
32. Tamibmaniam J, Hussin N, Cheah WK, Ng KS, Muninathan P. Proposal of a clinical decision tree algorithm using factors associated with severe dengue infection. PLoS One. 2016;11(8):e0161696.
33. The TD. Clinical features of dengue in a large Vietnamese cohort: Instrinsically lower platelet counts and greater risk for bleeding in adults than children. 2012;6(6):e1679. PLOS Neglected Tropical Diseases.
34. Rao SM. Internal Medicine Inside. Herbert Open Access Journals; 2013.
35. Khan MI, Anwar E, Agha A, Hassanien NS, Ullah E, Syed IA, Raja A. Factors predicting severe dengue in patients with dengue fever. Mediterranean journal of hematology and infectious diseases. 2013;5(1):e2013014.
36. Vasanwala FF, Puvanendran R, Fook-Chong S, Ng JM, Suhail SM, Lee KH. Could peak proteinuria determine whether patient with dengue fever develop dengue hemorrhagic/dengue shock syndrome?–a prospective cohort study. BMC Infect Dis. 2011;11:212.
37. Laoprasopwattana K, Pruekprasert P, Dissaneewate P, Geater A, Vachvanichsanong P. Outcome of dengue hemorrhagic fever-caused acute kidney injury in Thai children. J Pediatr. 2010;157(2):303 9.
38. Mallhi TH, Khan AH, Adnan AS, Sarriff A, Khan YH, Jummaat F. Incidence, characteristics and risk factors of acute kidney injury among dengue patients: a retrospective analysis. PLoS One. 2015;10(9):e0138465.
39. Mallhi TH, Sarriff A, Adnan AS, Khan YH, Hamzah AA, Jummaat F, Khan AH. Dengue-induced acute kidney injury (DAKI): a neglected and fatal complication of dengue viral infection–a systematic review. J Coll Physicians Surg Pak. 2015;25(11):828–34.
40. Oliveira JF, Burdmann EA. Dengue-associated acute kidney injury. Clin Kidney J. 2015;8(6):681–5.
41. Gan VC, Lye DC, Thein TL, Dimatatac F, Tan AS, Leo YS. Implications of discordance in world health organization 1997 and 2009 dengue classifications in adult dengue. PLoS One. 2013;8(4):e60946.
42. Basuki PS, Budiyanto, Puspitasari D, Husada D, Darmowandowo W, Ismoedijanto SS, Yamanaka A. Application of revised dengue classification criteria as a severity marker of dengue viral infection in Indonesia. The Southeast Asian journal of tropical medicine and public health. 2010;41(5):1088–94.
43. WHO. World Health Organization:Dengue guidelines for diagnosis, treatment, prevention and control. In: Dengue: Guidelines for Diagnosis, Treatment, Prevention and Control, New Edition. edn. Geneva edn. Geneva: World Health Organization; 2009.
44. Cao XT, Ngo TN, Wills B, Kneen R, Nguyen TT, Ta TT, Tran TT, Doan TK, Solomon T, Simpson JA, et al. Evaluation of the World Health Organization standard tourniquet test and a modified tourniquet test in the diagnosis of dengue infection in Viet Nam. Tropical medicine & international health : TM & IH. 2002;7(2):125–32.
45. Hammond SN, Balmaseda A, Perez L, Tellez Y, Saborio SI, Mercado JC, Videa E, Rodriguez Y, Perez MA, Cuadra R, et al. Differences in dengue severity in infants, children, and adults in a 3-year hospital-based study in Nicaragua. The American journal of tropical medicine and hygiene. 2005;73(6):1063–70.
46. Mayxay M, Phetsouvanh R, Moore CE, Chansamouth V, Vongsouvath M, Sisouphone S, Vongphachanh P, Thaojaikong T, Thongpaseuth S, Phongmany S, et al. Predictive diagnostic value of the tourniquet test for the diagnosis of dengue infection in adults. Tropical medicine & international health : TM & IH. 2011;16(1):127–33.
47. Carter MJ, Emary KR, Moore CE, Parry CM, Sona S, Putchhat H, Reaksmey S, Chanpheaktra N, Stoesser N, Dobson AD, et al. Rapid diagnostic tests for dengue virus infection in febrile Cambodian children: diagnostic accuracy and incorporation into diagnostic algorithms. PLoS Negl Trop Dis. 2015;9(2):e0003424.

3

Health-related quality of life of the parents of children hospitalized due to acute rotavirus infection

Gunta Laizane[1*], Anda Kivite[2], Inese Stars[2], Marita Cikovska[1], Ilze Grope[1] and Dace Gardovska[1]

Abstract

Background: Rotavirus is the leading cause of severe diarrhea in young children and infants worldwide, representing a heavy public health burden. Limited information is available regarding the impact of rotavirus gastroenteritis on the quality of life of affected children and their families.

The objectives of study were to estimate the impact of rotavirus infection on health-related quality of life (HRQL), to assess the social and emotional effects on the families of affected children.

Methods: This study enrolled all ($n = 527$) RotaStrip®-positive (with further PCR detection) cases (0–18 years of age) hospitalized from April 2013 to December 2015 and their caregivers. A questionnaire comprising clinical (filled-in by the medical staff) and social (filled by the caregivers) sections was completed per child.

Results: Main indicators of emotional burden reported by caregivers were compassion (reported as severe/very severe by 91.1% of parents), worry (85.2%), stress/anxiety (68.0%). Regarding social burden, 79.3% of caregivers reported the need to introduce changes into their daily routine due to rotavirus infection of their child. Regarding economic burden, 55.1% of parents needed to take days off work because of their child's sickness, and 76.1% of parents reported additional expenditures in the family's budget.

Objective measures of their child's health status were not associated with HRQL of the family, as were the parent's subjective evaluation of their child's health and some sociodemographic factors. Parents were significantly more worried if their child was tearful ($p = 0.006$) or irritable ($p < 0.001$). Parents were more stressful/anxious if their child had a fever ($p = 0.003$), was tearful ($p < 0.001$), or was irritable ($p < 0.001$). Changes in parents' daily routines were more often reported if the child had a fever ($p = 0.02$) or insufficient fluid intake ($p = 0.04$).

Conclusion: Objective health status of the child did not influence the emotional, social or economic burden, whereas the parents' subjective perception of the child's health status and sociodemographic characteristics, were influential. A better understanding of how acute episodes affect the child and family, will help to ease parental fears and advise parents on the characteristics of rotavirus infection and the optimal care of an infected child.

Keywords: Rotavirus gastroenteritis, Health-related quality of life, Latvia, Childhood, Acute, Impact, Family

* Correspondence: lgunta@inbox.lv
[1]Department of Paediatrics, Riga Stradins University, Vienibas gatve 45, Riga LV-1004, Latvia

Background

Rotavirus is known to be the leading cause of severe gastroenteritis among infants and young children worldwide [1]. Rotavirus gastroenteritis is frequently associated with severe disease symptoms (vomiting, diarrhea, dehydration, etc.) and increased hospitalization episodes compared to other types of acute gastroenteritis caused by infectious agents [2].

Rotavirus gastroenteritis represents a heavy public health burden [3]. From 2010 to 2015, an average of 3000 registered rotavirus cases per year are reported in the age group of 0–6 years, being responsible for an average of approximately 1000 hospitalizations per year in Latvia [4].

The epidemiology of rotavirus gastroenteritis is well documented [5], but these data are not the only indicators of disease burden. Limited information is available regarding the impact of rotavirus gastroenteritis on the quality of life of affected children and their families [5].

Health-related quality of life (HRQL) refers to the subjective and objective impact of dysfunction associated with an illness or injury, medical treatment, and health care policy [6] and integrates physical, emotional and social well-being and functioning as perceived by the individual [7]. In pediatric research, HRQL measure has received an increasing attention and is recognized as a substantial health outcome [8]. Pediatric HRQL research is necessary to examine broader psychosocial outcomes and provide an in-depth understanding of the effects of disease and treatment on children's health status [9]. Nerveless, this measure is primarily used in children with various chronic diseases [8].

In the case of pediatric disease, assessment of HRQL of the family is becoming increasingly important because a child's illness affects the whole family as a holistic system. Studies in this area provide information on family needs, responses to the child's disease, coping strategies and changes in family functioning. Most studies are related to childhood chronic diseases, such as congenital heart disease [7], bleeding disorders [10], atopic dermatitis [11], attention deficit/hyperactivity disorder [12], chronic kidney disease [13], and juvenile idiopathic arthritis [14], etc., in association with the quality of family life because of the long-term progression of such diseases and their impact on quality of life.

Less information is available regarding associations between temporary health conditions, such as acute rotavirus gastroenteritis, and HRQL. However, as childhood rotavirus gastroenteritis is a public health problem, it should be evaluated beyond clinical trials with respect to the psychological, social and economic consequences of the disease.

Studies that evaluated the effect of acute childhood rotavirus gastroenteritis on the family have revealed negative effects on family function and parental psycho-emotional wellbeing [5, 15–17]. Parents indicated economic impact, such as lost work days lost due to the child's disease [5] and additional direct costs [17], disruption of schedules and restrictions on daily activities [15–17], high distress and worries due to symptoms [5, 15–17], exhaustion and helplessness [16], need for additional childcare and the use of more nappies [5].

The aim of this study was to estimate the impact of rotavirus infection on HRQL and to assess the social and emotional impacts on the families of affected children. In addition, the factors associated with HRQL characteristics will be clarified.

This article reports the family impact of rotavirus gastroenteritis requiring hospitalization of a child based on individual interviews with parents or legal caregivers and objective data from patient files.

Methods

Study design

To investigate the quality of life of families where child is suffering from acute rotavirus infection, a quantitative cross-sectional study was carried out among caregivers of children who had been hospitalized in the Children's Clinical University Hospital in Riga from April 2013 to December 2015.

Inclusion and exclusion criteria

The study enrolled all hospital cases of rotavirus-positive children (0–18 years of age) and their caregivers (parents or legal family representatives). Caregivers had to be willing to participate and provide written consent. As exclusion criteria included the absence of caregivers or caregivers not providing signed consent.

Data collection

Parents, of the laboratory confirmed rotavirus positive children, were invited to participate in individual interviews. The interviewer collected data regarding the clinical status of the child from patient files, and interviewed parents about emotional, social and economic factors pertaining to their child affecting their daily lives. All results and answers were collated in a questionnaire.

Instruments used

A questionnaire was developed to estimate the impact of rotavirus infection on parents of affected children.

The questionnaire consisted of two general parts: clinical (filled-in by the medical staff) and social (filled by the caregivers) parts. The clinical part posed questions regarding the demographic data of the patient and family, and objective and subjective signs and symptoms to determine the clinical severity of the case. To categorize clinical severity, the Vesikari score [18] was used. The social part of the questionnaire was developed based on concepts and research methods used in previous similar studies [5, 15–17] and covered the following domains of the impact of pediatric rotavirus on the family: 1) parental emotional wellbeing and feelings (distress; helplessness; mental exhaustion; worry; anxiety for the child; fear of being infected; feelings of guilt); 2) social burden of disease (or the disease impact on parents' daily activities (work schedule, training plans (syllabus), leisure time activities, domestic works (household)); 3) economic burden of the disease (working days lost due to child disease, additional financial expenditures); 4) parental opinion about the child's physical symptoms (diarrhea, vomiting, fever, abdominal pain, dehydration, loss of appetite) and changes in behavior (apathy, sleeping disorders, irritability, anxiety); 5) parental opinion about rotavirus vaccine use (awareness of vaccine existence (yes/no); use of vaccine (yes/no; if answered "no", the parents were asked about their motives for refusal).

Five-hundred twenty-seven hospitalized RotaStrip®-positive subjects further confirmed by PCR were enrolled in the study from April 2013 to December 2015. Totally 3301 hospitalized cases were registered from 2013 to 2015. As all enrolled patients were rotavirus-positive, the study did not have a rotavirus negative control group, but that can be considered in future research.

Statistical analysis

Descriptive statistics such as means for continuous variables and proportions for categorical variables were calculated. To evaluate the statistical significance of the differences of proportions of severe/very severe cases between subgroups, a Chi-square test or Fisher's exact test were used. Statistical significance was set at $p = 0.05$.

Data processing was performed using IBM SPSS Statistics (Statistical Package for the Social Science, Version 22.0).

Results

Demographic characteristics of study subjects and their parents

The characteristics of the subjects and their parents are summarized in Table 1 (uploaded as separate file). The children's mean age was 26.1 months, and the sex ratio was balanced between male and female subjects. The majority of responding parents where in the 25–34 year-old age group. Collected data on education levels revealed that majority of mothers had a higher education; among fathers - persons with secondary/vocational education and a higher education were equally represented. Most respondents had a stable social status, and were living in urban areas. Low income citizens are defined by Cabinet of Ministers of Latvia by regulation No.299. It determines that citizens with total monthly income less than 128.06 EUR per family member, can obtain status of low income person, and may apply for social support. Others have stable social status [19].

Table 1 Demographic and clinical characteristics of the study subjects and their parents ($n = 527^a$)

Parameter	Number	Percent
Age of the child (months)		
Mean (range)	26.1 (1–209)	
≤ 12	156	29.7
13–24	168	31.9
25–36	89	16.9
≥ 37	113	21.5
Gender of the child		
Female	258	49.0
Male	269	51.0
Age of the mother (years)		
≤ 24	55	10.5
25–34	335	63.8
35–44	127	24.2
≥ 45	8	1.5
Age of the father (years)		
≤ 24	27	5.3
25–34	281	55.1
35–44	164	32.2
≥ 45	38	7.5
Education of mother		
Primary	29	5.6
Secondary/vocational	189	36.2
Higher	304	58.2
Education of father		
Primary	36	7.2
Secondary/vocational	245	48.7
Higher	222	44.1
Place of residence		
Urban	449	87.2
Rural	66	12.8
Social status		
Low-income	28	5.4
Socially stable	491	94.6

[a]The sum of the stratified numbers can differ according to the parameters due to missing values

Objective and subjective appraisal of child's health status

Clinical symptoms were categorized as severe according to the Vesikari score [18] in 93% patients ($n = 463$) and moderate in 7% ($n = 35$); no mild cases were detected. The objective and subjective appraisals of the health status of the included children are summarized in Table 2 (uploaded as separate file). Three symptoms most often notified by parents as very severe were diarrhea (mentioned by 53.6% ($n = 280$) of parents), insufficient fluid intake (49.6%, $n = 259$) and loss of appetite (41.5%, $n = 215$).

Table 2 Objective and subjective appraisal of the child's health status ($n = 527^a$)

Parameter	Number	Percent
Maximal number of vomiting episodes per day		
Mean (range)	2.1 (0–3)	
Number of diarrhea episodes per 24 h		
Mean (range)	2.5 (1–3)	
Severity (assessed by Vesikari score)		
Mild	0	0
Moderate	35	7.0
Severe	463	93.0
Severity of symptoms (assessed by parent)		
Diarrhea		
Not at all	16	3.1
Mild	17	3.3
Moderate	77	14.8
Severe	132	25.3
Very severe	280	53.6
Vomiting		
Not at all	82	15.7
Mild	61	11.7
Moderate	87	16.7
Severe	111	21.3
Very severe	181	34.7
Fever		
Not at all	78	15.0
Mild	65	12.5
Moderate	110	21.2
Severe	109	21.0
Very severe	158	30.4
Abdominal pain		
Not at all	92	18.1
Mild	71	14.0
Moderate	135	26.6
Severe	108	21.3
Very severe	102	20.1
Insufficient fluid intake		
Not at all	40	7.7
Mild	34	6.5
Moderate	84	16.1
Severe	105	20.1
Very severe	259	49.6
Loss of appetite		
Not at all	45	8.7

Table 2 Objective and subjective appraisal of the child's health status ($n = 527^a$) *(Continued)*

Parameter	Number	Percent
Mild	44	8.5
Moderate	106	20.1
Severe	108	20.5
Very severe	215	41.5
Apathy		
Not at all	43	8.4
Mild	42	8.2
Moderate	106	20.6
Severe	139	27.0
Very severe	184	35.8
Inflamed bottom		
Not at all	203	39.2
Mild	81	15.6
Moderate	87	16.8
Severe	67	12.9
Very severe	80	15.4
Interrupted sleep mode		
Not at all	167	32.2
Mild	94	18.1
Moderate	121	23.3
Severe	82	15.8
Very severe	55	10.6
Tearfulness		
Not at all	78	15.0
Mild	75	14.4
Moderate	153	29.4
Severe	131	25.2
Very severe	83	16.0
Anxiety, irritability		
Not at all	124	23.9
Mild	95	18.3
Moderate	121	23.4
Severe	104	20.1
Very severe	74	14.3

[a]The sum of the stratified numbers can differ according to the parameters due to missing values

Assessment of emotional, social and economic impact of the disease on the family quality of life

Emotional, social, and economic impact of the disease is summarized in Table 3 (uploaded as separate file). Speaking about emotional burden of rotavirus infection - a very high level of compassion was found, mentioned as very severe in 76.4% ($n = 402$) of questionnaires, followed by a very high level of worry in 59.6% ($n = 311$) of cases and stress/anxiety (37.8% ($n = 199$) of cases). Social burden was analyzed by

Table 3 Assessment of emotional, social and economic impact of the disease on the family quality of life ($n = 527^a$)

Parameter	Number	Percent
Emotional burden		
Stress, anxiety		
Not at all	15	2.9
Mild	46	8.7
Moderate	112	21.3
Severe	154	29.3
Very severe	199	37.8
Helplessness, despair		
Not at all	108	20.6
Mild	77	14.7
Moderate	130	24.8
Severe	95	18.1
Very severe	114	21.8
Exhaustion		
Not at all	55	10.5
Mild	62	11.8
Moderate	149	28.4
Severe	110	21.0
Very severe	148	28.2
Worry		
Not at all	10	1.9
Mild	18	3.4
Moderate	53	10.2
Severe	130	24.9
Very severe	311	59.6
Compassion		
Not at all	8	1.5
Mild	4	0.8
Moderate	30	5.7
Severe	82	15.6
Very severe	402	76.4
Fear to get infected		
Not at all	265	50.4
Mild	91	17.3
Moderate	75	14.3
Severe	44	8.4
Very severe	51	9.7
Guilt		
Not at all	199	38.0
Mild	82	15.6
Moderate	94	17.9
Severe	60	11.5
Very severe	89	17.0

Table 3 Assessment of emotional, social and economic impact of the disease on the family quality of life ($n = 527^a$) *(Continued)*

Parameter	Number	Percent
Social burden		
Changes in daily routine		
Yes	413	79.0
No	110	21.0
Economic burden		
Days off work		
None	173	33.1
1–2	117	22.4
3–4	96	18.4
5+	76	14.5
Not employed	61	11.7
Other expenditures		
Yes	380	75.2
No	125	24.8

[a]The sum of the stratified numbers can differ according to the parameters due to missing values

changes in daily routines, and the analyzed data showed that 79.0% ($n = 413$) of families had changes in their daily routine. Economic impact was analyzed by describing parental work day loss directly related to episodes of their child's illness. It revealed that only 33.1% ($n = 173$) of parents did not need to take any days off work. Additionally - 75.2% ($n = 380$) of respondents had extra expenditures due to the disease (symptomatic drugs, diapers, etc.).

Factors associated with the impact of the disease on the family quality of life

To evaluate the emotional burden of the disease, the three most common indicators of emotional burden were chosen for the further analysis, i.e., compassion, worry and stress/anxiety. To better perceive and interpret the data for further analysis the categories "severe" and "very severe" were combined, and the categories "mild" and "not at all" were combined.

In Table 4 (uploaded as separate file) the independent factors (sociodemographic, subjective and objective health status indicators) associated with the emotional burden of the disease are summarized.

None of the sociodemographic factors showed a significant association with the indicators of emotional burden of rotavirus infection. The only factor showing a significant association with compassion was education of the father, i.e., fathers with higher education corresponded to a higher proportion reporting high or very high levels of compassion ($p = 0.01$).

None of the indicators of emotional burden showed a statistically significant association with the objective health status variables as well as with most of the subjective

Table 4 Emotional burden (stress/anxiety, worry, compassion) of the disease stratified by the associated factors ($n = 527^{a}$)

Factor	Not at all / mild		Moderate		Severe / very severe		*p*
	Number	%	Number	%	Number	%	
STRESS / ANXIETY							
Sociodemographic factors							
Gender							
Female	33	12.8	46	17.9	178	69.3	0.16
Male	28	10.4	66	24.5	175	65.1	
Age							
≤ 12 months	15	9.6	37	23.7	104	66.7	0.24
13–24 months	16	9.5	34	20.2	118	70.2	
25–36 months	9	10.2	21	23.9	58	65.9	
37+ months	21	18.6	20	17.7	72	63.7	
Age of the mother							
≤ 24 years	5	9.1	12	21.8	38	69.1	0.78
25–34 years	35	10.4	73	21.8	227	67.8	
35–44 years	20	15.9	24	19.0	82	65.1	
45+ years	1	12.5	2	25.0	5	62.5	
Age of the father							
≤ 24 years	2	7.4	7	25.9	18	66.7	0.99
25–34 years	35	12.5	59	21.0	187	65.5	
35–44 years	19	11.6	35	21.3	110	67.1	
45+ years	4	10.8	8	21.6	25	67.6	
Education of the mother							
Primary	4	13.8	5	17.2	20	69.0	0.95
Secondary / vocational	23	12.2	38	20.1	128	67.7	
Higher	34	11.2	67	22.1	202	66.7	
Education of the father							
Primary	7	19.4	6	16.7	23	63.9	0.57
Secondary / vocational	25	10.2	55	22.5	164	67.2	
Higher	28	12.6	47	21.2	147	66.2	
Family structure							
Both parents	58	11.8	106	21.6	327	66.6	0.20
Single parent	1	3.6	4	14.3	23	82.1	
Place of residence							
Urban	55	12.3	96	21.4	297	66.3	0.74
Rural	6	9.1	14	21.2	46	69.7	
Objective evaluation of the health status							
Vomiting (times per 24 h)							
0	1	33.3	0	0	2	66.7	0.36
1	12	12.4	18	18.6	67	69.1	
2	28	12.4	58	25.7	140	61.9	
3	18	10.8	30	18.0	119	71.3	
Diarrhea (times per 24 h)							
1	9	14.3	12	19.0	42	66.7	0.95

Table 4 Emotional burden (stress/anxiety, worry, compassion) of the disease stratified by the associated factors ($n = 527^{a}$) *(Continued)*

Factor	Not at all / mild		Moderate		Severe / very severe		*p*
	Number	%	Number	%	Number	%	
2	13	10.6	27	22.0	83	67.5	
3	37	11.9	68	21.8	207	66.3	
Severity of episode (Vesikari)							
Moderate	4	11.4	6	17.1	25	71.4	0.79
Severe / very severe	55	11.9	101	21.9	306	66.2	
Subjective evaluation of the health status							
Severity of diarrhea							
Not at all / mild	5	15.2	5	15.2	23	69.7	0.41
Moderate	13	17.1	17	22.4	46	60.5	
Severe / very severe	43	10.4	89	21.6	280	68.0	
Severity of vomiting							
Not at all / mild	15	10.5	35	24.5	93	65.0	0.33
Moderate	6	6.9	21	24.1	60	69.0	
Severe / very severe	40	13.7	56	19.2	195	67.0	
Severity of fever							
Not at all / mild	22	15.4	44	30.8	77	53.8	0.003
Moderate	10	9.2	22	20.2	77	70.6	
Severe / very severe	29	10.9	45	16.9	193	72.3	
Severity of abdominal pain							
Not at all / mild	24	14.7	34	20.9	105	64.4	0.61
Moderate	14	10.4	32	23.9	88	65.7	
Severe / very severe	21	10.0	44	21.0	145	69.0	
Severity of insufficient fluid intake							
Not at all / mild	8	10.8	16	21.6	50	67.6	0.74
Moderate	11	13.1	22	26.2	51	60.7	
Severe / very severe	42	11.6	73	20.1	248	68.3	
Severity of loss of appetite							
Not at all / mild	13	14.6	19	21.3	57	64.0	0.07
Moderate	9	8.5	33	31.1	64	60.4	
Severe / very severe	39	12.1	59	18.3	224	69.6	
Severity of apathy							
Not at all / mild	7	8.2	20	23.5	58	68.2	0.37
Moderate	17	16.0	25	23.6	64	60.4	
Severe / very severe	36	11.2	64	19.9	222	68.9	
Severity of inflamed bottom							
Not at all / mild	38	13.4	66	23.2	180	63.4	0.35
Moderate	10	11.6	14	16.3	62	72.1	
Severe / very severe	13	8.8	30	20.4	104	70.7	
Severity of interrupted sleep mode							
Not at all / mild	36	13.8	54	20.8	170	65.4	0.19

Table 4 Emotional burden (stress/anxiety, worry, compassion) of the disease stratified by the associated factors ($n = 527^{a}$) *(Continued)*

Factor	Not at all / mild		Moderate		Severe / very severe		p
	Number	%	Number	%	Number	%	
Moderate	14	11.6	32	26.4	75	62.0	
Severe / very severe	11	8.0	25	18.2	101	73.7	
Severity of tearfulness							
Not at all / mild	35	22.9	30	19.6	88	57.5	< 0.001
Moderate	12	7.9	43	28.3	97	63.8	
Severe / very severe	14	6.5	39	18.2	161	75.2	
Severity of anxiety / irritability							
Not at all / mild	44	20.2	47	21.6	127	58.3	< 0.001
Moderate	9	7.4	36	29.8	76	62.8	
Severe / very severe	8	4.5	27	15.2	143	80.3	
WORRY							
Sociodemographic factors							
Gender							
Female	12	4.7	20	7.8	224	87.5	0.16
Male	16	6.0	33	12.4	217	81.6	
Age							
≤ 12 months	6	3.9	16	10.4	132	85.7	0.12
13–24 months	6	3.6	15	8.9	147	87.5	
25–36 months	5	5.7	6	6.9	76	87.4	
37+ months	11	9.8	16	14.3	85	75.9	
Age of mother							
≤ 24 years	4	7.3	1	1.8	50	90.9	0.21
25–34 years	15	4.5	35	10.5	283	85.0	
35–44 years	9	7.3	14	11.3	101	81.5	
45+ years	0	0	2	25.0	6	75.0	
Age of father							
≤ 24 years	1	3.7	1	3.7	25	92.6	0.81
25–34 years	15	5.4	27	9.6	238	85.0	
35–44 years	9	5.6	18	11.1	135	83.3	
45+ years	1	2.8	5	13.9	30	83.3	
Education of mother							
Primary	0	0	2	6.9	27	93.1	0.58
Secondary / vocational	11	5.9	16	8.6	159	85.5	
Higher	17	5.6	33	10.9	252	83.4	
Education of father							
Primary	3	8.3	0	0	33	91.7	0.30
Secondary / vocational	12	5.0	26	10.8	203	84.2	
Higher	11	5.0	24	10.9	186	84.2	
Family structure							
Both parents	26	5.3	49	10.0	413	84.6	0.92
Single parent	1	3.6	3	10.7	24	85.7	
Place of residence							

Table 4 Emotional burden (stress/anxiety, worry, compassion) of the disease stratified by the associated factors ($n = 527^a$) *(Continued)*

Factor	Not at all / mild		Moderate		Severe / very severe		*p*
	Number	%	Number	%	Number	%	
Urban	25	5.6	48	10.8	372	83.6	0.27
Rural	3	4.6	3	4.6	59	90.8	
Objective evaluation of the health status							
Vomiting (times per 24 h)							
0	1	33.3	0	0	2	66.7	0.21
1	6	6.3	6	6.3	84	87.5	
2	11	4.9	26	11.6	187	83.5	
3	6	3.6	19	11.4	141	84.9	
Diarrhea (times per 24 h)							
1	6	9.5	3	4.8	54	85.7	0.13
2	5	4.1	10	8.1	108	87.8	
3	13	4.2	38	12.3	257	83.4	
Severity of episode (Vesikari)							
Moderate	2	5.7	2	5.7	31	88.6	0.64
Severe / very severe	22	4.8	49	10.7	387	84.5	
Subjective evaluation of the health status							
Severity of diarrhea							
Not at all / mild	2	6.1	5	15.2	26	78.8	0.07
Moderate	9	11.8	6	7.9	61	80.3	
Severe / very severe	17	4.2	41	10.0	350	85.8	
Severity of vomiting							
Not at all / mild	7	4.9	13	9.2	122	85.9	0.09
Moderate	1	1.1	14	16.1	72	82.8	
Severe / very severe	20	6.9	25	8.7	243	84.4	
Severity of fever							
Not at all / mild	11	7.8	13	9.2	117	83.0	0.14
Moderate	5	4.6	17	15.7	86	79.6	
Severe / very severe	12	4.5	22	8.3	232	87.2	
Severity of abdominal pain							
Not at all / mild	13	8.0	18	11.0	132	81.0	0.34
Moderate	8	6.1	14	10.7	109	83.2	
Severe / very severe	7	3.3	19	9.1	183	87.6	
Severity of insufficient fluid intake							
Not at all / mild	5	6.8	6	8.1	63	85.1	0.89
Moderate	3	3.6	9	10.7	72	85.7	
Severe / very severe	20	5.6	37	10.3	302	84.1	
Severity of loss of appetite							
Not at all / mild	5	5.6	9	10.1	75	84.3	0.57
Moderate	3	2.9	14	13.5	87	83.7	
Severe / very severe	19	5.9	29	9.0	273	85.0	

Table 4 Emotional burden (stress/anxiety, worry, compassion) of the disease stratified by the associated factors (n = 527[a]) *(Continued)*

Factor	Not at all / mild		Moderate		Severe / very severe		p
	Number	%	Number	%	Number	%	
Severity of apathy							
Not at all / mild	1	1.2	12	14.3	71	84.5	0.24
Moderate	7	6.6	12	11.3	87	82.1	
Severe / very severe	19	5.9	28	8.8	273	85.3	
Severity of inflamed bottom							
Not at all / mild	20	7.1	34	12.0	229	80.9	0.13
Moderate	4	4.7	5	5.8	77	89.5	
Severe / very severe	4	2.8	13	9.0	128	88.3	
Severity of interrupted sleep mode							
Not at all / mild	19	7.4	26	10.1	213	82.6	0.33
Moderate	5	4.2	14	11.7	101	84.2	
Severe / very severe	4	2.9	12	8.8	121	88.3	
Severity of tearfulness							
Not at all / mild	16	10.5	19	12.5	117	77.0	0.006
Moderate	6	4.0	16	10.6	129	85.4	
Severe / very severe	6	2.8	16	7.5	191	89.7	
Severity of anxiety / irritability							
Not at all / mild	21	9.7	26	12.0	170	78.3	< 0.001
Moderate	2	1.7	19	15.8	99	82.5	
Severe / very severe	5	2.8	7	4.0	165	93.2	
COMPASSION							
Sociodemographic factors							
Gender							
Female	3	1.2	15	5.8	239	93.0	0.25
Male	9	3.3	15	5.6	245	91.1	
Age							
≤ 12 months	3	1.9	4	2.6	149	95.5	0.21
13–24 months	6	3.6	9	5.4	153	91.1	
25–36 months	1	1.1	6	6.8	81	92.0	
37+ months	2	1.8	11	9.7	100	88.5	
Age of mother							
≤ 24 years	1	1.8	1	1.8	53	96.4	0.68
25–34 years	8	2.4	17	5.1	310	92.5	
35–44 years	3	2.4	10	7.9	113	89.7	
45+ years	0	0	1	12.5	7	87.5	
Age of father							
≤ 24 years	0	0	1	3.7	26	96.3	0.43
25–34 years	7	2.5	11	3.9	263	93.6	
35–44 years	5	3.0	11	6.7	148	90.2	
45+ years	0	0	4	10.8	33	89.2	
Education of mother							
Primary	0	0	1	3.4	28	96.6	0.36

Table 4 Emotional burden (stress/anxiety, worry, compassion) of the disease stratified by the associated factors ($n = 527^a$) *(Continued)*

Factor	Not at all / mild		Moderate		Severe / very severe		p
	Number	%	Number	%	Number	%	
Secondary / vocational	7	3.7	8	4.2	174	92.1	
Higher	5	1.7	20	6.6	278	91.7	
Education of father							
Primary	4	11.1	2	5.6	30	83.3	0.01
Secondary / vocational	4	1.6	13	5.3	227	93.0	
Higher	4	1.8	11	5.0	207	93.2	
Family structure							
Both parents	12	2.4	27	5.5	452	92.1	0.67
Single parent	0	0	2	7.1	26	92.9	
Place of residence							
Urban	11	2.5	27	6.0	410	91.5	0.79
Rural	1	1.5	3	4.5	62	93.9	
Objective evaluation of the health status							
Vomiting (times per 24 h)							
0	0	0	0	0	3	100.0	0.22
1	4	4.1	10	10.3	83	85.6	
2	4	1.8	9	4.0	213	94.2	
3	2	1.2	10	6.0	155	92.8	
Diarrhea (times per 24 h)							
1	1	1.6	6	9.5	56	88.9	0.54
2	4	3.3	6	4.9	113	91.9	
3	5	1.6	17	5.4	290	92.9	
Severity of episode (Vesikari)							
Moderate	0	0	4	11.4	31	88.6	0.24
Severe / very severe	10	2.2	25	5.4	427	92.4	
Subjective evaluation of the health status							
Severity of diarrhea							
Not at all / mild	0	0	2	6.1	31	93.9	0.48
Moderate	3	3.9	2	2.6	71	93.4	
Severe / very severe	8	1.9	26	6.3	378	91.7	
Severity of vomiting							
Not at all / mild	2	1.4	12	8.4	129	90.2	0.32
Moderate	3	3.4	2	2.3	82	94.3	
Severe / very severe	6	2.1	16	5.5	269	92.4	
Severity of fever							
Not at all / mild	3	2.1	11	7.7	129	90.2	0.84
Moderate	2	1.8	6	5.5	101	92.7	
Severe / very severe	6	2.2	13	4.9	248	92.9	
Severity of abdominal pain							
Not at all / mild	6	3.7	12	7.4	145	89.0	0.31
Moderate	1	0.7	6	4.5	127	94.8	

Table 4 Emotional burden (stress/anxiety, worry, compassion) of the disease stratified by the associated factors (n = 527[a]) *(Continued)*

Factor	Not at all / mild		Moderate		Severe / very severe		p
	Number	%	Number	%	Number	%	
Severe / very severe	4	1.9	10	4.8	196	93.3	
Severity of insufficient fluid intake							
Not at all / mild	0	0	5	6.8	69	93.2	0.41
Moderate	2	2.4	2	2.4	80	95.2	
Severe / very severe	9	2.5	23	6.3	331	91.2	
Severity of loss of appetite							
Not at all / mild	2	2.2	4	4.5	83	93.3	0.98
Moderate	2	1.9	6	5.7	98	92.5	
Severe / very severe	7	2.2	20	6.2	295	91.6	
Severity of apathy							
Not at all / mild	3	3.5	7	8.2	75	88.2	0.60
Moderate	3	2.8	5	4.7	98	92.5	
Severe / very severe	5	1.6	18	5.6	299	92.9	
Severity of inflamed bottom							
Not at all / mild	6	2.1	22	7.7	256	90.1	0.12
Moderate	3	3.5	4	4.7	79	91.9	
Severe / very severe	2	1.4	3	2.0	142	96.6	
Severity of interrupted sleep mode							
Not at all / mild	4	1.5	16	6.2	240	92.3	0.73
Moderate	4	3.3	5	4.1	112	92.6	
Severe / very severe	3	2.2	9	6.6	125	91.2	
Severity of tearfulness							
Not at all / mild	3	2.0	12	7.8	138	90.2	0.46
Moderate	5	3.3	7	4.6	140	92.1	
Severe / very severe	3	1.4	10	4.7	201	93.9	
Severity of anxiety / irritability							
Not at all / mild	4	1.8	15	6.9	199	91.3	0.53
Moderate	3	2.5	9	7.4	109	90.1	
Severe / very severe	4	2.2	6	3.4	168	94.4	

indicators of the child's health status. A significant correlation was found only between stress/anxiety and fever (more severe fever corresponded to a higher level of severe stress/anxiety ($p = 0.003$)), between stress/anxiety and irritability of the child, between worry and irritability of the child (more intense irritability corresponded to a higher proportion of caregivers reporting severe or very severe stress ($p < 0.001$) or feelings of worry ($p < 0.001$)), and between stress or worry and tearfulness of the child (more severe tearfulness corresponded to a higher proportion of parents reporting severe or very severe stress ($p < 0.001$) or worry ($p = 0.006$)).

Table 5 (find uploaded as separate file) shows the social burden of the acute rotavirus infection and its associations with different independent variables. No statistically significant associations were found between the necessity to introduce changes in the caregiver's daily routine and the objective health status indicators. The social burden showed statistically significant associations with different sociodemographic factors - older age of the child ($p < 0.001$), older age of the mother ($p < 0.001$) or the father ($p = 0.03$) and higher education level of the mother ($p < 0.001$) corresponded to larger proportions of caregivers reporting a need to introduce changes in their

Table 5 Social burden (changes in daily routine) of the disease stratified by the associated factors ($n = 527$)

Factor	Yes		No		p
	Number	%	Number	%	
Sociodemographic factors					
Gender					
Female	211	82.4	45	17.6	0.06
Male	202	75.7	65	24.3	
Age					
≤ 12 months	105	67.7	50	32.3	< 0.001
13–24 months	126	75.4	41	24.6	
25–36 months	79	89.8	9	10.2	
37+ months	102	91.1	10	8.9	
Age of the mother (years)					
≤ 24 years	31	56.4	24	43.6	< 0.001
25–34 years	264	79.3	69	20.7	
35–44 years	111	88.8	14	11.2	
45+ years	5	62.5	3	37.5	
Age of the father (years)					
≤ 24 years	18	66.7	9	33.3	0.03
25–34 years	212	75.4	69	24.6	
35–44 years	137	85.1	24	14.9	
45+ years	32	86.5	5	13.5	
Education of the mother					
Primary	18	62.1	11	37.9	< 0.001
Secondary / vocational	133	71.1	54	28.9	
Higher	257	85.1	45	14.9	
Education of the father					
Primary	24	70.6	10	29.4	0.30
Secondary / vocational	190	78.2	53	21.8	
Higher	181	81.5	41	18.5	
Family structure					
Both parents	386	79.1	102	20.9	0.61
Single parent	21	75.0	7	25.0	
Place of residence					
Urban	350	78.5	96	21.5	0.57
Rural	53	81.5	12	18.5	
Objective evaluation of the health status					
Vomiting (times per 24 h)					
0	1	33.3	2	66.7	0.08
1	70	72.2	27	27.8	
2	178	79.1	47	20.9	
3	135	81.3	31	18.7	
Diarrhea (times per 24 h)					
1	48	77.4	14	22.6	0.07
2	87	71.3	35	28.7	

Table 5 Social burden (changes in daily routine) of the disease stratified by the associated factors ($n = 527$) *(Continued)*

Factor	Yes		No		p
	Number	%	Number	%	
3	254	81.4	58	18.6	
Severity of episodes (Vesikari)					
Moderate	24	68.6	11	31.4	0.13
Severe / very severe	366	79.6	94	20.4	
Subjective evaluation of the health status					
Severity of diarrhea					
Not at all / mild	24	72.7	9	27.3	0.36
Moderate	56	74.7	19	25.3	
Severe / very severe	330	80.3	81	19.7	
Severity of vomiting					
Not at all / mild	110	77.5	32	22.5	0.23
Moderate	63	73.3	23	26.7	
Severe / very severe	237	81.4	54	18.6	
Severity of fever					
Not at all / mild	102	71.8	40	28.2	0.02
Moderate	94	85.5	16	14.5	
Severe / very severe	215	80.8	51	19.2	
Severity of abdominal pain					
Not at all / mild	123	75.9	39	24.1	0.63
Moderate	105	78.9	28	21.1	
Severe / very severe	168	80.0	42	20.0	
Severity of insufficient fluid intake					
Not at all / mild	50	68.5	23	31.5	0.04
Moderate	63	76.8	19	23.2	
Severe / very severe	296	81.5	67	18.5	
Severity of loss of appetite					
Not at all / mild	64	72.2	24	27.3	0.06
Moderate	78	74.3	27	25.7	
Severe / very severe	264	82.2	57	17.8	
Severity of apathy					
Not at all / mild	60	71.4	24	28.6	0.14
Moderate	85	81.0	20	19.0	
Severe / very severe	260	81.0	61	19.0	
Severity of inflamed bottom					
Not at all / mild	219	77.9	62	22.1	0.60
Moderate	82	82.8	15	17.2	
Severe / very severe	117	80.1	29	19.9	
Severity of interrupted sleep mode					
Not at all / mild	199	77.1	59	22.9	0.48

Table 5 Social burden (changes in daily routine) of the disease stratified by the associated factors (n = 527) *(Continued)*

Factor	Yes		No		p
	Number	%	Number	%	
Moderate	96	79.3	25	20.7	
Severe / very severe	112	82.4	24	17.6	
Severity of tearfulness					
Not at all / mild	116	76.3	36	23.7	0.59
Moderate	123	80.9	29	19.1	
Severe / very severe	169	79.7	43	20.3	
Severity of anxiety / irritability					
Not at all / mild	168	77.4	49	22.6	0.64
Moderate	98	81.0	23	19.0	
Severe / very severe	142	80.7	34	19.3	

daily routine because of the rotavirus infection (such as sporting, educational or culture events/activities).

Out of all subjective health status indicators, only fever (similarly to the emotional burden) and insufficient fluid intake were significantly associated with the social burden of the disease. That is, a larger proportion of caregivers reported needing to introduce changes in their daily routine when their child had more severe fevers ($p = 0.02$) or insufficient fluid intake ($p = 0.04$).

Finally, Table 6 (find uploaded as separate file) reveals the factors that increased the economic burden of rotavirus infection. None of the objective health status indicators significantly influenced the working abilities of the parents. Only two sociodemographic factors showed a significant impact on the economic burden of the disease: a higher age of the child ($p = 0.01$) and higher level of education of the mother ($p = 0.02$) corresponded to a larger proportion of respondents reporting the need to be absent from work for at least 1 day.

Out of all subjective health status indicators, only insufficient fluid intake (like the social burden) and inflamed bottom seems to increase the economic burden of the infection. A larger proportion of caregivers reported the need to be absent from work for cases of more severe insufficient fluid intake ($p = 0.02$) or inflamed bottom ($p = 0.03$) of their child.

Therefore, it can be concluded that the objective health status of the child does not influence the emotional, social or economic burden of the rotavirus infection, whereas the parents' subjective perceptions of the child's health status and some sociodemographic characteristics, such as the age of the child and the age or education of parents do influence the burden.

Discussion

This study reveals the impact of rotavirus gastroenteritis on HRQL of families whose children are affected. As the disease is characterized by a sudden onset, it can disrupt daily routine, require unexpected changes, and thus, can affect the physical, emotional and social wellbeing of the child and family. The results show that an acute illness negatively effects the family and increases their emotional, social and economic disease burden. Parents reported moderate or severe parental distress, worry and anxiety, as well as intense feelings of an exhaustion, helplessness and despair. This is consistent with the results of other studies that also reported parental emotions and feelings due to a child's illness. Parents reported high distress levels during the episode of rotavirus gastroenteritis [5, 17, 18] and felt exhausted and helpless [18]. Our study concludes that parents of hospitalized children are faced with disruptions of their daily routine and social activities. This fact has also been established in similar studies [17]. The economic burden of disease is related to lost days of work and additional expenditures. In our study and other studies, parents experienced lost work days [5, 20] and additional expenditures. [17, 21].

Current research has shown that stress, anxiety, worry and compassion are the most often (and more intense) feelings experienced by parents due a child's illness. Based on a subjective assessment of disease symptoms, parents reported that severe fever of the child, irritability and tearfulness promoted higher parental stress levels. Emotional reactions, to a certain extent, are socially formatted and structured [22]. Parental responses to a child's symptoms and their subsequent emotional feelings can be incorporated and interpreted in a cultural framework. In Latvia, fever in children is possibly overestimated as an abnormal and potentially life-threatening condition. This, in turn, can lead to excessive parental stress reactions. Cultural and personal beliefs held by parents also influence perceptions of how a "healthy child" should look and behave [23]. Tearfulness and irritability are usually not associated with the image of a healthy child in Latvia, and these symptoms can provoke more intense levels of parental distress, worry and anxiety. Cultural factors regarding the impact of rotavirus gastroenteritis on families were analyzed in an ethnographic study in Taiwan and Vietnam [21]; another study also compared the emotional reactions of Spanish, Italian and Polish parents due to childhood acute rotavirus gastroenteritis. To help parents manage their child's health needs during an acute illness and their own perceptions and reactions toward their child's symptoms, sufficient parental health education is required [24]. A successful and mutual physician-parent communication, as the foundation of the therapeutic relationship, is an essential tool for better social support [25]; otherwise,

Table 6 Economic burden (days off work) of the disease stratified by the associated factors ($n = 527^{a}$)

Factor	None		At least one		Not employed		p
	Number	%	Number	%	Number	%	
Sociodemographic factors							
Gender							
Female	81	31.6	148	57.8	27	10.5	0.49
Male	92	34.5	141	52.8	34	12.7	
Age							
≤ 12 months	67	43.8	61	39.9	25	16.3	0.01
13–24 months	56	33.3	96	57.1	16	9.5	
25–36 months	22	24.7	57	64.0	10	11.2	
37+ months	28	25.0	74	66.1	10	8.9	
Age of the mother							
≤ 24 years	17	31.5	28	51.9	9	16.7	0.84
25–34 years	110	32.9	188	56.3	36	10.8	
35–44 years	41	32.8	69	55.2	15	12.0	
45+ years	4	50.0	3	37.5	1	12.5	
Age of the father							
≤ 24 years	11	42.3	11	42.3	4	15.4	0.48
25–34 years	95	33.9	152	54.3	33	11.8	
35–44 years	54	33.1	92	56.4	17	10.4	
45+ years	7	18.9	25	67.6	5	13.5	
Education of the mother							
Primary	14	48.3	12	41.4	3	10.3	0.02
Secondary / vocational	73	39.0	85	45.5	29	15.5	
Higher	85	28.1	188	62.3	29	9.6	
Education of the father							
Primary	12	35.3	16	47.1	6	17.6	0.41
Secondary / vocational	82	33.6	140	57.4	22	9.0	
Higher	71	32.1	120	54.3	30	13.6	
Family structure							
Both parents	159	32.6	271	55.5	58	11.9	0.64
Single parent	11	39.3	15	53.6	2	7.1	
Place of residence							
Urban	145	32.6	245	55.1	55	12.4	0.53
Rural	23	34.8	38	57.6	5	7.6	
Objective evaluation of the health status							
Vomiting (times per 24 h)							
0	3	1000.	0	0	0	0	0.28
1	32	33.3	50	52.1	14	14.6	
2	78	34.7	123	54.7	24	10.7	
3	52	31.1	95	56.9	20	12.0	
Diarrhea (times per 24 h)							
1	23	36.5	33	52.4	7	11.1	0.95
2	40	32.5	66	53.7	17	13.8	

Table 6 Economic burden (days off work) of the disease stratified by the associated factors ($n = 527^a$) *(Continued)*

Factor	None		At least one		Not employed		p
	Number	%	Number	%	Number	%	
3	104	33.5	170	54.8	36	11.6	
Severity of episodes (Vesikari)							
Moderate	14	40.0	17	48.6	4	11.4	0.70
Severe / very severe	152	33.0	252	54.8	56	12.2	
Subjective evaluation of the health status							
Severity of diarrhea							
Not at all / mild	13	39.4	17	51.5	3	9.1	0.43
Moderate	31	40.8	39	51.3	6	7.9	
Severe / very severe	128	31.2	232	56.6	50	12.2	
Severity of vomiting							
Not at all / mild	55	38.7	71	50.0	16	11.3	0.26
Moderate	27	31.0	46	52.9	14	16.1	
Severe / very severe	90	30.9	171	58.8	30	10.3	
Severity of fever							
Not at all / mild	54	38.0	70	49.3	18	12.7	0.19
Moderate	27	24.8	69	63.3	13	11.9	
Severe / very severe	90	33.7	150	56.2	27	10.1	
Severity of abdominal pain							
Not at all / mild	61	37.4	84	51.5	18	11.0	0.12
Moderate	51	38.3	71	53.4	11	8.3	
Severe / very severe	57	27.1	124	59.0	29	13.8	
Severity of insufficient fluid intake							
Not at all / mild	32	43.8	28	38.4	13	17.8	0.02
Moderate	30	35.7	43	51.2	11	13.1	
Severe / very severe	110	30.4	216	59.7	36	9.9	
Severity of loss of appetite							
Not at all / mild	39	44.3	39	44.3	10	11.4	0.06
Moderate	39	36.8	54	50.9	13	12.3	
Severe / very severe	93	29.0	192	59.8	36	11.2	
Severity of apathy							
Not at all / mild	33	39.8	39	47.0	11	13.3	0.20
Moderate	34	32.4	55	52.4	16	15.2	
Severe / very severe	99	30.7	192	59.4	32	9.9	
Severity of inflamed bottom							
Not at all / mild	81	28.7	174	61.7	27	9.6	0.03
Moderate	37	42.5	38	43.7	12	13.8	
Severe / very severe	53	36.3	74	50.7	19	13.0	
Severity of interrupted sleep mode							
Not at all / mild	89	34.4	148	57.1	22	8.5	0.33
Moderate	37	30.6	66	54.5	18	14.9	
Severe / very severe	45	33.1	72	52.9	19	14.0	

Table 6 Economic burden (days off work) of the disease stratified by the associated factors ($n = 527^{a}$) *(Continued)*

Factor	None		At least one		Not employed		*p*
	Number	%	Number	%	Number	%	
Severity of tearfulness							
Not at all / mild	53	34.9	80	52.6	19	12.5	0.92
Moderate	47	30.7	88	57.5	18	11.8	
Severe / very severe	71	33.5	118	55.7	23	10.8	
Severity of anxiety / irritability							
Not at all / mild	69	31.7	121	55.5	28	12.8	0.27
Moderate	34	28.1	76	62.8	11	9.1	
Severe / very severe	67	38.1	90	51.1	19	10.8	

[a]The sum of the stratified numbers can differ according to the parameters due to missing values

lack of communication with a child's parents can lead to misunderstandings and cause additional stress. The social burden of disease is an essential domain of HRQL. This study revealed that older mothers and fathers more often reported the need to unexpectedly change their daily routine because of their child's acute illness, which was also true for mothers with higher education levels. This finding could be explained by the group of parents aged 35 or more as having more social duties and activities. Parents reported that severe fever and insufficient fluid intake were the most prevalent symptoms of their child that caused disruption of their daily schedule. This could be linked to cultural issues, parental education and health communication. In Latvia, information on child dehydration is broadly released, and the notion that children should drink fluids is strongly embodied in public discourses and practices.

Our study revealed that the main aspect of economic burden is the loss of work days. The larger proportion of parents (caregivers) experienced absence from work for at least 1 day due to a childhood rotavirus gastroenteritis when the child was of higher age. This finding could be explained by paid parental leave in Latvia, that covers first year of life. As children grow older, both parents usually are employed and sick-leave usually is required. Mothers with the higher educational levels more often reported the need to be absent from work at least 1 day. A possible explanation could be related to job specificity (duties, responsibility, etc.) and/or better social insurance and social security system. Parents reported that an inflamed bottom and insufficient fluid intake were the most prevalent symptoms of their child that led to lost work days, which could be linked to cultural and informational issues regarding symptom perception and management.

This study confirmed that acute childhood rotavirus gastroenteritis places a considerable burden on families. It affects all domains of HRQL. This study provides in-depth insight into parental subjective evaluation of their child's symptoms and their reactions to these symptoms. These results are important for promoting better communication between physicians and parents.

Additional research may be necessary to identify more profound factors and to measure the associations among factors in considering the current development of conceptual frameworks for HRQL assessment in acute gastroenteritis [26].

This study has several limitations. First, the results are not fully generalizable, as only hospitalized children and their families were included. Thus, the results may not be relevant upon extrapolation to milder cases of rotavirus infection.

Conclusions

In this study, we found that the objective health status of the child did not influence the emotional, social or economic burden of rotavirus infection, but rather parents' subjective perceptions of their child's health status and sociodemographic characteristics such as the age of the child or the age or education of parents did affect their burden.

A better understanding of how acute episode affect the child and the child's family could help to ease parental fears and advice parents on the characteristics of rotavirus infection and the optimal care of an affected child.

Abbreviations

CI: Confidence interval; HRQL: Health-related quality of life; n: Absolute number; OR: Odds ratio; PCR: Polymerase chain reaction

Acknowledgements

Authors would like to thank Riga Stradins University for granting the project "Clinical peculiarities of Rota viral infection, molecular epidemiology and health-associated life quality for hospitalized children and their family members". This manuscript was drafted as part of a project.

Funding

Project was granted by Riga Stradins University (Grant No. RSU ZP 06/2013/2-3/155). Manuscript was drafted as part of a project.

Authors' contributions
GL developed the clinical and social demographic parts of the questionnaire and was responsible for patient involvement, data collection, and preparation and submission of the manuscript. MC participated in patient involvement and data entry. AK participated in the development of the questionnaire, developed the platform for data entry, drafted the manuscript and performed the statistical analysis. IS participated in the development of the questionnaire and preparation of the manuscript. IG participated in the development of the clinical and social demographic parts of the questionnaire and preparation of the manuscript. DG was the project manager and supervisor. All authors read and approved the final manuscript.

Competing interests
Financial competing interests: Project was granted by Riga Stradins University (Grant No. RSU ZP 06/2013/2–3/155). Manuscript was drafted as part of a project.
Non-financial competing interests: This manuscript is part of the doctoral Thesis of the corresponding author Gunta Laizane.

Author details
[1]Department of Paediatrics, Riga Stradins University, Vienibas gatve 45, Riga LV-1004, Latvia. [2]Department of Public Health and Epidemiology, Riga Stradins University, Kronvalda boulevard 9, Riga LV-1010, Latvia.

References

1. Parashar UD, Nelson EA, Kang G. Diagnosis, management, and prevention of rotavirus gastroenteritis in children. BMJ. 2013;347:f7204. https://doi.org/10.1136/bmj.f7204.
2. Gimenez-Sanchez F, Delgado-Rubio A, Martinon-Torres F, Bernaola-Iturbe E. Rotascore research group. Multicenter prospective study analysing the role of rotavirus on acute gastroenteritis in Spain. Acta Paediatr. 2010;99:738–42. https://doi.org/10.1111/j.1651-2227.2010.01684.x.
3. Soriano-Gabarró M, Mrukowicz J, Vesikari T, Verstraeten T. Burden of rotavirus disease in European Union countries. Pediatr Infect Dis J. 2006;25: S7–S11. https://doi.org/10.1097/01.inf.0000197622.98559.01.
4. The center for disease Prevention and controle of Latvia. https://www.spkc.gov.lv/en.
5. Van der Wielen M, Giaquinto C, Gothefors L, Huelsse C, Huet F, Littmann M, et al. Impact of community-acquired paediatric rotavirus gastroenteritis on family life: data from the REVEAL study. BMC Fam Pract. 2010;11:22. https://doi.org/10.1186/1471-2296-11-22.
6. Spieth LE, Harris CV. Assessment of health-related quality of life in children and adolescents: an integrative review. J Pediatr Psychol. 1996;21:175–93. https://doi.org/10.1093/jpepsy/21.2.175.
7. Goldbeck L, Melches J. Quality of life in families of children with congenital heart disease. Qual Life Res. 2005;14:1915 24. https://doi.org/10.1007/s11136-005-4327-0
8. Grootenhuis MA, Koopman HM, Verrips EG, Vogels AG, Last BF. Health-related quality of life problems of children aged 8-11 years with a chronic disease. Dev Neurorehabil. 2007;10:27–33. https://doi.org/10.1080/13682820600691017.
9. Matza LS, Swensen AR, Flood EM, Secnik K, Leidy NK. Assessment of health-related quality of life in children: a review of conceptual, methodological, and regulatory issues. Value Health. 2004;7:79–92. https://doi.org/10.1111/j.1524-4733.2004.71273.x.
10. Bullinger M, Von Mackensen S, Haemo-QoL Group. Quality of life in children and families with bleeding disorders. J Pediatr Hematol Oncol. 2003; 25(Suppl 1):S64–7. https://doi.org/10.1097/00043426-200312001-00015.
11. Ben-Gashir MA, Seed PT, Hay RJ. Are quality of family life and disease severity related in childhood atopic dermatitis? J Eur Acad Dermatol Venereol. 2002;16:455–62. https://doi.org/10.1046/j.1468-3083.2002.00495.x.
12. Harpin VA. The effect of ADHD on the life of an individual, their family, and community from preschool to adult life. Arch Dis Child. 2005;90(Suppl 1):i2–7. https://doi.org/10.1136/adc.2004.059006.
13. Tong A, Lowe A, Sainsbury P, Craig JC. Experiences of parents who have children with chronic kidney disease: a systematic review of qualitative studies. Pediatrics. 2008;121:349–60. https://doi.org/10.1542/peds.2006-3470.
14. Mawani N, Amine B, Rostom S, El Badri D, Ezzahri M, Moussa F, et al. Moroccan parents caring for children with juvenile idiopathic arthritis: positive and negative aspects of their experiences. Pediatr Rheumatol Online J. 2013;11:39. https://doi.org/10.1186/1546-0096-11-39
15. Javier Diez D, Patrzalek M, Cantarutti L, Arnould B, Meunier J, Soriano-Gabarro M, et al. The impact of childhood acute rotavirus gastroenteritis on the parents quality of life: prospective observational study in European primary care medical practices. BMC Pediatr. 2012;12:58.
16. Huppertz HI, Forster J, Heininger U, Roos R, Neumann HU, Hammerschmidt T. The parental appraisal of the morbidity of diarrhea in infants and toddlers (PAMODI) survey. Clin Pediatr. 2008;47:363–71. https://doi.org/10.1177/0009922807310933.
17. Mast TC, DeMuro-Mercon C, Kelly CM, Floyd LE, Walter EB. The impact of rotavirus gastroenteritis on the family. BMC Pediatr. 2009;9:11. https://doi.org/10.1186/1471-2431-9-11.
18. Vesikari Clinical Severity Scoring System Manual Version 1.3, for external circulation. PATH A catalyst for global health, Kristen Lewis. 2011.
19. Cabinet of Ministers of Latvia. https://www.mk.gov.lv/. Accesed 15 Jan 2018.
20. Sénécal M, Brisson M, Lebel MH, Yaremko J, Wong R, Gallant LA, et al. Measuring the impact of rotavirus acute gastroenteritis episodes (MIRAGE): a prospective community-based study. Can J Infect Dis Med Microbiol. 2008;19:397–404.
21. O'Brien MA, Rojas-Farreras S, Lee HC, Lin LH, Lin CC, Hoang PL, et al. Family impact of rotavirus gastroenteritis in Taiwan and Vietnam: an ethnographic study. BMC Infect Dis. 2015;15:240. https://doi.org/10.1186/s12879-015-0968-y.
22. Von Scheve C. Emotion and social structures: the affective foundations of social order. Routledge; 2013.
23. Barr DA. Health disparities in the United States: social class, race, ethnicity, & health. Baltimore: Johns Hopkins University Press; 2008.
24. Betz CL, Ruccione K, Meeske K, Smith K, Chang N. Health literacy: a pediatric nursing concern. Pediatr Nurs. 2008;34:231–9.
25. Levetown M, American Academy of Pediatrics Committee on Bioethics. Communicating with children and families: from everyday interactions to skill in conveying distressing information. Pediatrics. 2008;121:e1441–60. https://doi.org/10.1542/peds.2008-0565.
26. Johnston BC, Donen R, Pooni A, Pond J, Xie F, Giglia L, et al. Conceptual framework for health-related quality of life assessment in acute gastroenteritis. J Pediatr Gastroenterol Nutr. 2013;56:280–9. https://doi.org/10.1097/MPG.0b013e3182736f49.

4

A novel mutation of WFS1 gene in a Chinese patient with Wolfram syndrome

Min Li[1†], Jia Liu[1†], Huan Yi[1], Li Xu[1], Xiufeng Zhong[2*] and Fuhua Peng[1*]

Abstract

Background: Wolfram syndrome (WS), caused by mutations of the Wolfram syndrome 1 (WFS1) gene on chromosome 4p16.1, is an autosomal recessive disorder characterized by diabetes insipidus (DI), neuro-psychiatric disorders, hearing deficit, and urinary tract anomalies.

Case presentation: Here we report a 11-year-old Chinese boy who presented with visual loss, was suspected with optic neuritis (ON) or neuromyelitis optica (NMO) and referred to our department for further diagnosis. Finally he was diagnosed with WS because of diabetes mellitus (DM) and optic atrophy (OA). Eight exons and flanking introns of WFS1 gene were analyzed by sequencing. A novel mutation c.1760G > A in WFS1 gene of exon 8 was identified.

Conclusion: This report reviews a case of WS associated with a novel mutation, c.1760G > A in WFS1 gene of exon 8, and emphasizes that WS should be taken into account for juveniles with visual loss and diabetes mellitus.

Keywords: Wolfram syndrome, WFS1 gene, Mutation

Background

Wolfram syndrome (WS) is a rare autosomal recessive disorder, mainly associated with juvenile-onset type 1 diabetes mellitus (T1DM) and optic atrophy (OA). Diabetes insipidus (DI), neuro-psychiatric disorders, hearing deficit, and urinary tract anomalies develop in many patients [1, 2].

Mutations of the WFS1 gene on chromosome 4p16.1 are in charge of the clinical manifestations in majority of patients with WS [3, 4]. WFS1 gene encodes wolframin, an 890-amino acid glycoprotein localized primarily in the endoplasmic reticulum (ER) [5]. Genetic analyses in WS have identified a wide spectrum of mutations, including mis-sense, frame shifting, nonsense, and splicing mutations, predominantly located in exon 8 (80–90%) [6].

Here we report a WS case onset with OA and T1DM in a Chinese juvenile. A novel mutation c.1760G > A in WFS1 gene of exon 8 was found, which was never reported before.

* Correspondence: xzhong13@qq.com; pfh93@163.com
† Equal contributors
[2] State Key Laboratory of Ophthalmology, Zhongshan Ophthalmic Center, Sun Yat-sen Univeristy, Guangzhou, Guangdong 510060, China
[1] Multiple Sclerosis Center, Department of Neurology, the Third Affiliated Hospital of Sun Yat-Sen University, Guangzhou, Guangdong 510630, China

Case presentation

A 11-year-old boy was admitted to our department with a 1-year history of progressive visual loss. He was initially taken as pseudomyopia without treatment. Four months ago, he was diagnosed with T1DM and found bilateral OA by brain magnetic resonance image (MRI), optic coherence temography (OCT) and visual evoked potential (VEP) (no pictures provided) in the local hospital. And he was treated with compound anisodine hydrobromide injection and mouse nerve factor injection for one and a half months without alleviating. Then the boy was referred to our department with suspicious of ON or NMO.

The patient was hospitalized in local hospital because of a sudden faint in school 4 months ago. Some of his laboratory tests were as follows: finger point blood glucose test > 33.3 mmol/L, blood glucose 38 mmol/L, HbAc 15.8%, and positive urine sugar and ketone. His mother recallded that he was polydipsia, polyphagia and polyuria with weight loss for 1 month. So he was diagnosed with 'type 1 diabetes mellitus (DM1), ketoacidosis and coma', and treated with insulin pump of Medtronic in the local hospital.

Some of his main investigations in our hospital revealed as follows. ANA+ENA + ANCA, TSH in serum, AQP4 and OCB in serum and cerebrospinal fluid were

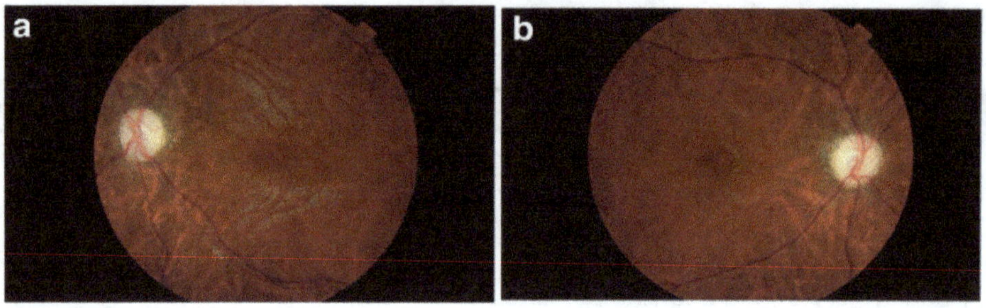

Fig. 1 Photographic images of eyes. Fundus image discloses marked left (**a**) and right (**b**) atrophic optic discs with temporal pallor

negative. His HbAc was 5.9% and blood glucose was 4.88 mmol/L. His anti-GAD antibody and anti-insulin antibody in serum was negative. Regular urinalysis and hearing was normal. The photographic images of the patient's eyes showed bilateral papillary atrophy (Fig. 1). OCT measure around the disc showed thin retina (Fig. 2). Brain MRI showed bilateral optic nerve atrophy thinner (Fig. 3). OA and DM1 in a young patient suggested his clinically diagnose of WS.

The patient was the first child, and had one little sister. Both his little sister and his parents had no signs or symptoms. And his parents were non-consanguineous.

For further confirmation of the diagnosis, we got the consent to sequence WFS1 gene for the patient and his parents without his other family members. The patient's number 587 codon, c.1760G > A, located in exon 8, mutated and changed from arginine to glutamine. He was homozygote while his parents were both heterozygote of mutant genes. We used the Human Gene Mutation Database (HGMD) to assess that this was a novel mutation. Exome sequencing disclosed a novel mutation in WFS1 gene (the novel variant c.1760G > A) (Fig. 4), confirming WS.

Discussion and conclusions

WS is a rare progressive neurodegenerative hereditary disease, known as DI-DM-OA-D which stands for diabetes insipidus, diabetes mellitus, optic atrophy, and deafness [1]. The coexistence of T1DM and OA in juvenile suggests WS but molecular confirmation is mandatory [7]. Patients usually present with DM followed by OA in the first decade. DM is often the first clinical sign of WS, but differ from classical T1DM in normal autoimmune laboratory parameters. Patients with WS usually demonstrate progressive ophthalmologic symptoms. Deafness in WS is commonly a high frequency, symmetric hearing loss, usually detected in the second or third decade with a relatively slow rate of deterioration [8, 9]. Some studies have reported urological abnormalities which were expected about 58% in patients with WS [10].

Studies showed that WS was caused by loss-of-function mutations in the WFS1 gene, encoding wolframin [6]. Wolframin is abundantly expressed in pancreas, brain, heart, and muscle, with lesser amounts being present in liver and kidneys [11]. Although no function has yet been attributed to wolframin. Recently, it has been shown that WFS1 gene has a crucial role in the negative regulation of a feedback loop of the ER stress signaling network and preventing secretory cells. For example, wolframin deficiency in mice leads to progressive loss of B cells and impaired glucose tolerance [12]. Yamamoto H et al. concluded that dual dysfunction of wolframin in optic nerve glial cells and retinal ganglion cells in the cynomolgus monkey might explain the progressive optic nerve atrophy in WS [13].

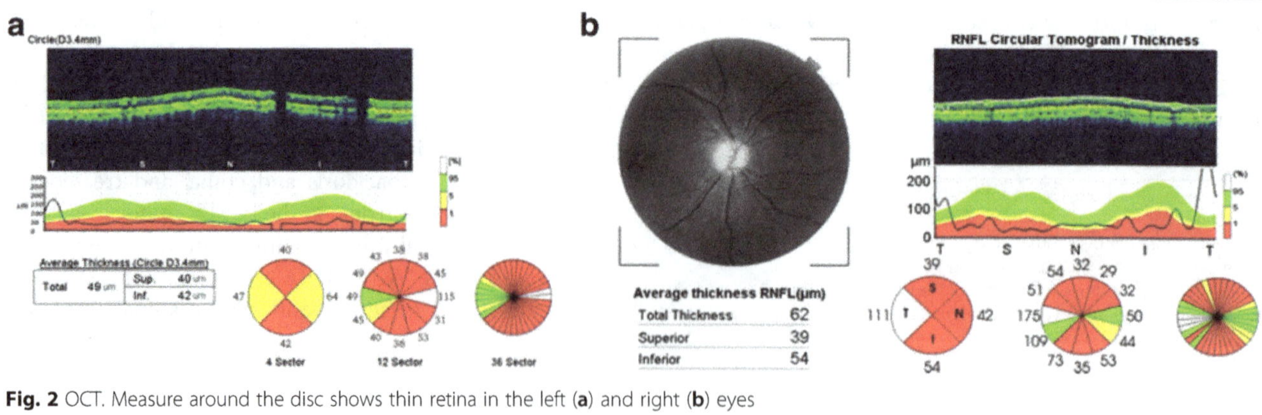

Fig. 2 OCT. Measure around the disc shows thin retina in the left (**a**) and right (**b**) eyes

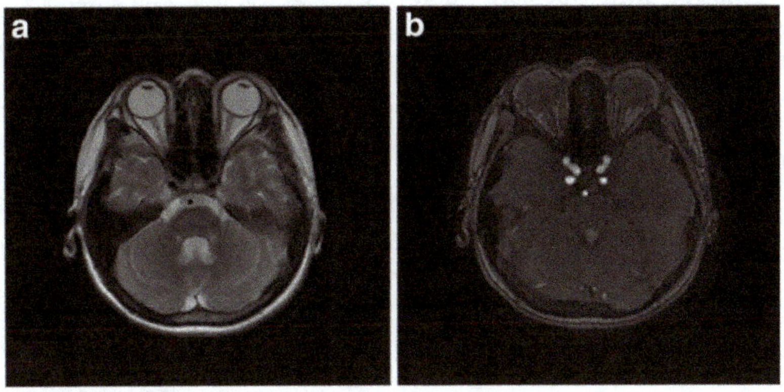

Fig. 3 Cranium MRI. MRI shows bilateral optic nerve atrophy on T2WI (**a**) and T1W+C (**b**)

The prognosis of WS is currently poor as most patients die at the age of 30s (range, 25–49 years) because of respiratory failure as a result of brain stem atrophy [1, 10].

But our case demonstrates an unusual presentation. The boy reported here onset with OA and T1DM, and both deafness and urological abnormalities were not found. His parents were non-consanguineous and were found mutant heterozygote while he was mutant homozygote. His condition was stable with a follow-up of 12 months.

Vision loss in Neurology was usually associated with ON or NMO. NMO can be associated with other autoimmune disease, such as T1DM [14]. So it is necessary to differentiate WS from NMO with T1DM in children.

Based on the findings of the present case, we should be aware of WS in adolescence patients presenting with T1DM (non-autoimmune) and OA without any signs of diabetic retinopathy. And it is mandatory to perform direct sequencing analysis of the WFS1 gene to confirm

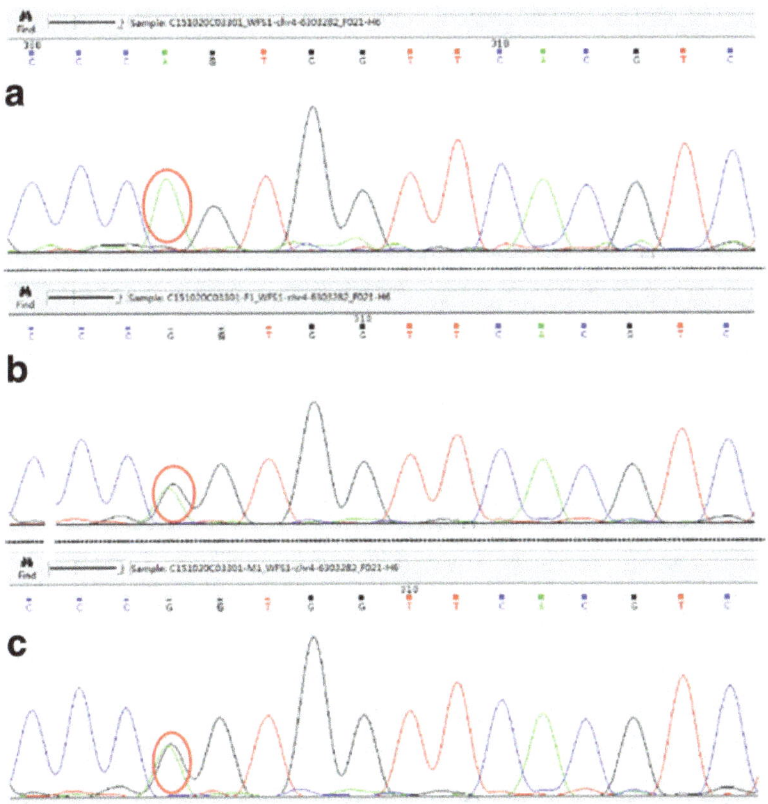

Fig. 4 Exome sequencing. WFS1 exon 8 forward sequences of a homozygote for the patient (**a**), and heterozygotes for his father (**b**) and mother (**c**)

the clinical diagnosis. No genotype-phenotype correlation has been identified [6]. Although our study increases the spectrum of WFS1 gene mutations with a novel variant c.1760G > A, whether the novel mutation relates with mild clinical symptoms or just involves vision and blood glucose remains to be further studied and confirmed.

Abbreviations

ANA: Anti-nuclear anti-body; ANCA: Anti-neutrophil cytoplasmic antibodies; AQP4: Aquaporin 4; D: Deafness; DI: Diabetes insipidus; DM: Diabetes mellitus; ENA: Extracted nuclear antigens; ER: Endoplasmic reticulum; HbAc: Glycosylated hemoglobin; HGMD: Human Gene Mutation Database; MRI: Magnetic resonance image; NMO: Neuromyelitis optica; OA: Optic atrophy; OCB: Oligoclonal bands; OCT: Optic coherence tomography; ON: Optic neuritis; TSH: Thyroid stimulating hormone; VEP: Visual evoked potential; WFS1: Wolfram syndrome 1; WS: Wolfram syndrome

Acknowledgments

The authors would like to thank the patient's family for their participation and help.

Funding

This study was supported by National Science Foundation of Guangdong Province (No. 2015A03013167), Science & Technology Project of Guangzhou (No. 201510010251) and National Science Foundation of China (No. 81271327).

Authors' contributions

ML and JL conceived the study and revised the manuscript critically for important intellectual content. HY and LX collected the raw data from our hospital work system and critically reviewed the manuscript. ML and JL interpreted the results for the case report, drafted, wrote and revised the report, and provided important intellectual review. XZ and FP analysed the data and reviewed the manuscript. All authors have read and approved the final manuscript.

Competing interests

The authors declare that they have no competing interests.

References

1. Barrett TG, Bundey SE, Macleod AF. Neurodegeneration and diabetes: UK nationwide study of Wolfram (DIDMOAD) syndrome. Lancet. 1995;346:1458–63.
2. Marshall BA, Permutt MA, Paciorkowski AR, Hoekel J, Karzon R, Wasson J, et al. Phenotypic characteristics of early Wolfram syndrome. Orphanet J Rare Dis. 2013;8:64. https://doi.org/10.1186/1750-1172-8-64.
3. Chaussenot A, Bannwarth S, Rouzier C, Vialettes B, Mkadem SA, Chabrol B, et al. Neurologic features and genotype-phenotype correlation in Wolfram syndrome. Ann Neurol. 2011;69:501–8. https://doi.org/10.1002/ana.22160.
4. Rigoli L, Di Bella C. Wolfram syndrome 1 and Wolfram syndrome 2. Curr Opin Pediatr. 2012;24:512–7. https://doi.org/10.1097/MOP.0b013e328354ccdf.
5. Takeda K, Inoue H, Tanizawa Y, Matsuzaki Y, Oba J, Watanabe Y, et al. Wfs1 (Wolfram syndrome 1) gene product: predominant subcellular localization to endoplasmic reticulum in cultured cells and neuronal expression in rat brain. Hum Mol Genet. 2001;10:47–84.
6. Rigoli L, Lombardo F, Di Bella C. Wolfram syndrome and WFS1 gene. Clin Genet. 2011;79:103–17. https://doi.org/10.1111/j.1399-0004.2010.01522.x.
7. Zmyslowska A, Borowiec M, Fichna P, Iwaniszewska B, Majkowska L, Pietrzak I, et al. Delayed recognition of Wolfram syndrome frequently misdiagnosed as type 1 diabetes with early chronic complications. Exp Clin Endocrinol Diabetes. 2014;122:35–8. https://doi.org/10.1055/s-0033-1357160.
8. Pennings RJ, Huygen PL, van den Ouweland JM, Cryns K, Dikkeschei LD, Van Camp G, et al. Sex-related hearing impairment in Wolfram syndrome patients identified by inactivating WFS1 mutations. Audiol Neurooto. 2004;9: 51–62. https://doi.org/10.1159/000074187
9. Plantinga RF, Pennings RJ, Huygen PL, Bruno R, Eller P, Barrett TG, et al. Hearing impairment in genotyped Wolfram syndrome patients. Ann Otol Rhinol Laryngol. 2008;117:494–500. https://doi.org/10.1177/000348940811700704.
10. Barrett TG, Bundey SE. Wolfram (DIDMOAD) syndrome. J Med Genet. 1997; 34:838–41.
11. Ribeiro MR, Crispim F, Vendramini MF, Moisés RS. Wolfram syndrome: from definition to molecular bases. Arq Bras Endocrinol Metabol. 2006;50:839–44.
12. Fonseca SG, Ishigaki S, Oslowski CM, Lu S, Lipson KL, Ghosh R, et al. Wolfram syndrome 1 gene negatively regulates ER stress signaling in rodent and human cells. J Clin Invest. 2010;120:744–55. https://doi.org/10.1172/JCI39678.
13. Yamamoto H, Hofmann S, Hamasaki DI, Yamamoto H, Kreczmanski P, Schmitz C, et al. Wolfram syndrome 1 (WFS1) protein expression in retinal ganglion cells and optic nerve glia of the cynomolgus monkey. Exp Eye Res. 2006;83:1303–6. https://doi.org/10.1016/j.exer.2006.06.010.
14. Kawazoe T, Araki M, Lin Y, Ogawa M, Okamoto T, Yamamura T, et al. New-onset type I diabetes mellitus and anti-aquaporin-4 antibody positive optic neuritis associated with type I interferon therapy for chronic hepatitis C. Intern Med. 2012;51:2625–9. https://doi.org/10.2169/internalmedicine.51.7771.

5

Sucking behaviour using feeding teats with and without an anticolic system

Marina Kreitschmann[1], Lea C. Epping[2], Ariane Hohoff[3], Cristina Sauerland[4] and Thomas Stamm[3*]

Abstract

Background: This study aimed to investigate differences in sucking behavior of infants bottle-fed with vented (so-called anticolic) teats (VTs) and nonvented teats (NVTs).

Methods: Trial design: Prospective, randomized clinical trial. Ninety-six term, healthy infants (aged 1–8 months) were assessed for eligibility. Seventy-three infants remained for intention-to-treat (ITT) and 65 infants (vented group: $n = 31$; nonvented group: $n = 34$) for the per-protocol (PP) analysis. During bottle-feeding, sucks/min, pauses/min, amount of formula intake (mL), feeding time (min), heart rate (bpm), respiratory rate (bpm), and oxygen saturation (%) were recorded. In addition, a parental survey was carried out to reveal possible symptoms of infantile colic. Sample-size calculation and confirmatory and exploratory analyses were performed using the Mann-Whitney *U* test and Fisher's exact test.

Results: Except for the parameter sucking pauses per minute (NVTs > VTs, $p = .03$), no differences between groups were found with the ITT and PP analysis. After excluding infants with a disproportionately complementary diet (subgroup analysis, infants aged 1–6 months, $n = 54$) the primary outcome (sucks per minute) showed significant differences (NVTs > VTs, $p = .01$). The amount of formula intake, feeding time, and cardiorespiratory parameters were similar in both groups. The parental survey did not show any relation between types of feeding teats and possible symptoms of infantile colic.

Conclusions: Compared with an NVT group, infants aged 1–6 months need fewer sucks and pauses when fed with VTs. In both groups, equal amounts of feeding medium and feeding time were observed. With NVT feeding, disruption occurs when the bottle vacuum is released by air from the oral cavity. Therefore, higher sucking frequency is needed to rebuild the oral vacuum for bottle milk flow, which implies higher risk of aerophagia. Overall, we suggest that the VTs provided a more coordinated drinking pattern than did the NVTs, which may have a positive effect on gastric distress.

Keywords: Vented teat, Bottle-feeding, Infants, Infantile colic, Feeding-teat, Aerophagia

* Correspondence: stammt@uni-muenster.de
[3]Department of Orthodontics, University of Münster, Albert-Schweitzer-Campus 1, 48149 Münster, Germany

Background

Infantile colic portrays a widespread problem with an uncertain prevalence of 5%–40% [1] within the first 4 [2] or 6 months [1] of an infant's life. The occurrence is difficult to identify due to differences in classification, methods of data collection, study design, and parents' perception of defining colic [1].

Although the history of research now reaches over 115 years, based on the paper of Zahorsky [3], the etiology of infantile colic still remains unknown [4]. As a result, therapeutic interventions to reduce the severity of symptoms and crying episodes are lacking their effectiveness [4, 5] and stressed parents seeking alternative methods to cope with their suffering infants. In this situation parents are susceptible to promises made by manufacturers of feeding bottles. Numerous bottle-nipple systems (BNSs) are available on the market, advertised to reduce infantile colic. The idea behind those so-called "anticolic" teats is to prevent excessive air swallowing (aerophagia) during feeding. It is estimated that 70% of the gastrointestinal gas is swallowed [6] and it was hypothesized that a substantial proportion of air could accumulate, leading to symptoms of distension, discomfort [7, 8], or colic [9, 10].

Studies on the relationship between vented BNS and reduction of infant colic symptoms are limited. Available information is based on subjective assessments like expert opinion [11], parents' recordings of infant's level of arousal, sleep states [12] and questionnaires to rank infant's symptoms on a Likert-type scale [13].

Studies on direct measurement of air swallowing during bottle-feeding are not available. However, BNSs were assessed concerning suck-swallow-breath coordination in relation to breastfeeding [7, 14]. It was speculated that increased air swallowing leads to air accumulation in the stomach which may cause gastric upset and that pulse oximetry measures may help to clarify post feeding distress [7].

To examine the effect of a vented "anticolic" teat on suck-swallow-breath coordination we investigated the sucking behaviour of infants bottle-fed with vented teats (VTs) and nonvented teats (NVTs). We hypothesize that an uncoordinated random-like sucking behaviour implies more stress in terms of increased sucking frequency, oxygen desaturation, increased cardiorespiratory parameters, leading to a higher risk of aerophagia.

Methods

Trial design

The present study was a randomized controlled clinical trial conducted from November 2013 to July 2015 in Muenster (North-Rhine-Westphalia, Germany) and Berlin, Germany. We investigated two different feeding teats (Nuk First Choice Plus and Nuk Classic, Mapa, Zeven, Germany), one of which was specifically developed (according to the manufacturer) to prevent infantile colic. It has a device (an "anticolic valve") at the base of the teat through which air can pass into the bottle during drinking, thus preventing vacuum formation. The other feeding teat has no anticolic system, serving for the control group (Fig. 1). Both teats have a so-called orthodontic shape. Cardiorespiratory parameters during feeding were recorded by an ECG monitor.

Changes to trial design

Recording of the cardiorespiratory parameters—heart and respiratory rates and oxygen saturation—was changed from once during the drinking process to 5 min prior to the feeding procedure and 10 min after feeding to consider potential differences in the initial situation of the infants. Due to a disappointing recruitment rate in Muenster, we finally had to choose an additional location for recruitment, namely, the Department of Orthodontics in Berlin.

Participants

Eligibility criteria were as follows: (i) Caucasian neonates whose mothers delivered in the 38th week of gestation or later, (ii) healthy neonates, (iii) neonates whose parents decided in advance to feed by bottle exclusively or whose breast-feeding had terminated at least 8 weeks prior, (iv) postnatal age of 1–8 months, (v) dietary supplement was allowed, (vi) medication was permitted, but had to be noted precisely by the parents.

Exclusion criteria were as follows: (i) upper respiratory infection (ii) anomalies of the oro-facial region (iii) known suckling or swallowing disorders, (iv) already known intolerances to food components, (v) twins or other multiples.

Eligibility determination as well as the measurements took place at the orthodontic departments of the University Clinic of Muenster and Charité, University Clinic of Berlin.

Interventions

Written informed consent was obtained from both parents of each infant who participated in the study. For the purpose of the study, parents received randomly allocated feeding teats with corresponding bottles, and the infants were given 2–3 weeks of acclimatization during which

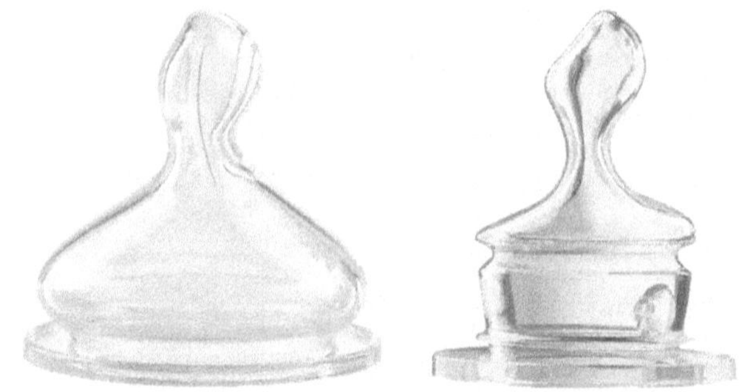

Fig. 1 Used feeding teats. Left: Vented teat Nuk First Choice Plus. Right: Nonvented teat Nuk Classic. Both, Nuk, Mapa, Zeven, Germany

Table 1 Questionnaire Items Group B - vented teat and nonvented teat groups

Item	Nonvented Teat Group ($n = 29$)	Vented Teat Group ($n = 25$)
1. My/our infant chokes while drinking (*n*).		
Never	6	3
Rarely	20	18
Always	3	4
2. My/our child spits out a significant amount of milk after drinking.		
Never	4	5
Rarely	18	15
Always	7	5
3. My/our child cries at least 3 days per week and 3 h or more per day.		
Yes	1	2
No	28	23
4.The intervals in which the child cries or screams begin abruptly.		
Yes	6	3
No	23	22
5. My/our child has a bloated, hard stomach after feeding.		
Never/rarely	24	15
Occasionally/often	5	10
6. I/we notice increased muscle tension, clenched fists, and drawn-up legs against the child's abdomen.		
Never/occasionally	24	22
Often	4	3
No information	1	0
7. I/we notice flatulence in our child.		
Never	7	2
Rarely	8	10
Occasionally/often	14	13
8. During the phases of excessive crying, the child's cries are more piercing, brighter, or shriller than usual.		
Yes	5	4
No	24	21
9. My/our child is inconsolable during the phases of excessive crying and cannot be calmed.		
Yes	3	3
No	26	22
10. The phases during which the child cries excessively and is difficult or impossible to soothe are timed.		
Throughout the day	7	2
Especially in the late afternoon and evening	1	2
Especially in the evening and at night	2	4
At other times	3	3
No information /no evaluation	16	14
11. Our child was administered the following medications during the study phase (please note all medications, even nonprescription).		
No evaluation	3	3
None	7	9
Others	16	9
Antibiotics	1	1
Gastrointestinal therapeutics (Sab Simplex, Lefax)	2	3
12. If a complementary diet was given, please state exactly what was given and at what time.		
No evaluation	1	2
Yes	13	7
No	15	16
13. We experienced problems with the feeding teat.		
Yes	13	6
No	16	19

they were to be fed exclusively by the feeding teats received prior to the appointment for measurement. Randomization was stratified by gender and a random integer list of 0 and 1 (random.org). Parents were instructed to complete a self-administered, non-validated questionnaire (Table 1) after 1 week of the acclimatization phase to reveal possible symptoms of infantile colic.

Following acclimatization, the parents made a one-time appointment at one of the clinics mentioned above. Here, the children were connected to an ECG monitor (Vitaguard VG 3100, Getemed Medizin und Informationstechnik AG, Teltow, Germany), which recorded their heart and respiratory rates and oxygen saturation (Fig. 2). The recording and feeding were done in a quiet, closed room to minimize disturbances. Infants were fed in a supine, semi-upright position by their parents (Fig. 3).

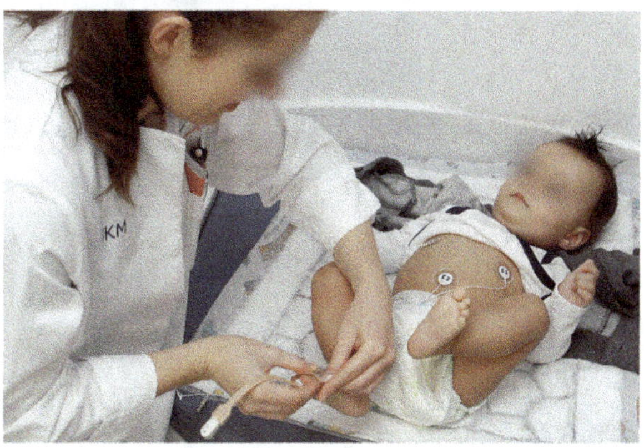

Fig. 2 Electrodes placed on the infant and connected to the ECG monitor according to the manufacturer's information

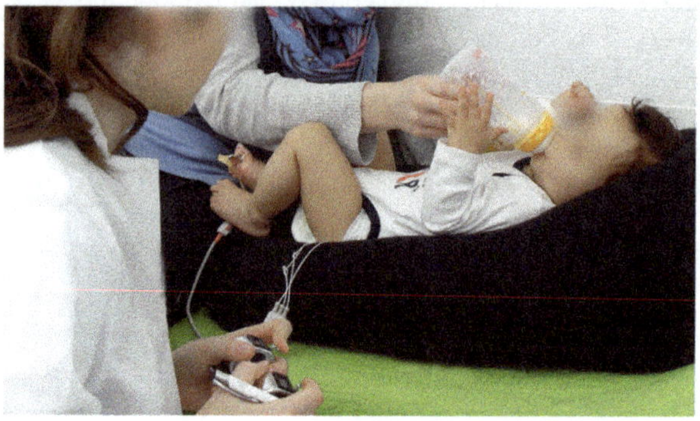

Fig. 3 Examiner records sucks and pauses by direct observation

Two examiners, not blinded to the study, were involved to take all records. Both defined and agreed on the characteristics what constitutes sucking and swallowing before the study. Since the lifting of the larynx was difficult to detect (the chin of the child laid on the chest during drinking) sucks were defined as the rhythmic forward and backward motion of the lower jaw [15]. Interruption of this rhythmic movement was defined as a pause.

During each study session one examiner took the records three times: (t1) 5 min before feeding, (t2) during feeding with parallel observation and documentation of sucking and swallowing patterns, and (t3) 10 min after feeding (Fig. 4). During the feeding procedure, the children themselves determined the time and amount of feeding until the infant had stopped drinking by himself. Following that, results from observation of the drinking patterns the cardiorespiratory parameters and the information from the parents' questionnaire were examined for possible associations.

Statistical methods

Statistical analyses were performed using SAS software, version 9.4 of the SAS System for Windows (SAS Institute, Cary, NC) and IBM SPSS Statistics 23 for Windows (IBM Corp, Somers, NY).

According to the intervention's objectives, the primary outcome of the trial was the number of sucks/min while pauses/min, feeding time, heart rate, respiratory rate, oxygen saturation, volume of milk intake, and data from the questionnaire were secondary outcomes.

Sample size calculation was performed under the assumption of a mean number of 70 sucks/min and a standard deviation of 9 sucks/min [16]. Differences in the primary outcome variable (sucking frequency) were considered relevant if they were in the order of a magnitude of at least 10%. Based on this information and a significance level of 5%, the necessary sample size comprised 29 evaluable cases per group to detect relevant differences in the two-sided Mann-Whitney *U* test with 80% statistical power.

The data were described for categorical variables by absolute and relative frequencies and for continuous variables by mean, standard deviation, median, and range. Categorical variables were compared between groups by Fisher's exact test and for continuous variables using the Mann-Whitney *U* test. *P* values <.05 were considered to be statistically significant. All *p* values reported were two-sided.

Results

Subjects

Of a total of 96 enrolled infants, 21 interrupted their contributions due to nonacceptance of the conventional

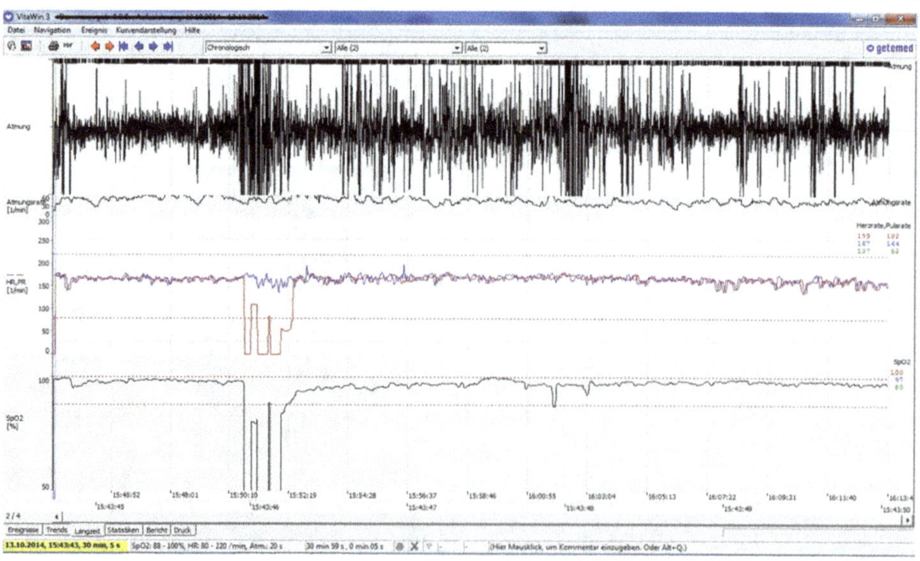

Fig. 4 Graphical representation of heart and respiratory rates and oxygen saturation with VitaWin 3 (Getemed Medizin-und Informationstechnik AG, Teltow, Germany)

NVT. One participant with a VT discontinued because of mistrust in the study and another missed the agreed appointment (Fig. 5).

Seventy-three infants remained for the intention-to-treat (ITT) analysis (NVT, $n = 40$; VT, $n = 33$). During the course of the study, a total of eight children (NVT, $n = 6$; VT, $n = 2$) were excluded because they did not want to drink or were restless, tired, or saturated; so, 65 infants remained for the per-protocol (PP) analysis.

Analysis of the questionnaire revealed a significant relationship between infant age (> 6 months) and the complementary diet ($p < .0001$). We therefore excluded infants older than 6 months for a subgroup analysis to assess the effect of a complementary diet.

Measurements

The ITT (Table 2) and PP analysis revealed no differences between the groups except the parameter "sucking pauses per minute". There was no difference in drinking time ($p = .13$, $p = .10$) and the amount of formula intake ($p = .15$, $p = .20$), but infants fed with nonvented teats needed more pauses ($p = .03$, $p = .02$) than did infants fed with vented teats. Neither gender nor age had an influence on the measurements obtained.

After excluding infants with a disproportionately complementary diet (subgroup B analysis, Table 3) the primary outcome (sucks/min) showed significant differences ($p = .01$) between the VT and NVT group (Fig. 6). The VT group showed significantly fewer pauses per minute than did the NVT group in the ITT and PP analysis, which is a trend ($p = .06$) only in the subgroup B analysis (Fig. 7). In Group B, 65.5% (19 / 29) of the infants with nonvented teats had ≤3 pauses/min. In contrast, this proportion was 88% (22/25) for infants with vented teats. Both the amount of formula intake (Fig. 8) and feeding time (Fig. 9) were similar in both groups.

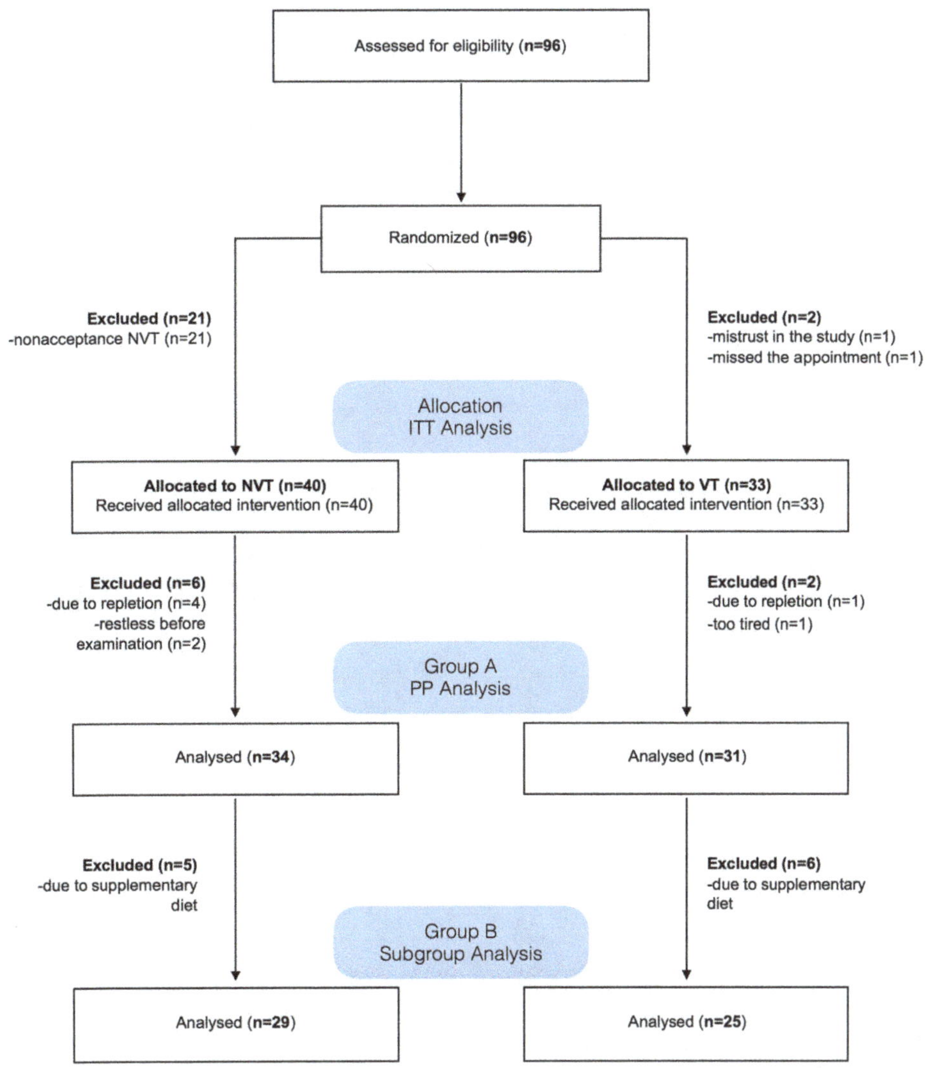

Fig. 5 Flow diagram according to the CONSORT statement

Table 2 Main group (intention-to-treat analysis). Baseline characteristics by vented teat group and nonvented teat group

	Total	Vented Teat Group	Nonvented Teat Group	*P* Value
Main Group, n (%)	73 (100)	33 (45)	40 (55)	
Age, months				0.72
Mean (SD)	4.6 (2.1)	4.5 (2.2)	4.7 (21.1)	
Median (Range)	5	4 (1–8)	5 (0–8)	
Gender, n (%)				0.64
Male	38 (52)	16 (48.5)	22 (55)	
Female	35 (48)	17 (51.5)	18 (45)	
Characteristics during bottle-feeding				
Sucks/min				0.63
Mean (SD)	40.0 (17.8)	38.7 (16.8)	41.1 (18.7)	
Median (Range)	38.2 (9.7–78.6)	36.3 (12.7–78.6)	40.7 (9.7–70.1)	
Pauses/ min				0.03
Mean (SD)	2.5 (1.3)	2.1 (1.3)	2.7 (1.2)	
Median (Range)	2.0 (0.0–6.0)	2.0 (0.0–6.0)	3 (0.5–6.0)	
Amount of formula intake (ml)				0.15
Mean (SD)	136.1 (57.2)	147.6 (58.2)	126.7 (55.4)	
Median (Range)	120.0 (25.0–250.0)	140.0 (50.0–250.0)	120 (25.0–230.0)	
Feeding time (minutes)				0.13
Mean (SD)	12.1 (6.5)	10.4 (3.7)	13.5 (7.8)	
Median (Range)	11.0 (3.5–37.0)	10.0 (5.5–19.6)	11.4 (3.5–37.0)	
Vital parameters				
Heart rate (bpm)				
Before feeding Median (Range)	143.0 (94.0–201.0)	141.0 (115.0–199.0)	144.0 (94.0–201.0)	0.74
During feeding Median (Range)	153.0 (130.0–184.0)	153.0 (139.0–178.0)	154.0 (130.0–184.0)	0.57
After feeding Median (Range)	148.0 (123.0–181.0)	146.0 (125.0–176.0)	148.0 (123.0–181.0)	0.77
Respiratory rate (bpm)				
Before feeding Median (Range)	41.0 (30.0–59.0)	40.0 (31.0–59.0)	41.0 (30.0–54.0)	0.35
During feeding Median (Range)	45.0 (36.4–61.0)	44.0 (38.0–61.0)	46.0 (36.4–60.0)	0.43
After feeding Median (Range)	41.0 (30.0–58.0)	39.0 (33.0–58.0)	41.5 (30.0–50.0)	0.52
Oxygen Saturation (%)				
Before feeding Median (Range)	98.0 (87.0–100.0)	99.0 (93.0–100.0)	98.0 (87.0–100.0)	0.01
During feeding Median (Range)	98.0 (88.0–100.0)	98.0 (88.0–100.0)	98.0 (90.0–100.0)	0.71
After feeding Median (Range)	98.0 (84.0–99.0)	98.0 (84.0–99.0)	98.0 (90.0–99.0)	0.82

Abbreviation: *ml* millilitre, *bpm* beats per minute, *bpm* breaths per minute

Table 3 Subgroup B analysis. Baseline characteristics by vented teat group and nonvented teat group

	Total	Vented Teat Group	Nonvented Teat Group	*P* Value
Subgroup, n (%)	54/73 (74)	25/33 (76)	29/40 (73)	
Age, months				0.52
Mean (SD)		3.76 (1.64)	4.03 (1.68)	
Median (Range)		4 (1–6)	4 (1–6)	
Gender, n				1.00
Male	27	12	15	
Female	27	13	14	
Chracteristics during bottle-feeding				
Sucks/min				0.01
Mean (SD)	43.0 (16.4)	36.7 (15.2)	48.4 (15.6)	
Median (Range)	39.0 (19.7–77.1)	32.4 (19.7–77.1)	50.4 (19.8–70.1)	
Pauses/ min				0.06
Mean (SD)	2.7 (1.3)	2.3 (1.3)	2.9 (1.3)	
Median (Range)	2.3 (0.0–6.0)	2.0 (0.0–6.0)	3.0 (0.7–6.0)	
Amount of formula intake (ml)				0.33
Mean (SD)	135.0 (54.2)	143.4 (56.4)	127.8 (52.2)	
Median (Range)	120.0 (50.0–250.0)	120.0 (50.0–250.0)	120.0 (50.0–230.0)	
Feeding time (minutes)				0.34
Mean (SD)	12.0 (6.1)	10.6 (3.5)	13.2 (7.5)	
Median (Range)	10.8 (5.2–37.0)	10.2 (5.5–19.6)	11.3 (5.2–37.0)	
Vital parameters				
Heart rate (bpm)				
Before feeding Median (Range)	144.5 (107.0–201.0)	142.0 (123.0–199.0)	147.0 (107.0–201.0)	0.33
During feeding Median (Range)	156.5 (130.0–183.0)	153.0 (140.0–177.0)	159.0 (130.0–183.0)	0.68
After feeding Median (Range)	149.5 (124.0–177.0)	146.0 (131.0–176.0)	153.0 (124.0–177.0)	0.34
Respiratory rate (bpm)				
Before feeding Median (Range)	41.5 (31.0–59.0)	41.0 (31.0–59.0)	42.0 (35.0–54.0)	0.16
During feeding Median (Range)	45.0 (38.0–61.0)	44.0 (38.0–61.0)	46.9 (38.0–60.0)	0.21
After feeding Median (Range)	42.7 (31.0–58.0)	42.0 (33.0–58.0)	43.0 (31.0–50.0)	0.6
Oxygen Saturation (%)				
Before feeding Median (Range)	99.0 (87.0–100.0)	99.0 (93.0–100.0)	98.0 (87.0–100.0)	0.16
During feeding Median (Range)	98.0 (88.0–100.0)	98.0 (88.0–100.0)	98.0 (90.0–100.0)	0.97
After feeding Median (Range)	98.0 (90.0–99.0)	98.0 (91.0–99.0)	98.0 (90.0–99.0)	0.83

Abbreviation: *ml* millilitre, *bpm* beats per minute, *bpm* breaths per minute

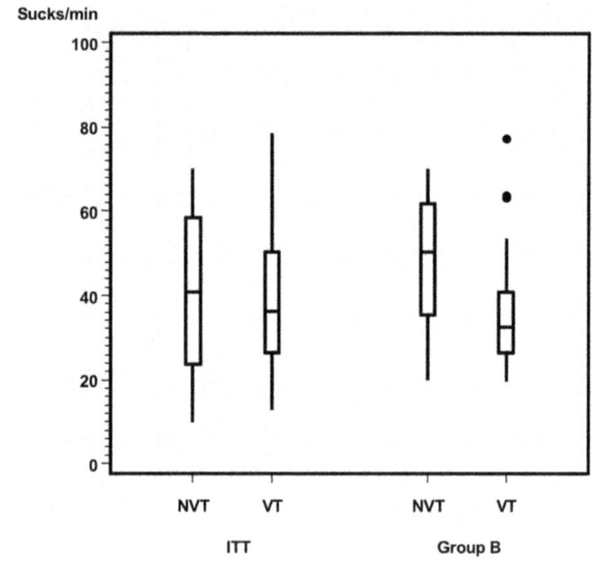

Fig. 6 Primary outcome sucks per minute between NVTs (ITT: 41.1 ± 18.7; Group B: 48.4 ± 15.6) and VTs (ITT: 38.7 ± 16.8; Group B: 36.7 ± 15.2). ITT ($p = .63$), Group B ($p = .01$)

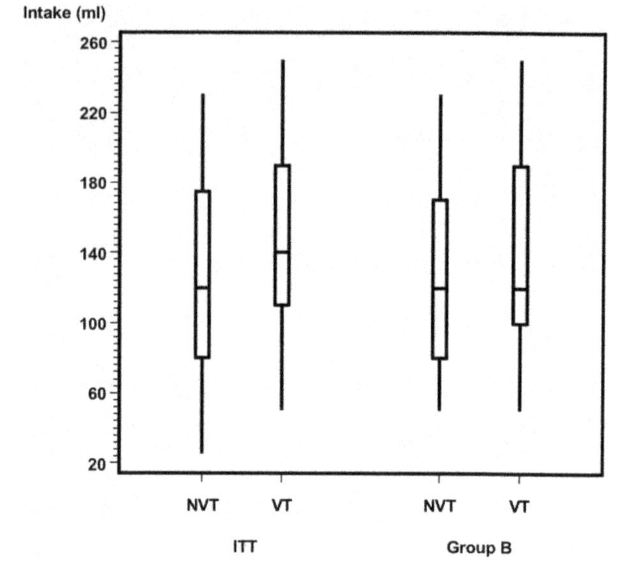

Fig. 8 Primary outcome formula intake (mL) between NVTs (ITT: 126.7 ± 55.4; Group B: 127.8 ± 52.2) and VTs (ITT: 147.6 ± 58.2; Group B: 143.4 ± 56.4). ITT ($p = .15$), Group B ($p = .33$)

Heart rates were within normal limits and showed a similar pattern in both groups (Fig. 10). Heart rates increased by 8.9 ± 10.9 bpm during feeding (from t1 to t2) and decreased by 6.1 ± 7.4 bpm after feeding (from t2 to t3). The VT group showed consistently lower median bpm values than did the NVT group at each recording time, but not to a significant extent.

Respiratory rate had similar characteristics. On average, the rate increased by 3.9 ± 4.8 bpm during feeding (from t1 to t2) and decreased by 4.2 ± 5.2 bpm after feeding (from t2 to t3). Again, with respect to recording times, the VT group showed consistently lower median breaths/min than did the NVT group but also not to a significant extent (Fig. 11).

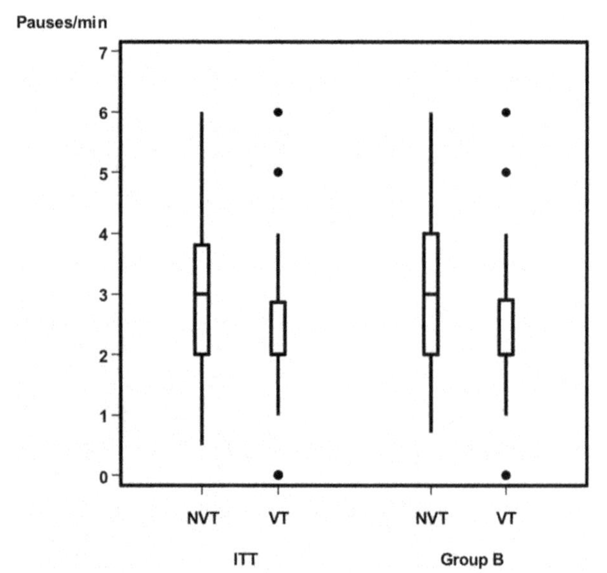

Fig. 7 Pauses per minute between NVTs (ITT: 2.7 ± 1.2; Group B: 2.9 ± 1.3) and VTs (ITT: 2.1 ± 1.3; Group B: 2.3 ± 1.3). ITT ($p = .03$), Group B ($p = .06$)

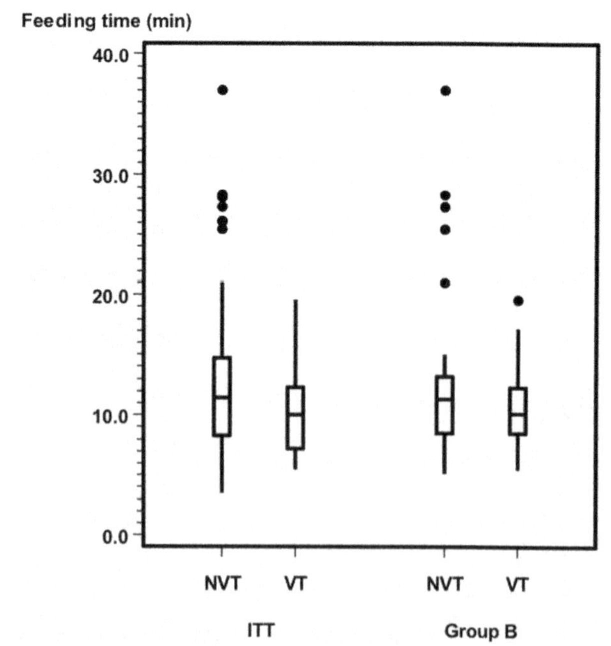

Fig. 9 Feeding time in minutes for the NVT (ITT: 13.5 ± 7.8; Group B: 13.2 ± 7.5) and VT group (ITT: 10.4 ± 3.7; Group B: 10.6 ± 3.5). ITT ($p = .13$), Group B ($p = .34$)

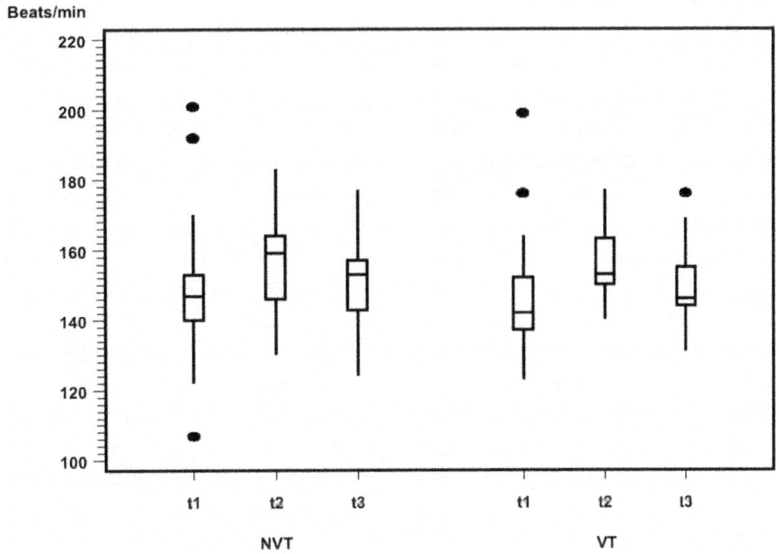

Fig. 10 Heart rates in beats per minute (bpm) before, during, and after feeding

Oxygen saturation was consistently in the normal range, at approximately 97% at any recording time. There was no difference between the groups.

Questionnaire

The questionnaire by itself did not show any differences in the ITT, PP, or subgroup B analysis between both types of feeding teats regarding possible symptoms of infantile colic (Table 1). There was no difference in any parameters in infants who took medication and those who did not.

Discussion

The aim of this study was to investigate differences in sucking behaviour of infants bottle-fed with vented and nonvented teats. We hypothesized that possible differences of milk flow may result in uncoordinated sucking, implying more stress in terms of oxygen desaturation, increased heart and respiratory rates, and increased sucking frequency, leading to a higher risk of aerophagia. We used a mixed approach consisting of a parents' self-administered, non-validated questionnaire and a monitoring of infants' heart and

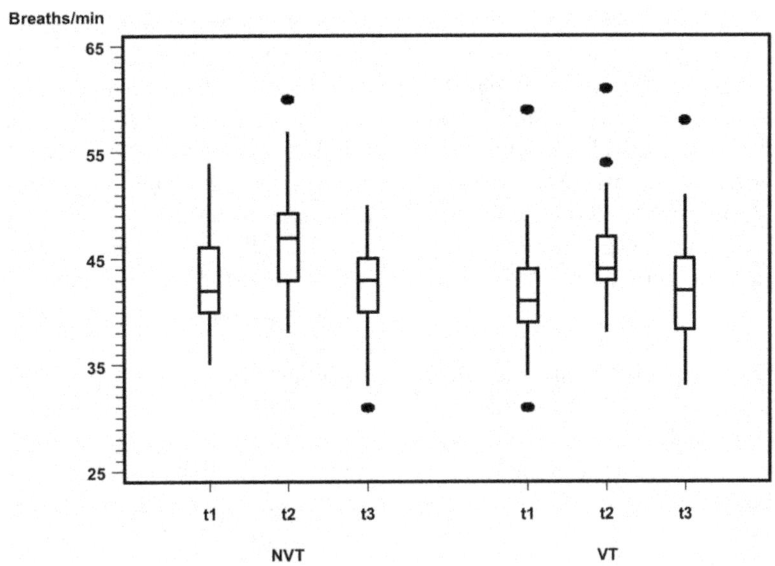

Fig. 11 Respiratory rate in breaths per minute (bpm) before, during, and after feeding. The VT group showed consistently slightly lower median bpm values than did the NVT group at each recording time, but not to a significant extent

respiratory rates and oxygen saturation before, during, and after feeding.

Various studies have investigated topics related to nutritive and nonnutritive sucking and their mechanisms and various BNSs and how they influenced the infant, but as far as we are aware, no previous studies have been published, comparing the sucking behaviour in full term infants using vented and nonvented teats. For this reason, our results cannot be discussed in view of comparable investigations.

One focus of research is the comparison of breast- and bottle-feeding. Despite high variability in breastfeeding studies, sucking behaviour improves with maturation [14] and bottle fed term infants show lower breathing frequency [17], lower oxygen saturation [7, 17], higher heart rate and lower blood pressure [18], lower suck frequency [15, 17], less coordinated (random) sucks [7], and less sucking pauses [15].

Nipple units differ in size, shape, consistency and mechanics and these factors are thought to influence suck-swallow-breath coordination in both term and preterm infants [7, 16, 19–21].

We found that sucking frequency using VTs was lower in the ITT analysis and significantly lower in the subgroup B analysis ($p = .01$). A comparative investigation of vented and nonvented bottles in preterm infants showed results nearly similar to ours [21]. The authors observed that sucking frequency is lower in a vacuum-free bottle system which confirmed "a more mature stage of sucking" [21]. The preterm infants showed a sucking frequency of 0.6 sucks/s with a vacuum-free bottle system and 0.9 sucks/s with a standard bottle, which corresponds to 36 sucks/min with a vacuum-free bottle system and 54 sucks/min using a standard bottle, closely matching our results (Table 3).

Moral and coworkers used the same VT as in our study when comparing breast- and bottle-feeding [15]. They found in a group of exclusively bottle-fed infants 37.9 ± 13.5 sucks/min which corresponds closely to our findings (Tables 2, 3). Infants 3–5 months of age showed significantly less pauses during bottle-feeding compared to breast-feeding [15]. In contrast, other studies found higher sucking values when different nonvented nipples were used [16].

Various studies focus on the influence of a specific bottle or nipple design on a particular health parameter of the infant. These studies comparing BNSs focused, inter alia, on vital parameters such as oxygen saturation during bottle-feeding with a particular feeding teat design [7, 20, 22] and sucking skills [7, 21].

Fucile et al. investigated skills of suck-swallow-respiration coordination and observed higher sucking stages when fed with the VT bottle [21]. This more mature sucking [21] corresponds to our own findings: We found no differences between the amount of formula intake and feeding time throughout the feeding procedure, meaning that, with the same amount of feeding medium for the same time, subgroup B needed fewer sucks and less pauses with the VTs than with the NVTs. Clinically, lower mean suck frequency suggests that the nipple enables to lengthen the intrasuck interval to allow the time necessary for swallowing larger volume of milk [22]. Our findings indicate that, on the one hand, the VTs did not hasten the formula flow nor did they increase formula intake. On the other hand, they did foster a more constant nonrandom drinking process.

Even though the drinking process is different between the VT and NVT group, we found no differences concerning cardiorespiratory measurements. Our results support the findings of Fadavi et al. who observed no differences in oxygen saturation when term neonates were bottle-fed with different nipples [22]. This is in contrast to other studies that found decreased oxygenation saturation during feeding of term neonates [7, 17]. One possible explanation for our results may be that we included older infants who maintained stable oxygen saturation.

Preterm infants have significant desaturation during bottle-feeding [23], but it could be shown that oxygen saturation increases significantly if a vented BNS is used [20]. Interestingly, some authors reported significantly lower SpO2 after feeding and attribute this to aerophagia in terms of burping and gastric distress [7, 24]. In general, higher oxygen levels during bottle-feeding is seen as a more coordinated sucking, swallowing, and breathing pattern [7]. The authors stated, "If a system can be designed that promotes less swallowing, babies can feed more like the natural physiologic norm of breast-feeding." [7].

Results from the literature and our own findings suggest that nonvented teats have a higher risk for aerophagia. The mechanism behind nonvented teats is the vacuum that builds up within the bottle and results in a net decrease of milk flow [21]. The infant tries to compensate for the negative pressure by increasing sucking frequency or amplitude until nipple release after air reflux from the oral cavity. Vented teats allow the nipple to deliver formula in an uninterrupted process [20].

The hypothesis that aerophagia causes colic symptoms [3, 10, 25] is unproven, and the evidence of vented BNS on infant colic is very low. Subjective assessments like expert opinion [11] and questionnaires [12, 13] attribute a positive effect of vented BNS on infant colic. Other studies found that aerophagia could be seen as a consequence of increased sucking frequency, which may cause gastric upset [7, 24]. Our own results also support the findings that increased sucking implies the risk of aerophagia which could be reduced by using vented BNSs. In our investigation, the used questionnaire by itself did not show any differences between the two types of feeding teats in connection with colic symptoms. However, valid tools to assess infant colic are not available [26] and further studies are needed to prove the relation between aerophagia and infant colic.

The age of the infants is a confounding factor and a potential limitation of this study. Sucking behaviour improves with age and the inclusion of infants older than 6 months may have biased the sample. We included older infants due to a disappointing recruitment rate of exclusively bottle-fed healthy infants. Complementary diet increased with age and showed an effect on the ITT and PP analysis. Therefore, 6 to 8 months old infants were excluded.

Maturation may also be the reason why both groups maintain stable cardiorespiratory parameters and the effect of a ventilation is too small to create significant differences between the groups. Preterm or other impaired infants may be more vulnerable to this effect.

Specific bottle or nipple designs have an influence on sucking behaviour. We therefore used the same "orthodontic" shape of one manufacturer for both groups. The different base size may have an effect but lip resting was not disturbed with both teats.

Conclusions

Our hypothesis that an uncoordinated sucking behaviour implies more stress in terms of increased sucking frequency could be confirmed, whereas the effect of oxygen desaturation and cardiorespiratory parameters must be rejected. Compared with an NVT group, infants aged 1–6 months need fewer sucks and pauses when fed with VTs. In both groups, equal amounts of feeding medium and feeding time was observed. With NVT feeding, disruption occurs when the bottle vacuum is released by air from the oral cavity. Therefore, higher sucking frequency is needed to rebuild the oral vacuum for bottle milk flow, which implies a higher risk of aerophagia. The role of aerophagia in the occurrence of infantile colic is vague and must be investigated further. Overall, we suggest that the VTs provided a more coordinated drinking pattern than did the NVTs, which may have a positive effect on gastric distress.

Abbreviations

BNS: Bottle-nipple system; ITT: Intention- to- treat; NVT: Nonvented teat; PP: Per-protocol; VT: Vented teat

Acknowledgments

We thank Prof Dr. Jost-Brinkmann and Mrs Milkereit from the Charité-Universitätsmedizin Berlin for supporting the participants' examination at the Charité. We also acknowledge the participation of the parents and their infants.

Funding

The study was funded by:
MAPA GmbH.
Industriestraße 21-25.
27404 Zeven.
Germany.
E-mail:info@mapa.de
URL:http://www.mapa.de/

Authors' contributions

TS and AH suggested the original idea for the paper and developed the study design. MK and LE wrote the study protocol, registered the study, recruited the patients, collected the data, and wrote parts of the manuscript. CS made the statistical analysis and contributed to the interpretation of the results. TS contributed to the statistical analysis and data handling and wrote the main part of the manuscript. AH, LE, and MK wrote parts of the paper, did the literature search, and reviewed the paper for content, including the final version of the manuscript. All authors read and approved the final manuscript.

Competing interests

All authors declare that they have no competing interests.

Author details

[1]Private Practice Dr. Thomas Hinz, Dr. Uta Neumann, Stoeckstraße 106, 44649 Herne, Germany. [2]Private Practice, Weststraße 1, 49176 Hilter, Germany. [3]Department of Orthodontics, University of Münster, Albert-Schweitzer-Campus 1, 48149 Münster, Germany. [4]Institute of Biostatistics and Clinical Research, University of Münster, Schmeddingstraße 56, 48149 Münster, Germany.

References

1. Lucassen PL, Assendelft WJ, van Eijk JT, Gubbels JW, Douwes a C, van Geldrop WJ. Systematic review of the occurrence of infantile colic in the community. Arch Dis Child. 2001;84(5):398–403. https://doi.org/10.1136/adc.84.5.398.
2. Wessel MA, Cobb JC, Jackson EB, Harris GS, Detwiler AC. Paroxysmal fussing in infancy, sometimes called colic. Pediatrics. 1954;14(5):421–35.
3. Zahorsky J. Mixed feeding of infants. Pediatrics. 1901;11:208–15.
4. Pace CA. Infantile colic: what to know for the primary care setting. Clin Pediatr (Phila). 2017;56(7):616–8.
5. Biagioli E, Tarasco V, Lingua C, Moja L, Savino F. Pain-relieving agents for infantile colic. Cochrane Database Syst Rev. 2016;9:CD009999.
6. Stone RT, Morgan MC. Aerophagia in children. Am Fam Physician [Internet]. 1971;3:94–5.
7. Goldfield EC, Richardson MJ, Lee KG, Margetts S. Coordination of sucking, swallowing, and breathing and oxygen saturation during early infant breast-feeding and bottle-feeding. Pediatr Res. 2006;60(4):450–5. https://doi.org/10.1203/01.pdr.0000238378.24238.9d.
8. Dowling DA, Tycon L. Bottle/nipple systems: helping parents make informed choices. Nurs Womens Health. 2010;14(1):61–6. https://doi.org/10.1111/j.1751-486X.2010.01508.x.
9. HUTH EF. Aerophagy in infancy. Kinderarztl Prax. 1959;27(5):219–22.
10. Leung A. Infantile colic: a review. J R Soc Promot Heal. 2004;124(4):162–6.
11. Waddell L. A topic in 10 questions: managing infantile colic. J Fam Health Care. 2013;23(1):24–5.
12. Cirgin Ellett ML, Perkins SM. Examination of the effect of Dr. Brown's natural flow baby bottles on infant colic. Gastroenterol Nurs. 2006;29(3):226–31. https://doi.org/10.1097/00001610-200605000-00004.
13. Tikochinski Y, Kukliansky I. Examination of the effect of BornFree ActiveFlow baby bottles on infant colic. Gastroenterol Nurs. 2013;36(2):123–7. https://doi.org/10.1097/SGA.0b013e318288d13a.
14. Sakalidis VS, McClellan HL, Hepworth AR, Kent JC, Lai CT, Hartmann PE, et al. Oxygen saturation and suck-swallow-breathe coordination of term infants during breastfeeding and feeding from a teat releasing milk only with vacuum. Int J Pediatr. 2012;2012:1–10.

15. Moral A, Bolibar I, Seguranyes G, Ustrell JM, Sebastia G, Martinez-Barba C, Rios J. Mechanics of sucking: comparison between bottle feeding and breastfeeding. BMC Pediatr. 2010;10:6–2431.
16. Mathew OP, Belan M, Thoppil CK. Sucking patterns of neonates during bottle feeding: comparison of different nipple units. Am J Perinatol. 1992; 9(4):265–9. https://doi.org/10.1055/s-2007-994786.
17. Mathew OP, Bhatia J. Sucking and breathing patterns during breast- and bottle-feeding in term neonates. Am J Dis Child. 1989;143:588–92.
18. Butte NF, Smith EOB, Garza C. Heart rates of breast-fed and formula-fed infants. J Pediatr Gastroenterol Nutr. 1991;13:391–6.
19. Mathew OP. Breathing patterns of preterm infants during bottle feeding: role of milk flow. J Pediatr [Internet]. 1991;119:960–5.
20. Jenik A, Fustiñana C, Marquez M, Mage D, Fernandez G, Mariani G. A new bottle design decreases hypoxemic episodes during feeding in preterm infants. Int J Pediatr. 2012;2012:531608. https://doi.org/10.1155/2012/531608.
21. Fucile S, Gisel E, Schanler RJ, Lau C. A controlled-flow vacuum-free bottle system enhances preterm infants' nutritive sucking skills. Dysphagia. 2009; 24(2):145–51. https://doi.org/10.1007/s00455-008-9182-z.
22. Fadavi S, Punwani IC, Jain L, Vidyasagar D. Mechanics and energetics of nutritive sucking: a functional comparison of commercially available nipples. J Pediatr. 1997;130(5):740–5.
23. Poets CF, Langner MU, Bohnhorst B. Effects of bottle feeding and two different methods of gavage feeding on oxygenation and breathing patterns in preterm infants. Acta Paediatr [Internet]. 1997;86:419–23.
24. Hammerman C, Kaplan M. Oxygen saturation during and after feeding in healthy term infants. Biol Neonate. 1995;67(2):94–9.
25. Leung AK, Chan PY, Cho HYCM. An updated review of infantile colic. Can J Clin Med. 1997;4(10):16–9.
26. García Marques S, Chillón Martínez R, González Zapta S, Rebollo Salas M, Jiménez Rejano JJ. Tools assessment and diagnosis to infant colic: a systematic review. Child Care Health Dev. 2017;43(4):481–8. https://doi.org/10.1111/cch.12454. Epub 2017 Mar 5

6

Factors associated with congenital anomalies in Addis Ababa and the Amhara Region, Ethiopia

Molla Taye[1*], Mekbeb Afework[2], Wondwossen Fantaye[3], Ermias Diro[4] and Alemayehu Worku[5]

Abstract

Background: The early stage of embryo development is extremely vulnerable to various teratogenic factors, leading to congenital anomalies. In Ethiopia, a significant number of babies are born with congenital anomalies, but the risk factors for the anomalies have never been studied. Understanding the specific risk factors for congenital anomalies is very essential to provide health education that aims at creating awareness and establishing preventive strategic plan/s. The main objective of this study was to assess the risk factors associated with congenital anomalies in Addis Ababa and the Amhara Region, Ethiopia.

Methods: A case-control study was conducted from January 1- June 30, 2015. The participants were recruited at the purposively selected hospitals in Addis Ababa and the Amhara Region. A total of 207 cases and 207 controls were included in the study. Cases were neonates, infants, and children 0-11 months of age with external and internal major congenital anomalies diagnosed by pediatricians. Controls were neonates, infants, and children 0-11 months of age without external and internal anomalies. Data on sociodemographic characteristics, exposure to risk factors, and reproductive history were collected by face to face interviews with children's mothers/caregivers using a structured questionnaire. Binary logistic regression was employed to explore risk factors associated with the occurrence of the problems.

Results: About 87.4% of the children were below 6 months, and 12.6% were between 6 and 11 months. The majority (59.9%) of the children were male, with the M: F sex ratio of 1.49. The mean age of the mothers was 26 years (16-45 years). Unidentified medication use during early pregnancy (AOR = 4.595; 95% CI: 1.868-11.301, *P*-value = 0.001), maternal alcohol drinking (AOR = 2.394; 95% CI: 1.212-4.726, *P*-value = 0.012), and exposure to chemicals (AOR = 9.964; 95% CI = 1.238-80.193, *P*-value = 0.031) were significantly associated with the occurrence of congenital anomalies. Iron folate use (AOR = 0.051; 95% CI: 0.010-0.260, *P*-value = < 0.001) before and during early pregnancy had a protective effect on congenital anomaly.

Conclusion: Unidentified medication use, alcohol drinking during early pregnancy, and exposure to chemicals had a significant association with the occurrence of congenital anomalies, whereas iron folate use before and during early pregnancy had a protective effect from congenital anomalies.

Keywords: Congenital anomaly, Case-control, Teratogen, Risk/Associated factors

* Correspondence: mollataye2@gmail.com
[1]Department of Anatomy, School of Medicine, College of Medicine and Health Sciences, the University of Gondar, Gondar, Ethiopia

Background

The early stages of embryo development are a critical period which may mark vulnerability to disruption by teratogenic agents that lead to congenital anomaly [1–3]. Congenital anomaly (CA) is defined as a structural or functional defect that may be detected during pregnancy or be visible at birth or later in life. CAs are the major cause of new born/infant morbidity, mortality, and disability in addition to adding to the burden of the health care system [4]. It is estimated that about 20–30% of infant deaths occur due to CAs [5]; severe CAs occur in 3% of live [6, 7], and 20% of still births [8], and 7.9 million children are born with serious CAs, accounting for 6% of all births globally [9].

According to literature, genetic and environmental factors play a major role in causing CAs during the first trimester [10]. Approximately, 7.6 million children are born with CAs worldwide due to genetic factors [11]. Although there is a better understanding of the etiology of CA in the literature, the causes of most of the CAs are still unknown. However, they are believed to be caused by several etiologic factors [12, 13].

The occurrence of certain risk factors, such as maternal chronic diseases, like diabetes, family history, and viral infections during early pregnancy increase the risk of having a baby with CAs [14–17]. Furthermore, risk factors linked to the occurrence of CAs include unidentified medication/illicit/prescribed drug/s use, alcohol consumption, smoking cigarettes, exposure to radiation, chemical agents, parental age, parental occupation, nutritional deficiencies, and chromosomal mutations as well as socio-economic factors [7, 14, 15, 18–20]. Hence, exposure to all of these factors can influence the organogenesis processes of the embryo [7, 12].

Moreover, some studies showed that maternal use of folic acid and multivitamins containing folic acid around conception and the first 3 months of pregnancy have a protective effect against certain types of CAs [21, 22].

In general, the prevalence of CAs varies with race, ethnicity, and geographical regions across the world [7, 11, 16, 23, 24]. In Ethiopia, a significant number of babies are born with CAs, but the causes of these CAs have never been studied. In fact, whether the causes are environmental or genetic factors or interactions between environmental and genetic factors are not known. In addition, there are no preventive strategic plans to reduce or control the occurrence of these problems. It is obvious that children born with major CA are prone to die or even if they survive, they may confront a long-term morbidity and disability and may also undergo repeated surgical interventions. Evidence based information about specific risk factors for CAs are very essential to provide health education to communities, especially to females in the reproductive age. This could not only help to create awareness so as to reduce the occurrence of anomalies but also assists policy makers/responsible bodies to develop preventive strategic plans.

The main objective of this study was to assess the risk factors for CAs in Addis Ababa and the Amhara Region. The results are believed to provide information for public health actions and to create awareness about CAs and their etiologic factors. They may also be used as baseline for further investigations.

Methods

Study sites

The study was carried out in Addis Ababa and the Amhara region, Ethiopia.

Addis Ababa, the capital of Ethiopia, has 10 sub-cities with an estimated total population of 3,273,001(47.4% male, 52.6% female). The population of Addis is diverse by ethnicity. The majority of the people are Christians, followed by Muslims and some followers of other religions [25]. The city is subject to population increase through continuous migrations [25]. All of the hospitals in the city provide inpatient, outpatient, and delivery services, except Cure Ethiopia International Children's Hospital, which does not provide delivery services.

The Amhara Region, the second largest northwest region of the country has a population of 20,399,004 (50. 1% male, 49.9% female). The majority of the people live in rural areas and the minority in large and small towns. Most of the Amhara people are Christians, with a good number of Muslims and some followers of other faiths [25]. All of the hospitals in the regional state provide various inpatient and outpatient services including delivery.

Selection of study hospitals

Five public hospitals in Addis Ababa and three in the Amhara Region were purposively selected for this study on the basis of case load. All of the hospitals are referral with high patient flow and various specialized departments or units, which provide various services to neonates, infants, children, and adults.

Study design and sample size

A case-control design was used to investigate exposure status to risk factors for CAs in the case and control children.

A sample of 414 children (207 cases, 207 controls) was recruited for this study. The sample size was calculated by using a ratio of 1:1, power of 90%, a 5% significance level and 38.81% of likelihood of an event in controls (i.e. exposure in controls) [17], and assuming the Odds ratio to be 2. The study children were matched by age. Cases were neonates, infants, and children 0-11 months of age with external and internal major CAs. Major CAs are defined as anomalies that have partial or complete organ/ organ system absence/defects, resulting in functional, health, and cosmetic effects, which require surgical repair and rehabilitations [4]. The cases were selected from live births at the study hospitals, neonate units and under five clinics. The type of CAs were classified as major by using WHO/CDC/ICBDSR manual 2014 [4]. Based on WHO/ CDC/ICBDSR classification method, the cases with neural tube, orofacial region, musculoskeletal system and genitourinary system defects and less than 12 months of age were purposively selected and included in the study. Children aged 12 months and above and had major and minor CA were excluded. All cases had isolated CAs except one child who had multiple anomalies. The diagnoses of the cases were confirmed through physical examinations and echocardiography (i.e. for cases with heart defects) by pediatricians. The cases were selected purposively. The controls were neonates, infants, and children 0-11 months of age without external and internal CAs. The controls were randomly selected in the same hospitals where children with CAs were identified. All children aged 0-11 months constituted the source population.

Data collection method

The data were collected by a face to face interview of the children's mothers/caregivers by using a structured questionnaire and checklists. The questionnaire prepared in English and translated to Amharic was pretested at other hospitals and amended according to the results. Data were collected on residence, sociodemo graphic characteristics, reproductive/pregnancy history and adverse outcomes, family history of CAs, socioeconomic status, parental ethnicity, parental occupation, maternal educational level, maternal nutritional status/ history, parental exposures to risk factors and/or teratogenic agents, such as radiation, chemicals, pesticides, etc. for CAs, maternal illness/disease, medication/illicit drug use, substance abuse (alcohol consumption, smoking), blood relationships among parents, antenatal care visits, folic acid and multivitamin use, and birth order of children. The data were gathered at delivery rooms/ wards, neonatal units, and under five clinics. Prior to data collection, data collectors (nurses, midwifes) were trained for 2 days. The data were collected from January 1- June 30, 2015.

Data management and analysis

Data were checked on daily basis by collectors and further overseen by the principal investigator and supervisors for completeness and correctness during collection periods. It was also rechecked during data entry. The data were coded and entered into Epi-Info version 3.5.1 and then transferred to SPSS version 21 for analysis. Data cleaning, error checking, and analysis were conducted by using SPSS version 21. Data were calculated by using frequency, cross tabulation, and binary logistic regression. Significance level was considered at less than 0.05 *p*-value. Crude Odds ratio and confidence level were calculated. After the crude Odds ratios were identified, adjusted Odds ratios were computed to assess risk factors associated with the occurrence of CAs by using backward stepwise logistic regression. Exposure variables with P-value ≤0.2 in the crude Odds ratio were entered into the multivariable logistic regression model to observe their relationships and CAs (i.e. to observe associated variables with CAs in the adjusted Odds ratio). The characteristics of cases and controls were explained in percentages and numbers. The crude and adjusted Odds ratios, confidence intervals, *p*-values and the overall findings are presented in the result section in the form of texts and tables.

Ethical clearance

Ethical clearance was obtained from Addis Ababa University, College of Health Sciences Institutional Review Board, the National Research Ethics Review Committee, Addis Ababa City Administration Health Bureau Ethical Clearance Committee, and the Amhara National Regional State Health Bureau Regional Health Research Laboratory Center. Supportive letters were written to all zonal health departments and study hospitals by the health bureaus. Ethical and supportive letters were submitted to all hospital administrators. The purpose of the study was explained to the participant children's mothers/caregivers. Data collection began after permissions were obtained from hospital managers/medical directors and after a written consent was obtained from children's mothers/caretakers. Data collected from the participants were kept in secured and locked cabinets in order to maintain confidentiality.

Results

Socio-demographic characteristics of the study participants

The sample consisted of 414 (207 cases, 207 controls) children. The age of children ranged from 1 day to 11 months. About 87.4% of the children were below 6 months and 12. 6% between 6 and 11 months. The majority (59.9%) of the children were male and 40.1% female with a sex ratio of 1. 49, respectively. The mean age of the children's mothers was 26 years (range 16-45). Among the participants, 63.3% were urban and 36.7% rural dwellers. In terms of income, 47.8% had middle and 37.2% low economic status as stated by the mothers/respondents. The majority (93.5%) of the children's mothers were married; about 37.4% had no formal education; 31.9% had primary education, and 30.7% secondary and higher level of education. By religious affiliation, 72.2, 27.3, and 0.5% of the parents were Christian, Muslim, and others, respectively. Among the mothers, 53% were housewives, 17.9% government, private, or self-employed, 14.3% farmers, and 14% jobless. Similarly, 49.3, 38.9, and 11.8% of the children's fathers were employees, farmers, and jobless, respectively. The major (62.1%) ethnic group in this study were Amhara, 23.2% Oromo, 5.6% Guragie, 3.6% Tigre, and 3.6% Seltie. The other socio-demographic characteristics of the participants are shown in Table 1.

About 12 (5.8%) and 13 (6.3%) of mothers whose children had and had no CAs, respectively, were in the 15-19 years of age group. Besides, 49 (23%) and 68 (32.9%) of mothers whose children were exposed and not exposed to CAs, respectively, were 20-24 years of age. Similarly, 69 (33.3%) and 68 (32.9%) of the mothers who had children with and without CAs, respectively, were in the 25–29 years of age group, whereas 49 (23.7%) and 31 (15%) mothers who had and free children, respectively, were in the 30–34 years of age group. Likewise, 28 (13.5%) and 27 (13%) of the mothers who had affected and non-affected children, respectively, were 35–39 years of age.

About 99.5% of the CAs identified were isolated/single, while 1 (0.5%) was multiple. The frequency of CAs by organ/organ system is shown in Table 2.

Reproductive, obstetric, and offspring background/history

As far as the birth order of children was concerned, 32.9, 19.8, and 47.3% were first, second, third and above (3+) children to their families, respectively. Among the controls, about 48.3, 22.7, and 29% were first, second, third and above (3+) children, respectively, to their parents. About 16.4% of mothers whose children had CAs and 9. 2% of the mothers who had children without CAs, had no antenatal care (ANC) visits. The total number of pregnancy history, preterm, miscarriage, stillbirth, gravidity, gestational age at first ANC, number of live births, and neonate/infant/child deaths are presented in Table 3.

Risk factors associated with congenital anomalies

There were maternal/medical illnesses (i.e. infections or chronic diseases such as diseases with fever, chronic disorders) in 24 (11.6%) of the mothers who had children with CAs and 13 (6.3%) of mothers whose children were not affected with CAs. Passive smokers were observed in 37 (17.9%) and 28 (13.5%) of mothers who had children with and without CAs, respectively. Among the participants, unidentified medication use in early pregnancy by mothers whose children had and had no CAs were 16.9 and 3.9%, respectively. Contraceptive (both pill and injection) use around conception was 11.6% in the mothers who had children with CAs and 2.4% in the mothers who had no children with CAs. In addition, anemia was observed in 55 (26.6%) of the affected children's mothers and 37 (17.9%) of mothers whose children had no CAs (Table 4).

Blood relationships among parents were reported in 4. 8% of children's the exposed mothers and 1.0% of not exposed children's mothers. Family history of CA as seen in the children was also reported in 4.3% of the affected children's parents and 1.4% of the parents whose children had no CAs. Exposure to chemicals among mothers who had children with and without CAs was 6. 3 and 0.5%, respectively. On the other hand, two (0.97%) of mothers whose children had CAs used fertility enhancing drugs. Again, one (0.5%) of the affected child mother had diabetes during pregnancy. On the contrary, mothers who had children without CAs reported no use of fertility enhancing drugs around conception and had no diabetes during and before pregnancy. In addition, none of the affected children's mothers took multivitamins before they got pregnant, while one (0.5%) of the mother who had child without CA used multivitamin before pregnancy. Moreover, about 25 (12.1%) of mothers whose children had CAs and 17 (8.2%) of the mothers who had children without CAs, had no food shortage before and during pregnancy (Table 4). However, the above-mentioned factors were not statistically significant in the multivariable analysis, the adjusted Odds Ratio. In addition, maternal age, parental ethnicity, mothers educational level, parental occupation (Table 1) and parity, birth order, preterm, still birth, and miscarriage (Table 3) were not statistically significant in the crude and adjusted Odds Ratio analysis.

Thirteen variables were entered into the COR analysis. Of these, unidentified medication used during the first 3 months of gestation (COR = 5.062; 95% CI: 2.286-11. 206, *P*-value = < 0.001), alcohol consumption during early/throughout pregnancy (COR = 3.256; 95% CI: 1. 823-5.816, *P*-value = < 0.001), anemia during early pregnancy (COR = 1.663; 95% CI: 1.038-2.662, *p*-value = 0. 034), contraceptive use around conception (COR = 5. 298; 95% CI: 1.980- 14.175, *P*-value = 0.001), and chemical exposure during early pregnancy (COR = 13.804; 95% CI; 1.789-106.522, *P*-value = 0.012), and blood relation among parents (COR = 5.203; 95% CI:1.126-24.046, *P*-value = 0.035) were associated with CAs in the crude Odds ratio analysis. On the other hand, folic acid/iron folate (COR = 0.082; 95% CI: 0.019-.354, *P*-value = 0.001) and vegetable servings/use during early pregnancy (COR = 0.536; 95% CI: 0.344-0.835, *P*-value = 0.006) was protective against the occurrence of CAs (Table 4). However, vegetable serving was not associated with the occurrence of CAs in the adjusted Odds ratio analysis.

Twelve variables (alcohol drinking, anemia, iron folate/ folic acid, unidentified medication, contraceptive, exposure to chemicals, vegetable serving, blood relationship between child parents, exposure to radiation, maternal illness, family history, and food shortage during early pregnancy) whose value ended up with 0.2 and below in the crude Odds ratio were entered into the multivariable logistic regression model to observe exposure variables

Table 1 The socio-demographic characteristics of the study participants, Addis Ababa and the Amhara Region, Ethiopia, 2016

Characteristics		Cases ($n = 207$)		Controls ($n = 207$)		Total ($n = 414$)	
		Frequency	%	Frequency	%	Frequency	%
Study Site	Addis Ababa	106	51.2	107	51.7	213	51.4
	Amhara Region	101	48.8	100	48.3	201	48.6
Infant/Child Age	Below 6 months	181	87.4	181	87.4	362	87.4
	6-11 months	26	12.6	26	12.6	52	12.6
Infant/Child Sex	Male	123	59.4	125	60.4	248	59.9
	Female	84	40.6	82	39.6	166	40.1
Child Mother Age	< 20 years	11	5.3	11	5.3	22	5.3
	20-34 years	167	80.7	169	81.6	336	81.2
	> 34 years	29	14.0	27	13.0	56	13.5
Child Mother Marital status	Married	190	91.8	197	95.2	387	93.5
	Never married	17	8.2	10	4.8	27	6.5
Religion	Christian	139	67.1	160	77.3	299	72.2
	Muslim	66	31.9	47	22.7	113	27.3
	Other	2	1.0	0	0	2	0.5
Child Mother Education	No education	101	48.8	54	26.1	155	37.4
	Primary	59	28.5	73	35.3	132	31.9
	Secondary and higher	47	22.7	80	38.6	127	30.7
Monthly income	Regular	84	40.6	74	35.7	158	38.2
	Irregular	123	59.4	133	64.3	256	61.8
Child Mother Ethnicity	Oromo	63	30.4	33	15.9	96	23.2
	Amhara	122	58.9	135	65.2	257	62.1
	Guragie	7	3.4	17	8.2	24	5.8
	Others[a]	15	7.3	22	10.6	37	8.7
Child Mother Occupation	House wife	122	58.9	101	48.8	223	53.9
	Employed	28	13.5	46	22.2	74	17.9
	Farmer/Agriculture	32	15.5	27	13.0	59	14.3
	No job/unemployed	25	12.1	33	15.9	58	14.0
Residence	Urban	97	46.9	165	79.7	262	63.3
	Rural	110	53.1	42	20.3	152	36.7
Economic Status	Low	89	43.0	65	31.4	154	37.2
	Middle	100	48.3	98	47.3	198	47.8
	higher	18	8.7	44	21.3	62	15.0
Child Father Ethnicity	Oromo	63	30.4	33	15.9	96	23.2
	Amhara	116	56	133	64.3	249	60.1
	Guragie	8	3.9	15	7.2	23	5.6
	Others[a]	20	9.6	26	12.6	46	10.9
Child Father Occupation	Employed	72	34.8	132	63.8	204	49.3
	Farmer/Agriculture	107	51.7	54	26.1	161	38.9
	No job/unemployed	28	13.5	21	10.1	49	11.8
Region originated	Amhara	106	51.2	101	48.8	207	50.0
	Oromia	45	21.7	18	8.7	63	15.2
	Addis Ababa	35	16.9	80	38.6	115	27.8
	Other regions [b]	21	10.3	8	3.9	29	7.0

[a]Others = Tigre, Somali, Afar, Seltie, Benishangul, Agew, Gamo, Hadya, Argob
[b]Other regions = Southern Nations Nationalities and People, Tigray, Afar, Benishangul-Gumuz, Harari, Dire Dawa

Table 2 Frequency of congenital anomalies by organ/organ system among the study subjects, Addis Ababa and the Amhara Region, Ethiopia, 2016

Type of Congenital Anomalies	frequency	%
Neural Tube Defects (Spina bifida with and without hydrocephaly, clubfoot; encephalocele (occipital, frontal, and nasal))	124	30
Orofacial Clefts (cleft lip, cleft lip and palate, and cleft palate)	54	13
Masculoskeletal Defects (reduction defects of tibia, femur, ulna, and radial bones, talipes equinovarus, tracheoesophageal fistula, gastroschisis, and amelia of upper limb)	20	4.8
Heart Defects (ventricular septal defects)	5	1.2
Genitourinary Anomalies (hypospadias with sub-coronal and penile)	3	0.7
Bladder extrusion with cleft lip and palate	1	0.2
No Congenital Anomalies/Controls	207	50
Total	414	100

associated with CAs. As indicated in Table 4, unidentified medication use (AOR = 4.595; 95% CI: 1868-11.301, *P*-value = 0.001), maternal alcohol drinking in early pregnancy (AOR = 2.394; 95% CI: 1.212-4.726, *P*-value = 0.012) , and exposure to chemicals during early pregnancy (AOR = 9.964; 95% CI: 1.238-80.193, *P*-value = 0.031) were significantly associated with the occurrence of CAs. On the contrary, iron folate/folic acid supplementation (use) before and during early pregnancy (AOR = 0.051; 95% CI: 0.010-0.260, *P*-value = < 0.001) had a protective effect against CA.

Discussion

According to our findings, unidentified medication use, alcohol consumption during early pregnancy or throughout pregnancy, and exposure to chemicals during early pregnancy had significant associations with the occurrence of CAs in this study, whereas iron folate supplementation before and during early pregnancy showed a protective effect against CA.

Like our study, scientific literature reports that drug usage during pregnancy is associated with CAs [26–31]. In Ethiopia, drugs are being sold by private drug venders, stores, clinics, and some shops with and without prescriptions. This indicates that mothers are likely to use medications/over-the counter drugs during their early pregnancy. Therefore, responsible bodies should control over-the-counter.

The association of alcohol drinking during and before early pregnancy and CA was also reported by Grewal et al., [32], Zhang et al., [33], and O'Leary et al., [34, 35]. In the liver, alcohol is metabolized into acetaldehyde, a toxic chemical/substance. To convert this toxic substance into a non-toxic and usable chemical, enzyme acetaldehyde dehydrogenases that secreted converts the acetaldehyde into acetic acid, which is useable by the body. However, when the unconverted acetaldehyde accumulates in the body, it causes irritation of the cells and tissues and then damages the cells and tissues, leading to metabolism and cellular growth abnormalities [36]. Moreover, alcohol is capable of crossing the placenta membrane and being carried to all developing cells and tissues of the embryo and fetus, and as a result causes damages to the developing tissues and cells and subsequently leads to a structural abnormality. Furthermore, alcohol drinking during pregnancy results in a serious consequences which manifest with recognized characteristics of physical and mental abnormal features after a baby is born [36–44].

In Ethiopia, alcohol is consumed by the community [45, 46], particularly locally made alcoholic beverages known as "areki" and "tella" in Amharic are consumed by both men and women in rural communities, especially among Christians, more specifically Orthodox Christians, across the country, whereas some urban dwellers, including women drink beer and other alcoholic drinks. In this study, women who consumed alcohol daily and women who took alcohol to an increasing degree had children with CAs. Therefore, health education is essential for the community, particularly women in the 15-49 years of age group.

In the present study, exposure to chemicals had a significant association with CAs. Likewise, exposure to chemicals has been reported as having a significant association with the occurrence of CAs [47–51].

In this study, mothers of cases who reported maternal/medical illnesses during early pregnancy had higher odds of babies with CAs compared to mothers of controls. Similarly, maternal diseases or medical illnesses, such as syphilis, Rubella, measles, other viral infections, [52–56] and chronic diseases were reported by several researchers as known causes of CAs [14, 18, 52–59].

Many studies reported that iron folate/folic acid supplementation in the early pregnancy and before protected or reduced the occurrence of certain CAs. For example, neural defects can be reduced if a pregnant woman appropriately takes the recommended dose of iron folate/folic acid. Women who take iron folate/folic acid are less likely to have babies with CA compared to those who do not take folic acid during and before early pregnancy [14, 60–68]. Folic acid together with vitamin B12 plays a vital role in the synthesis of nucleic acid, lipids, and proteins, required for cell division. Iron folate/folic acid also has a role in amino acids metabolisms that are needed for DNA and RNA synthesis and plays an important role as an antioxidant agent. Therefore, it is essential to make it available to all pregnant women.

Table 3 Reproductive history of the study participants/children's mothers, Addis Ababa and the Amhara Region, Ethiopia, 2016

Characteristics		Cases		Controls		Total	
		(*n* = 207)	%	(*n* = 207)	%	(*n* = 414)	%
Birth order	First	68	32.9	100	48.3	168	40.6
	Second	41	19.8	47	22.7	88	21.3
	Third and above	98	47.3	60	29.0	158	38.2
Total number of pregnancy	1	67	32.4	100	48.3	167	40.3
	2-3	69	33.3	70	33.8	139	33.6
	4 and above	71	34.3	37	17.9	108	26.1
Full and post term pregnancy	Post term	12	5.8	5	2.4	17	4.1
	1-2	124	59.9	165	79.7	289	69.8
	3 and above	71	34.3	37	17.9	108	26.1
Preterm	None	158	76.3	178	86.0	336	81.2
	1	47	22.7	26	12.6	73	17.6
	2 and above	2	1.0	3	1.4	5	1.2
Elective termination	None	184	88.9	199	96.1	383	92.5
	1-2	23	11.1	8	3.9	31	7.5
Miscarriage	None	131	63.3	174	84.1	305	73.7
	1-2	76	36.7	31	15.0	107	25.8
	3 and above	0	0	2	1.0	2	0.5
Still birth	None	164	79.23	190	91.8	354	85.5
	1-2	42	20.29	17	8.2	59	14.3
	3 and above	1	0.5	0	0	1	0.2
Neonate/Infant/child death	None	178	86.0	189	91.3	367	88.9
	1-2	29	14.0	17	8.2	46	11.1
	3 and above	0	0	1	0.5	1	0.2
Living children	None	7	3.4	0	0	7	1.7
	1-2	129	62.3	169	81.6	298	72.0
	3 and above	71	34.3	38	18.4	109	26.3
Gravidity	Primigravida	70	33.8	100	48.3	170	41.1
	Multigravida	137	66.2	107	51.7	244	58.9
Gestational age at 1st ANC (antenatal care) visit	No ANC visit	34	16.4	19	9.2	53	12.8
	1-3 months	27	13.0	29	14.0	56	13.5
	4 months and above	146	70.5	159	76.8	305	73.7
Institution for ANC attended	Public hospital	27	13.0	23	11.1	50	12.1
	Public health center	130	62.8	147	71.0	277	66.9
	Private hospital	6	2.9	4	1.9	10	2.4
	Private clinic	7	3.4	13	6.3	20	4.8
	Health post	3	1.4	1	0.5	4	1.0
	No ANC visit	34	16.4	19	9.2	53	12.8

Various studies suggested that multivitamin or folic acid containing multivitamin use during/ before pregnancy reduces/protects against some CAs [60, 65–68]. Multivitamins are essential organic substances, which are required by the body for normal body metabolic functions, body building, and controlling chemical reactions, such as converting food substances into energy and living tissues, as well as for survival or living healthy. Some components of multivitamins act as antioxidant substances (i.e. protect cells from damage by free radicals), for example, vitamin "E" and "C". Moreover, some components of multivitamins are also important for body defense mechanisms, for

Table 4 Participant's response on risk factors for congenital anomaly: Results from multivariable analysis-adjusted for substance abuse/ behavioral, parental, and environmental factors, maternal illness, iron folate/folic acid, multivitamin, and vegetable use variables, Addis Ababa and the Amhara Region, Ethiopia, 2016

Characteristics		Cases		Controls		COR	AOR	95% CI		*P*-value
		Number	%	Number	%			lower	upper	
Iron folate/folic acid use	Yes	2	1	22	10.6	0.082	0.051	0.010	0.260	< 0.001
	No	205	99	185	89.4	1Ref				
Unidentified medication use	Yes	35	16.9	8	3.9	5.062	4.595	1.868	11.301	0.001
	No	172	83.1	199	96.1	1				
Drank alcohol (daily, occasionally and 1-3times in a week)	Yes	49	23.7	18	8.7	3.256	2.394	1.212	4.726	0.012
	No	158	76.3	189	91.3	1				
Exp. to chemical (mother)	Yes	13	6.3	1	0.5	13.804	9.964	1.238	80.193	0.031
	No	194	93.7	206	99.5	1				
Contraceptive use	Yes	24	11.6	5	2.4	5.298	4.840	1.647	14.224	0.004
	No	183	88.4	202	97.6	1				
Blood relationship between child parents	Yes	10	4.8	2	1	5.203	6.234	0.959	40.521	0.055
	No	197	95.2	205	99	1				
Family history	Yes	9	4.3	3	1.4	3.091	3.397	0.862	13.393	0.081
	No	198	95	204	98.6	1				
Vegetable Serving	Yes	139	67.1	164	79.2	0.536	0.644	0.392	1.059	0.083
	No	68	32.9	43	20.8	1				
Maternal illness	Yes	24	11.6	13	6.3	1.957	2.025	0.903	4.54	0.087
	No	183	88.4	194	93.7	1				
Exp. to radiation before conception (child father)	Yes	7	3.4	2	1	3.587	6.838	0.741	63.109	0.090
	No	200	96.6	205	99	1				

Exp exposure, *COR* crude odds ratio, *AOR* adjusted odds ratio, *CI* confidence interval, *Ref* reference

instance, zinc, vitamin "C", and vitamin "A" protect the body from diseases.

As observed in this study, in Ethiopia, health care providers might not have been providing folic acid or multivitamin containing folic acid supplementation to pregnant women until recent times. However, recently the Federal Ministry of Health recommended iron folate supplementation to all pregnant women although most such women have not been provided still. Moreover, research on folic acid supplementation and knowledge of women about folic acid use during pregnancy is limited in Ethiopia.

In this study, maternal age, ethnicity, sex of child, maternal education, and parity were not significantly associated with the occurrence of CAs. This finding is in agreement with that of a study conducted in Saudi Arabia by Salih et al., [18]. However, previous studies have shown a linkage to maternal age, (greater than 35) [14, 69], maternal education, and parity with the occurrence of CA [69].

In the present study, cigarette smoking and passive smoking were not associated with CAs although several researchers reported that smoking/passive smoking was associated with a specific types of CAs [32, 70–73]. In some societies, women in the reproductive age group smoke cigarettes. This may be due to cultural and personal habits. In addition, exposure to radiation had no statistically significant link in this study. Moreover, blood relationship, family history, and the Odds of having children with CA had no statistically significant associations in this study. To the contrary, other studies reported that a significant association occurred between blood relationship/family history and CA [18, 73–75]. This variation might be due to differences in the cultures of consanguinity marriage and genetic makeup. In addition, there were no associations between birth order, preterm, miscarriage, and CAs in the present study.

In general, the present study indicates that the characteristics of cases and controls are closer, except for a few variations, like maternal alcohol drinking and maternal illness. In addition, our findings are in line with some previous reports and at variance with others. The reason they are different from the reports of some studies may be differences in socio-demographic, geographic, study setting, methodological, and environmental characteristics.

Conclusion

The findings of this study showed that alcohol drinking, unidentified medication use, and exposure to chemicals had significant associations with the occurrence of CAs. Iron folate use before and during pregnancy indicated a protective effect on CAs. However, current iron folate and multivitamin supplementation to pregnant women has been inadequate and infrequent because only very few women are observed using them during pregnancy, while the majority of women in the reproductive age groups are not getting prior to conception and during early pregnancy. Therefore, we emphasize that the supplementation is required to reproductive age groups, particularly around conception and during early pregnancy.

Although the causes of CAs are unknown and not studied in Ethiopia, screening nutritional deficiencies, chronic diseases, such as anemia, diabetics, infections/diseases (i.e. viral infections and sexually transmitted diseases) and establishing preventive measures, for example, health education to the public, specifically to reproductive age women are very important. So, to understand and identify the risk factors for CAs, it is necessary to conduct further population based investigations in different parts of the country to further ascertain the presently observed risk factors in association with CAs, as well as fully explore factors, which are not associated with CAs.

Abbreviations
ANC: Antenatal care; CA: Congenital anomaly; CAs: Congenital anomalies; WHO/CDC/ICBDSR: World Health Organization/Centers for Disease Control and Prevention/International clearinghouse for Birth Defects Surveillance and Research

Acknowledgements
We would like to thank midwives, nurses, and other health professionals working at Tikur Anbesa General Specialized Hospital, Zewditu Memorial Hospital, Gandhi Memorial Hospital, St. Paul Specialized Millennium Hospital, Yekatit 12 Hospital, Desse Referral Hospital, Felege Hiwet Referral Hospital, and Gondar University Hospital for their support. We would like to appreciate and acknowledge the participants. We wish to thank the medical directors and managers of the respective hospitals for their support and permission. We would also like to thank all those who assisted us in one way or another during data collection. Lastly, we would like to acknowledge Addis Ababa University and the University of Gondar for their special support.

Funding
This study obtained fund from Addis Ababa University and the University of Gondar for data collection only. The authors declare that they have not received funds for the publication of this manuscript. The authors also declare that they have had no external source of grant/fund for both data collection and publication.

Authors' contributions
Conceived the idea: MT. Designed the methodology: MT, MA, WF, ED, AW. Conducted the study: MT, MA, WF, ED, AW. Interpreted data: MT, MA, WF, ED, AW. Data analysis: MT, AW. Wrote draft manuscript: MT. Wrote the final manuscript: MT, AW. Review and edit the manuscript: MT, MA, WF, ED, AW. All authors read and approved the final manuscript and agreed for submission: MT, MA, WF, ED, AW.

Ethics approval and consent to participate
The study was reviewed and approved by the College of Health Sciences Institutional Review Board, Addis Ababa University, Ref. No. 060/14, dated June 12, 2014; the National Research Ethics Review Committee, Ref. No. 3.10/781/07, dated October 16, 2014; HARI-ALERT Ethical Review Committee, Project Reg. No. PO58/14, dated December 23, 2014; Addis Ababa City Administration Health Bureau Ethical Clearance Committee, Ref. No. A/A/H/B/1972/25, dated 27/10/2014; and the Amhara National Regional State Health bureau Regional Health Research Laboratory Center Ref. No. ሳብ/20/4963, dated 27/01/2007(Ethiopian Calendar). Data were collected after verbal and written agreements to participate were secured from children's mothers/caregivers.

Competing interests
We declared that we have no financial and nonfinancial competing interests.

Author details
[1]Department of Anatomy, School of Medicine, College of Medicine and Health Sciences, the University of Gondar, Gondar, Ethiopia. [2]Department of Anatomy, School of Medicine, College of Health Sciences, Addis Ababa University, Addis Ababa, Ethiopia. [3]School of Dentistry, College of Health Sciences, Addis Ababa University, Addis Ababa, Ethiopia. [4]School of Medicine, College of Medicine and Health Sciences, the University of Gondar, Gondar, Ethiopia. [5]School of Public Health, College of Health Sciences, Addis Ababa University, Addis Ababa, Ethiopia.

References
1. Francine R, Psascale S, Aline H. Congenital anomalies: prevalence and risk factors. Universal J Public Health. 2014;2(2):58–63.
2. Yamada S, Nakashima T, Hirose A, Yoneyama A, Takeda T, Takakuwa T. In: Yamada S, editor. Developmental anatomy of the human embryo – 3D-imaging and analytical techniques, the human embryo; 2012. ISBN: 978-953-51-0124-6, InTech, Available from: http://www.intechopen.com/books/the-human-embryo/developmental-anatomy-of-the-human-embryo-3dimaging-and-analytical-techniques.
3. Taye M, Afework M, Fantaye W, Diro E, Worku A. Magnitude of birth defects in central and Northwest Ethiopia from 2010-2014: a descriptive retrospective study. PLoS One. 2016;11(10):e0161998. https://doi.org/10.1371/journal.pone.0161998.
4. World Health Organization/US-Center for Disease Control and Prevention/ International Clearance House on Birth Defects Surveillance and Research. Birth defects surveillance: a manual for programme managers. Geneva: World Health Organization; 2014.
5. Ahmed AM, el Kader SA, El Hamid A, Gaafar M. Assessment of risk factors for fetal congenital anomalies among pregnant women at Cairo University hospitals. J Am Sci. 2011;7(12):899–907.
6. Mohammed AR, Mohammed SA-R, AbdulFetah AMH. Congenital anomalies among children: knowledge and attitude of Egyptian and Saudi mothers. J Biol Agric Healthc. 2013;3(20):18–29.
7. Brent RL. Environmental causes of human congenital malformations: the pediatrician's role in dealing with these complex clinical problems caused by a multiplicity of environmental and genetic factors. J Am Acad Pediatr. 2004;113(4):957–68.
8. Serra-Juhe C, Rodriguez-Santiago B, Cusco I, Vendrell T, Camats N, Toran N, Perez-Jurado LA. Contribution of rare copy number variants to isolated human malformations. PLoS One. 2012;7(10):1–8.
9. Çanaku D, Toçi E, Roshi E, Burazeri G. Prevalence and factors associated with congenital malformations in Tirana Albania during 2011-201. Mater Sociomed. 2014;26(3):158–62.
10. Sun G, Xu ZM, Liang JF, Li L, Tang DX. Twelve-year prevalence of common neonatal congenital malformations in Zhejiang Province, China. World J Pediatr. 2011;7(4):331–6.
11. Kaur A, Singh JR. Chromosomal abnormalities: genetic disease burden in India. Int J Hum Genet. 2010;10(1-3):1–14.
12. Butt F, Shahzad R, Pasha I. Pattern and outcome of congenital anomalies and maternal risk factor association. Biomedica. 2013;29:234–9.

13. Basso O, Olsen J, Christensen K. Recurrence risk of congenital anomalies-the impact of paternal, social, and environmental factors: a population-based study in Denmark. Am J Epidemiol. 1999;150(6):598–604.
14. Kishimba RS, Mpembeni R, Mghamba J. Factors associated with major structural birth defects among newborns delivered at Muhimbili National Hospital and municipal hospitals in Dar Es Salaam, Tanzania 2011-2012. Pan Afr Med J. 2015;20:153. https://doi.org/10.11604/pamj.2015.20.153.4492. Available online at: http://www.panafrican-med-journal.com/content/article/11620/11153/full/
15. The McGraw-Hill Company. Congenital malformations. In: Kumar P, Burton B, editors. Evidence base evaluation and management. USA; 2008. https://doi.org/10.1036/0071471898.
16. Bailey LB, Berry RJ. Folic acid supplementation and the occurrence of congenital heart defects, orofacial clefts, multiple births, and miscarriage1–3. Am J Clin Nutr. 2005;81(Supp. 1):1213S–12137S.
17. Malik S, Cleves MA, Honein MA, Romitti PA, Botto LD, Yang S, et al. Maternal smoking and congenital heart defects. Pediatrics. 2008;121(4):E810–6. https://doi.org/10.1542/peds.2007-1519.
18. Salih MAM, Murshid WR, Mohamed AG, Ignacio LC, de Jesus JE, Baabbad R, HME B. Risk factors for neural tube defects in Riyadh City, Saudi Arabia: case-control study. Sudan J Paediatr. 2014;14(2):49–60.
19. Grandi DC, Maccarone MB, Luchtenberg G, Rittler YM. La obesidad materna como factor de riesgo para defectos congenitos. Rev Hosp Mat Inf Ramon Sarda. 2012;31(3):100–2.
20. Desrosiers TA, Herring AH, Shapira SK, Hooiveld M, Luben TJ, Herdt-Losavio ML, et al. Paternal occupation and birth defects: findings from the national birth defects prevention study. Occup Environ Med. 2013;69(8):534–42.
21. Rozendaal AM, van Essen AJ, te Meerman GJ, Bakker MK, van der Biezen JJ, Goorhuis-Brouwer SM, et al. Periconceptional folic acid associated with an increased risk of oral clefts relative to non-folate related malformations in the Northern Netherlands: a population based case-control study. Eur J Epidemiol. 2013; https://doi.org/10.1007/s10654-013-9849-0.
22. Mobasheri E, Keshtkar A, Golalipour MJ. Maternal folate and vitamin B12 status and neural tube defects in northern Iran: a case control study. Iran J Pediatr. 2010;20(2):167–73.
23. World Health Organization Regional Office for South-East Asia. Workshop on birth defects surveillance. Colombo; 2012. p. 10–3.
24. Prajapati V, Kacha AR, Kakkad KM, Damor PB, Nandaniya AM. Study of congenital malformation in neonates born at tertiary care hospital. National J Community Med. 2015;6(1):30–4.
25. Central Statistical Agency [Ethiopia]. Statistical abstracts: population projection of Ethiopia for all regions at wereda levels, from 2014-2017. Addis Ababa; 2013.
26. van Gelder MMHJ, Bos JHJ, Roeleveld N, de Jon-van den Berg LTW. Drugs associated with teratogenic mechanisms. Part I: dispensing rates among pregnant women in the Netherlands, 1998-2009. Hum Reprod. 2013;0(0):1–7. https://doi.org/10.1093/humrep/det1369. http://humrep.oxfordjournals.org/
27. van Gelder MMHJ, van Rooij IALM, Miller RK, Zielhuis GA, de Jong-van den Berg LTW, Roeleveld N. Teratogenic mechanisms of medical drugs. Hum Reprod Update. 2010;16(4):378–94. https://doi.org/10.1093/humupd/dmp052.
28. Mohammed MA, Ahmed JH, Workicho A, Aljadhey HS. Medications use among pregnant women in Ethiopia: a cross sectional study. J Appl Pharm Sci. 2013;3(04):116–23. https://doi.org/10.7324/JAPS.2013.3421. Available online at http://www.japsonline.com
29. Admasie C, Wasie B, Abeje G. Determinants of prescribed drug use among pregnant women in Bahir Dar city administration, Northwest Ethiopia: a cross sectional study. BMC Pregnancy Childbirth. 2014;14:325. http://www.biomedcentral.com/1471-2393/1414/1325
30. Abeje G, Admasie C, Wasie B. Factors associated with self-medication practice among pregnant mothers attending antenatal care at governmental health centers in Bahir Dar city administration, Northwest Ethiopia, a cross sectional study. Pan Afr Med J. 2015;20:276. https://doi.org/10.11604/pamj.2015.20.276.4243. Available online at: http://www.panafrican-med-journal.com/content/article/11620/11276/full
31. Kebede B, Gedif T, Getachew A. Assessment of drug use among pregnant women in Addis Ababa, Ethiopia. Pharmacoepidemiol Drug Saf. 2009;18: 462–8. https://doi.org/10.1002/pds.1732.
32. Grewal J, Carmichael SL, Ma C, Lammer EJ, Shaw GM. Maternal periconceptional smoking and alcohol consumption and risk for select congenital anomalies. Birth Defects Res A. 2008;82:519–26.
33. Zhang X, Li S, Wu S, Hao X, Guo S, Suzuki K, et al. Prevalence of birth defects and risk-factor analysis from a population-based survey in Inner Mongolia, China. BMC Pediatr. 2012;12:125. https://doi.org/10.1186/1471-2431-12-125. http://www.biomedcentral.com/1471-2431/1112/1125
34. O'Leary CM, Elliott EJ, Nassar N, Bower C. Exploring the potential to use data linkage for investigating the relationship between birth defects and prenatal alcohol exposure. Birth Defects Res A. 2013;97:497–504.
35. O'Leary CM, Nassar N, Kurinczuk JJ, de Klerk N, Geelhoed E, Elliott EJ, Bower C. Prenatal alcohol exposure and risk of birth defects. Pediatrics. 2010;126(4): e843–50. https://doi.org/10.1542/peds.2010-0256.
36. Yeigh T, Kean B. Drinking and congenital birth defects: alcohol awareness in the northern rivers region of new South Wales, Australia. Int Electron J Health Educ. 2005;8:153–66.
37. Assadi F. Effects of prenatal alcohol exposure on the developing kidneys. Iran J Pediatr. 2008;18(1):5–10.
38. Spagnolo A. Teratogenesis of alcohol. Ann 1st Super Sanita. 1993;29(1):89–96.
39. Ministry for Children and Families Edition. Parenting children affected by fetal alcohol syndrome. A guide for daily living. Ministry for children and families edition (British Columbia). Canada: Published by the society of special needs adoptive parents in cooperation with the B.C. Ministry for Children and Families Child Protection Division; 1999.
40. de Sanctis L, Memo L, Pichini S, Tarani L, Vagnarelli F. Fetal alcohol syndrome: new perspectives for an ancient and underestimated problem. The journal of maternal-fetal & neonatal medicine : the official journal of the European Association of Perinatal Medicine, the Federation of Asia and Oceania Perinatal Societies. Int Soc Perinat Obstet. 2011;24(Suppl 1):34–7. https://doi.org/10.3109/14767058.14762011.14607576.
41. Ornoy A, Ergaz Z. Alcohol abuse in pregnant women: effects on the fetus and newborn, mode of action and maternal treatment. Int J Environ Res Public Health. 2010;7(2):364–79. https://doi.org/10.3390/ijerph7020364.
42. Streissguth AP, Bookstein FL, Barr HM, Sampson PD, O'malley K, Young JK. Risk factors for adverse life outcomes in fetal alcohol syndrome and fetal alcohol effects. Dev Behav Pediatr. 2004;25(4):228–38.
43. Werk CM, Cui X, Tough S. Fetal alcohol spectrum disorder among aboriginal children under six years of age and living off reserve: first nations Child & Family Caring Society of Canada. First Peoples Child Fam Rev. 2013;8(1):7–13.
44. Maier SE, West JR. Drinking patterns and alcohol-related birth defects. Alcohol Res Health. 2001;25(3):168–74.
45. Anteab K, Demtsu B, Megra M. Assessment of prevalence and associated factors of alcohol use during pregnancy among the dwellers of Bahir-Dar City, Northwest Ethiopia. Int J Pharma Sci Res. 2014;5(12): 939–45. ISSN: 0975-9492
46. Central Statistical Agency [Ethiopia] and ICF International. Ethiopia demographic and health survey 2011. Addis Ababa and Calverton: Central Statistical Agency and ICF International; 2012.
47. Mitro SD, Johnson T, Zota AR. Cumulative chemical exposures during pregnancy and early development. Curr Environ Health Rep. 2015;2(4):367–78. https://doi.org/10.1007/s40572-40015-40064-x.
48. Bell E, Hertz-Picciotto I, Beaumont J. A case-control study of pesticides and fetal death due to congenital anomalies. Epidemiology. 2001;12(2):148–56.
49. Araneta MRG, Schlangen KM, Edmonds LD, Destiche DA, Merz RD, Hobbs CA, et al. Prevalence of birth defects among infants of gulf war veterans in Arkansas, Arizona, California, Georgia, Hawaii, and Iowa, 1989-1993. Birth Defects Res A. 2003;67:246–60.
50. Dolk H, Vrijheid M, Armstrong B, Abramsky L, Bianchi F, Garne E, et al. Risk of congenital anomalies near hazardous-waste landfill site in Europe: the EUROHAZCON study. Lancet. 1998;352:423–7.
51. Heeren GA, Tyler J, Mandeya A. Agricultural chemical exposures and birth defects in the eastern Cape Province, South Africa a case – control study. Environ Health. 2003;2:11. Available from: http://www.ehjournal.net/content/12/11/11
52. WHO fact sheet on rubella: includes key facts, definition, symptoms, congenital rubella syndrome, vaccination, WHO response; 2016. Available at: http://www.who.int/mediacentre/factsheets/fs367/en/
53. WHO Fact Sheet. The measles and rubella initiative is a global partnership committed to ensuring no child dies from measles or is born with congenital rubella syndrome, 2016. http://measlesrubellainitiative.org/resources/advocacy-tools/2016-fact-sheet/.
54. Centers for Disease Control and Prevention (US-CDC): Congenital syphilis - CDC fact sheet. 2015. www.cdc.gov/std/syphilis/stdfact-congenita

55. Ornoy A, Tenenbaum A. Pregnancy outcome following infections by coxsackie, echo, measles, mumps, hepatitis, polio and encephalitis viruses. Reprod Toxicol. 2006:1–12. https://doi.org/10.1016/j.reprotox.2005.1012.1007. Available at www.sciencedirect.com
56. De Santis M, De Luca C, Mappa I, Spagnuolo T, Licameli A, Straface G, Scambia GS. Syphilis infection during pregnancy: fetal risks and clinical management. Infect Dis Obstet Gynecol. 2012:1–4. https://doi.org/10.1155/2012/430585.
57. Li Z, Ren A, Liu J, Pei L, Zhang L, Guo Z, Li Z. Maternal flu or fever, medication use, and neural tube defects: a population-based case-control study in northern China. Birth Defects Res A Clin Mol Teratol. 2007;79(4): 295–300. https://doi.org/10.1002/bdra.20342.
58. Liu S, Joseph KS, Lisonkova S, Rouleau J, Van den Hof M, Sauve R, Kramer MS. Association between maternal chronic conditions and congenital heart defects: a population-based cohort study. Am Heart Assoc. 2013:1–20. https://doi.org/10.1161/CIRCULATIONAHA.1112.001054. http://circ.ahajournals.org/content/early/002013/001006/001027/CIRCULATIONAHA.001112.001054
59. Csaky-Szunyogh M, Vereczkey A, Kosa Z, Gerencser B, Czeizel AE. Risk and protective factors in the origin of conotruncal defects of heart–a population-based case-control study. Am J Med Genet A. 2013;161(10): 2444–52. https://doi.org/10.1002/ajmg.a.36118.
60. Fernandez N, Henao-Mejia J, Monterrey P, Perez J, Zarante I. Association between maternal prenatal vitamin use and congenital abnormalities of the genitourinary tract in a developing country. J Pediatr Urol. 2012;8:121–6. https://doi.org/10.1016/j.jpurol.2011.07.005.
61. Chan AC, Essen PV, Scott H, Haan EA, Sage L, Scott J, Gill TK, Nguyen A-MT. Folate awareness and the prevalence of neural tube defects in South Australia, 1966-2007. MJA. 2008;189(10):566–9.
62. De Wals P, Tairou F, Allen MIV, Soo-Hong U, Lowry RB, Sibbald B, et al. Reduction in neural-tube defects after folic acid fortification in Canada. N Engl J Med. 2007;357(2):135–42. www.nejm.org
63. Björklund NK, Gordon R. A hypothesis linking low folate intake to neural tube defects due to failure of post-translation methylations of the cytoskeleton. Int J Dev Biol. 2006;50:135–41. https://doi.org/10.1387/ijdb.052102nb.
64. Bortolus R, Blom F, Filippini F, van Poppel MN, Leoncini E, de Smit DJ, et al. Prevention of congenital malformations and other adverse pregnancy outcomes with 4.0 mg of folic acid: community-based randomized clinical trial in Italy and the Netherlands. BMC Pregnancy Childbirth. 2014;14:166. https://doi.org/10.1186/1471-2393-14-166. http://www.biomedcentral.com/1471-2393/1114/1166
65. Wilson R, Audibert F, Brock J, Carroll J, Cartier L, Gagnon A, et al. Pre-conception folic acid and multivitamin supplementation for the primary and secondary prevention of neural tube defects and other folic acid-sensitive congenital anomalies. J Obstet Gynaecol Can. 2015;37(6):534–52.
66. Musumeci G, Castrogiovanni P, Trovato F, Parenti R, Szychlinska M, Imbesi R. Pregnancy, embryo-fetal development and nutrition: physiology around fetal programming. J Histol Histopathol. 2015;2(1):1. https://doi.org/10.7243/2055-7091X-7242-7241. http://www.hoajonline.com/journals/pdf/2055-7091X-7242-7241.pdf
67. Munger RG, Sauberlich HE, Corcoran C, Nepomuceno B, Daack-Hirsch S, Solon FS. Maternal vitamin B-6 and folate status and risk of oral cleft birth defects in the Philippines. Birth Defects Res A Clin Mol Teratol. 2004;70(7): 464–71. https://doi.org/10.1002/bdra.20037.
68. Shaw G, Nelson V, Carmichael S, Lammer E, Finnell R, Rosenquist T. Maternal periconceptional vitamins: interactions with selected factors and congenital anomalies? Epidemiology. 2002;13(6):625–30.
69. Nili F, Jahangir T. Risk factors for neural tube defects A study at university affiliated hospitals in Tehran. Arch Iranian Med. 2006;9(1):20–5.
70. Alverson CJ, Strickland MJ, Gilboa SM, Correa A. Maternal smoking and congenital heart defects in the Baltimore-Washington infant study. Pediatrics. 2011;127(3):e647–53. https://doi.org/10.1542/peds.2010-1399. www.pediatrics.org/cgi/doi/1510.1542/peds.2010-1399
71. Little J, Arslan MT, Mossey PA. Smoking and orofacial clefts. A United Kingdom–based case-control study. Cleft Palate Craniofac J. 2004; 41(4):383–6.
72. Hackshaw A, Rodeck C, Boniface S. Maternal smoking in pregnancy and birth defects: a systematic review based on 173 687 malformed cases and 11.7 million controls. Hum Reprod Update. 2011;17(5):589–604. https://doi.org/10.1093/humupd/dmr022.
73. Honein MA, Paulozzi LJ, Moore CA. Family history, maternal smoking, and clubfoot: an indication of a gene-environment interaction. Am J Epidemiol. 2000;152(7):658–64.
74. Raza MZ, Sheikh A, Ahmed SS, Sajid A, Naqvi SMA. Risk factors associated with birth defects at a tertiary care center in Pakistan. Ital J Pediatr. 2012; 38(68):1–7.
75. Mosayebi Z, Movahedian AH. Pattern of congenital malformations in consanguineous versus nonconsanguineous marriages in Kashan, Islamic Republic of Iran. La Revue de Sante de la Mediterranee orientale. 2007;13(4): 868–74.

7

Chylopericardium in a child with IgA nephropathy

Yu-lin Kang[1], Yun Cui[2], Ying Wu[1], Shen Hao[1], Xin-yu Kuang[1], Yu-cai Zhang[2], Wen-yan Huang[1] and Guang-hua Zhu[1*]

Abstract

Background: Chylopericardium effusion is characterized by the accumulation of milky effusion in the pericardium. It is often idiopathic but it can be secondary to trauma, chest radiation, tuberculosis and malignancy. If cardiac tamponade ensues, it becomes life-threatening. Herein we describe chylopericardium tamponade in a child with IgA nephropathy. To the best of our knowledge, this is the first reported case of chylopericardium tamponade in IgA nephropathy.

Case presentation: A 6 years old boy with IgA nephropathy presented with dyspnea, orthopnea, pretibial pitting edema, ascites and fever. Muffled heart sounds and hepatomegaly were also noted. Echocardiography and thoracic CT revealed that there was a large volume of hydropericardium. Moreover, the pericardial milky fluid by pericardiocentesis was analyzed and chylopericardium effusion was eventually confirmed. Pericardial drainage was continued and his diet was modified to low fat, rich MCT and high protein. Complete remission was achieved after 3 weeks of this combined treatment.

Conclusion: Chylopericardial tamponade could be a rare and life-threatening complication of IgA nephropathy. Etiological analysis is critical for determining the therapeutic approach in patients with pericardial effusion.

Keywords: Chylopericardium tamponade, IgA nephropathy, Pericardiocentesis, Pericardium drainage, Middle chain triglyceride

Background

Pericardial effusion is a rare complication in renal diseases and could lead to hemodynamic compromise. Patients may initially present with clinical tamponade, characterized by dyspnea, tachycardia, jugular venous distension or even shock, while others may be asymptomatic if pericardial fluid accumulation is small [1, 2]. Pericardial effusion may be idiopathic or secondary to underlying diseases, such as acute myocardial infarction, end stage renal disease and autoimmune diseases [3–5]. Prompt diagnosis is critical. However, chylopericardial effusions may be difficult to diagnose unless the pericardial fluid undergoes chemical analysis. It is recognized that chylopericardium effusion may result from trauma, infection or blockage of the lymphatics [6]. In this paper, to the best of our knowledge, we are presenting the first case of chylopericardial tamponade in a child with IgA nephropathy.

Case presentation

A 6 years old boy with dyspnea, orthopnea, generalized pitting edema and fever, was admitted to the pediatric intensive care unit, Shanghai Children's Hospital. Three years before this episode, he presented to our hospital with acute onset of edema, hypoalbuminemia, heavy proteinuria and hyperlipidemia. The diagnosis of IgA nephropathy (Grade II) was made by percutaneous renal biopsy and in accordance with Lee's classification [7]. Initially he responded well to steroid therapy, but became steroid resistant after 2 years treatment. Immunosuppressive agents administered during this time period, included cyclophosphamide, mycophenolate mofetil and tacrolimus. He had no history of trauma, tuberculosis or radiation therapy.

Physical examination revealed tachypnea, orthopnea, anasarca and ascites. The heart sounds were muffled

* Correspondence: ghzhu301@sjtu.edu.cn
[1]Department of Nephrology and Rheumatology, Shanghai Children's Hospital, Shanghai Jiao Tong University, Shanghai, China

and hepatomegaly was also noted. Blood pressure ranged from 90/60 mmHg (systolic/diastolic blood pressure) to 130/70 mmHg. Blood cell count showed that white blood cells (WBC) was 14.49×10^9/L, neutrophils 79%, hemoglobin 11.5 g/dl, C-reactive protein 130 mg/L. Biochemistry analysis revealed total protein of 36 g/L, albumin 10 g/L, alanine aminotransferase (ALT) 10 U/L, aspartate aminotransferase (AST) 29 U/L, triglycerides 2.05 mmol/L, cholesterol 10.13 mmol/L. Serum electrolytes (Na^+, K^+, Ca^{2+} and Cl^-) were normal. Heavy proteinuria and hematuria were found on urinalysis (urinary protein: creatinine ratio 30.38). Serum creatinine was normal and estimated glomerular filtration rate (eGFR, calculated with Schwartz formula) was 147 ml/min/1.73m^2. Blood and urine cultures were sterile. T-spot for tuberculosis was negative. There was no ultrasound evidence of thrombosis in the superior vena cava or subclavian vein. Ultrasound also demonstrated that both kidneys were enlarged with a loss of cortico-medullary differentiation. Thoracic computed tomography (CT) found no evidence of congenital malformation or malignancies. Echocardiography revealed pericardial fluid of 4.6 cm at maximal thickness, suggesting a large volume hydropericardial effusion. The massive pericardial and pleural effusions were additionally confirmed by thoracic CT (Fig. 1a). Notably, milky fluid was obtained from the pericardial space by pericardiocentesis (Fig. 1b). Chyle test was positive. Cell counts and biochemistry in the pericardial effusion revealed WBC 405×10^6/L, lymphocytes count 92%, red blood cells 63×10^6/L, AST 8 U/L, lactate dehydrogenase (LDH) 58 U/L, Glucose 7.22 mmol/L, total protein 7 g/L, albumin 4 g/L, adenylate deaminase (ADH) 2.6 U/L, triglycerides 2.55 mmol/L, cholesterol 0.79 mmol/L. These findings confirmed the diagnosis of chylopericardial effusion.

Continuous renal replacement (CRRT) therapy was performed to alleviate the fluid overload. Meanwhile, pericardial drainage was performed and the diet was modified to low fat but rich in middle chain triglycerides and high protein. No side effects were encountered with this diet modification. The symptoms of cardiac tamponade subsided promptly, while the edema receded gradually over the subsequent 2 weeks. The indwelling pericardial catheter was removed when no fluid was drained after 3 weeks treatment and as shown in Fig. 1c, the chylopericardial effusion was removed successfully. Pericardial effusion has not recurred at 1 year of follow up, on follow up echocardiography.

Discussion and conclusions

Chylopericardium is characterized by a milky pericardial effusion, which is saturated with chyle and triglyceride. Clinical manifestations vary from asymptomatic to life threatening pericardial tamponade, depending on the extent of the effusion [8]. Our case highlights the importance of early diagnosis and treatment, as such patients can be easily misdiagnosed. Thoracic and pericardium effusion are seldom suspected to be chylous fluid in nephrotic syndrome unless the fluid sample is specifically analyzed for chyle and triglycerides. Thus, the awareness of chylopericardial tamponade needs to be heightened in renal or rheumatology diseases.

Chylopericardium can be idiopathic or secondary to trauma, tuberculosis, radiation, mediastinal tumor, venous thrombosis and congenital anomalies of the lymphatic duct [9]. Therefore, a history of blunt injury or thoracic operation needs to be reviewed. Neoplasm, thrombosis and congenital malformations should be looked for using CT scan, magnetic resonance imaging (MRI) or ultrasound. Tuberculosis can be excluded by the T-spot assay. Furthermore, lymphangiography and lymphoscintigraphy may be employed to exclude anatomic abnormities of thoracic lymphatic system [10, 11]. Additionally, it should be recognized that thrombosis and tuberculosis are two common complications seen in nephrotic syndrome and other glomerular diseases with nephrotic range proteinuria. As a

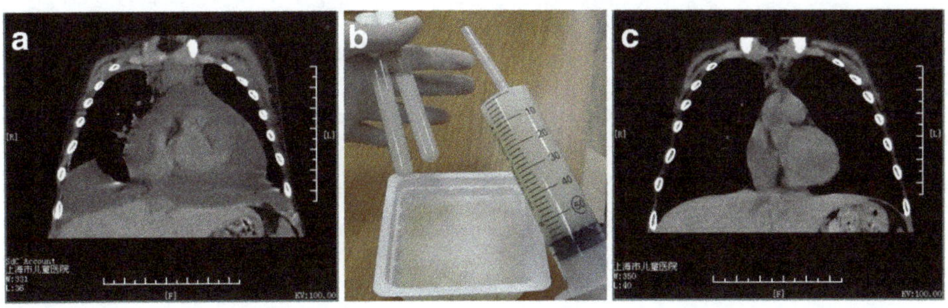

Fig. 1 a Thoracic CT demonstrating massive pericardial and pleural effusion. **b** The milky pericardial effusion was obtained from the child with IgA nephropathy. Laboratory tests revealed that this milky pericardial fluid was saturated chylous effusion. **c** The thoracic CT demonstrating resolution of pericardial effusion after pericardial drainage and modified diet therapy

result, chylopericardial effusion may occur if the integrity of the lymphatic duct was damaged by such conditions. However, no evidence of any of these causes was present in our case. The diagnosis of idiopathic chylopericardium may be made if no underlying cause is found. It has been reported that idiopathic chylopericardial effusion affects both genders equally and exists in different age groups [12, 13]. The etiology remains unclear, but it may due to elevated intrathoracic lymphatic pressure, increased permeability of lymphatic vessel walls, or valvular incompetence and ruptured lymphatic valves [6]. The most common manifestations of patients with idiopathic chylopericardial infusion range from absence of symptoms to cough, dyspnea and fatigue. Table 1 details clinical presentations of cases reported in the literature. Our case presented with life threatening dyspnea and orthopnea. Thus, chylopericardial effusion should be suspected, if patients with IgA nephropathy have hydropericardium, given the potential for life threatening complications despite its rarity.

Regarding therapeutic approaches, the most important step is to relieve the symptoms by urgent pericardiocentesis or pericardial drainage, if a life-threatening situation exists [14]. Drainage should not be terminated until the effusion recedes to a very small amount, as it may be helpful for self-repair of the damaged lymphatic tubule. In our case, it took 3 weeks for pericardial drainage to cease suggesting a relatively long duration for self-recovery. Meanwhile, some studies reported other surgical procedures such as ligature and excision of thoracic duct combined with partial pericardiectomy were necessary if pericardial effusion is recurrent [15]. Table 1 summarizes our review of the literature and details different treatments and outcomes. It also has been reported that administration of octreotide is effective in reducing intestinal absorption of fats [13].Most importantly it is necessary to remove any underlying causes for chylopericardial effusion. For instance, if thrombosis is the primary cause of chylopericardial effusion, thrombolytic therapy must be considered. In addition, conservative therapies are also required, including low fat diet based on middle chain triglycerides (MCT) or total parenteral nutrition. In our study, the combined therapy of pericardial drainage and modified diet with low fat but rich in MCT and high protein brought about complete remission. Prognosis is good if patients receive timely surgical intervention and medical management.

Chylopericardial effusion should be suspected in patients with IgA nephropathy, when signs of tamponade are present. It is critical to exclude underlying causes. Surgical procedures for draining chylous fluid and medical therapy such as a modified diet are effective therapeutic approaches. To date, the challenging issue in chylopericardium is identification of underlying causes. Hopefully, less invasive approaches will be developed in the near future. Additionally, long-term follow up is important to obtain data on the outcome and occurrence of this rare complication of common renal diseases such as IgA nephropathy.

Table 1 Clinical features of chylopericardium in children

Reference	Age	Gender	Symptoms and signs	Etiology	Treatment	Duration	Prognosis
Suri et al. [16]	4Y	Female	Orthopnea, anasarca, tachycardia, tachypnea, pulsusparadoxus, engorged neck vein, muffled heart sound	Superior vena cava thrombosis	Heparin infusion and oral warfarin; Modified diet with low fat but rich in MCT; Pericardial drainage.	15 days	No recurrence
Lope-castilla et al. [17]	2 M	Male	Dyspnea and anorexia	Idiopathic	Pericardiocentesis; Pericardial drainage and low-fat total parenteral nutrition enriched with MCT	36 days	No recurrence
Tan et al. [18]	5Y	Male	Cough and dyspnea, distant heart sounds.	Idiopathic	Ligation of the thoracic duct and the creation of a pericardial window	1 week	N/A
Rivera-Beltran et al. [15]	16Y	Male	Intermittent chest pain and dizziness	Idiopathic	Pericardiocentesis; MCT-rich diet; Octreotide; transabdominal ligation of the thoracic duct with pericardial-peritoneal shunting	Rapid recovery	No recurrence
Musemeche et al. [19]	12Y	Male	Orthopnea, distant heart tones	Lymphangiectasia	Total parenteral nutrition; Right thoracotomy with ligation of the thoracic duct	Rapid recovery	No recurrence
Attias et al. [20]	13Y	N/A	Chest pain and fatigue	Idiopathic	Ligation of thoracic duct and partial pericardectomy; MCT-rich diet	Rapid recovery	No recurrence

Abbreviations: *N/A* not available, *Y* year, *M* Month

Acknowledgements
We sincerely thank Dr. Fiona Mackie from Sydney Children's Hospital for English editing. We appreciate Dr. Li Shen from the department of cardiothoracic surgery and Dr. Jie Shen from the department of cardiology for their expertise assistant in patient's care. We also express gratitude to Dr. Weiwei Xia and Dr. Zhen Zhu from the department of radiology, Shanghai Children' Hospital for their help in interpreting CT images.

Funding
This study was financially supported by Shanghai medical excellent youth training program (2017YQ073).

Authors' contributions
YK was responsible for the design of the study, analyzing data and manuscript writing. YC cared for the patient and participated in the design of this study. YW participated in designing the study and analyzing data. SH cared for the patient and participating in manuscript writing. XK participated in the collecting and analyzing data. YZ participated in caring for the patient and manuscript writing. WH participated in the design of the study and revised the manuscript. GZ was responsible for the design of the study, analyzing data and revised the manuscript. All authors read and approved the final manuscript.

Competing interests
The authors declare that they have no competing interests.

Author details
[1]Department of Nephrology and Rheumatology, Shanghai Children's Hospital, Shanghai Jiao Tong University, Shanghai, China. [2]Pediatric Intensive Care Unit, Shanghai Children's Hospital, Shanghai Jiao Tong University, Shanghai, China.

References
1. Sagrista-Sauleda J, Merce AS, Soler-Soler J. Diagnosis and management of pericardial effusion. World J Cardiol. 2011;3(5):135–43.
2. Shakti D, Hehn R, Gauvreau K, Sundel RP, Newburger JW. Idiopathic pericarditis and pericardial effusion in children: contemporary epidemiology and management. J Am Heart Assoc. 2014;3(6):e001483.
3. Nugue O, Millaire A, Porte H, de Groote P, Guimier P, Wurtz A, Ducloux G. Pericardioscopy in the etiologic diagnosis of pericardial effusion in 141 consecutive patients. Circ. 1996;94(7):1635–41.
4. Figueras J, Juncal A, Carballo J, Cortadellas J, Soler JS. Nature and progression of pericardial effusion in patients with a first myocardial infarction: relationship to age and free wall rupture. Am Heart J. 2002; 144(2):251–8.
5. Posner MR, Cohen GI, Skarin AT. Pericardial disease in patients with cancer. The differentiation of malignant from idiopathic and radiation-induced pericarditis. Am J Med. 1981;71(3):407–13.
6. Mandarry MT, Ru XH, Wei ZQ, Ge MJ. Primary idiopathic chylopericardium: a rare case with a synopsis of the literature. Singap Med J. 2012;53(7):e156–8.
7. Lee SM, Rao VM, Franklin WA, Schiffer MS, Aronson AJ, Spargo BH, Katz AI. IgA nephropathy: morphologic predictors of progressive renal disease. Hum Pathol. 1982;13(4):314–22.
8. Silva MA, Martins AS, Campos NL, Andrade RR, Tohi LM, Hueb JC. Primary idiopathic chylopericardium–case report. Arq Bras Cardiol. 2009; 92(6):e40–3. e67-70
9. Mehrotra S, Peeran NA, Bandyopadhyay A. Idiopathic chylopericardium: an unusual cause of cardiac tamponade. Tex Heart Inst J. 2006;33(2):249–52.
10. Gallant TE, Hunziker RJ, Gibson TC. Primary chylopericardium: the role of lymphangiography. AJR Am J Roentgenol. 1977;129(6):1043–5.
11. Nanjo S, Yamazaki J, Tsubuku M, Ohyama T, Ohtsuka T, Nakano H. Primary idiopathic chylopericardium: report of two cases. Ann Nucl Med. 2004;18(6):537–9.
12. Groves LK, Effler DB. Primary chylopericardium. N Engl J Med. 1954;250(12): 520–3.
13. Mikroulis D, Didilis V, Bitzikas G, Bougioukas G. Octreotide in the treatment of chylothorax. Chest. 2002;121(6):2079–80. author reply 2080-2071
14. Han Z, Li S, Jing H, Liu H. Primary idiopathic chylopericardium: a retrospective case series. BMC Surg. 2015;15:61.
15. Rivera-Beltran S, Ortiz VN, Diaz R, Hernandez JA. Transabdominal ligation of the thoracic duct with pericardial-peritoneal shunting in a case of primary idiopathic chylous pericardial effusion. J Pediatr Surg. 2013;48(6):1434–7.
16. Suri D, Gupta N, Morigeri C, Saxena A, Manoj R. Chylopericardial tamponade secondary to superior vena cava thrombosis in a child with nephrotic syndrome. Pediatr Nephrol. 2009;24(6):1243–5.
17. Lopez-Castilla JD, Soult JA, Falcon JM, Munoz M, Santos J, Gavilan JL, Rodriguez A. Primary idiopathic chylopericardium in a 2 month old successfully treated without surgery. J Pediatr Surg. 2000;35(4):646–8.
18. Tan JX, Fu Y, Chen J. Primary idiopathic chylopericardium: a case report. Cardiol Young. 2013;23(5):773–5.
19. Musemeche CA, Riveron FA, Backer CL, Zales VR, Idriss FS. Massive primary chylopericardium: a case report. J Pediatr Surg. 1990;25(8):840–2.
20. Attias D, Ou P, Souillard P, Boudjemline Y, Sidi D, Bonnet D. Spontaneous idiopathic chylopericardium in childhood. Arch Mal Coeur Vaiss. 2006;99(5):529–31.

8

Patterns of paediatric end-of-life care: a chart review across different care settings in Switzerland

Karin Zimmermann[1,2,3*], Eva Cignacco[1,4], Sandra Engberg[5], Anne-Sylvie Ramelet[6,7], Nicolas von der Weid[8], Katri Eskola[1,9], Eva Bergstraesser[3], on behalf of the PELICAN Consortium, Marc Ansari, Christoph Aebi, Reta Baer, Maja Beck Popovic, Vera Bernet, Pierluigi Brazzola, Hans Ulrich Bucher, Regula Buder, Sandra Cagnazzo, Barbara Dinten, Anouk Dorsaz, Franz Elmer, Raquel Enriquez, Patricia Fahrni-Nater, Gabi Finkbeiner, Bernhard Frey, Urs Frey, Jeannette Greiner, Ralph-Ingo Hassink, Simone Keller, Oliver Kretschmar, Judith Kroell, Bernard Laubscher, Kurt Leibundgut, Reta Malaer, Andreas Meyer, Christoph Stuessi, Mathias Nelle, Thomas Neuhaus, Felix Niggli, Geneviève Perrenoud, Jean-Pierre Pfammatter, Barbara Plecko, Debora Rupf, Felix Sennhauser, Caroline Stade, Maja Steinlin, Lilian Stoffel, Karin Thomas, Christian Vonarburg, Rodo von Vigier, Bendicht Wagner, Judith Wieland and Birgit Wernz

Abstract

Background: Paediatric end-of-life care is challenging and requires a high level of professional expertise. It is important that healthcare teams have a thorough understanding of paediatric subspecialties and related knowledge of disease-specific aspects of paediatric end-of-life care. The aim of this study was to comprehensively describe, explore and compare current practices in paediatric end-of-life care in four distinct diagnostic groups across healthcare settings including all relevant levels of healthcare providers in Switzerland.

Methods: In this nationwide retrospective chart review study, data from paediatric patients who died in the years 2011 or 2012 due to a cardiac, neurological or oncological condition, or during the neonatal period were collected in 13 hospitals, two long-term institutions and 10 community-based healthcare service providers throughout Switzerland.

Results: Ninety-three (62%) of the 149 reviewed patients died in intensive care units, 78 (84%) of them following withdrawal of life-sustaining treatment. Reliance on invasive medical interventions was prevalent, and the use of medication was high, with a median count of 12 different drugs during the last week of life. Patients experienced an average number of 6.42 symptoms. The prevalence of various types of symptoms differed significantly among the four diagnostic groups. Overall, our study patients stayed in the hospital for a median of six days during their last four weeks of life. Seventy-two patients (48%) stayed at home for at least one day and only half of those received community-based healthcare.

(Continued on next page)

* Correspondence: karin.zimmermann@unibas.ch
[1]Department Public Health (DPH), Nursing Science, University of Basel, Bernoullistrasse 28, 4056 Basel, Switzerland
[2]Paediatric Palliative Care, University Children's Hospital Zurich, Children's Research Center CRC, Steinwiesstrasse 75, 8032 Zurich, Switzerland

(Continued from previous page)

Conclusions: The study provides a wide-ranging overview of current end-of-life care practices in a real-life setting of different healthcare providers. The inclusion of patients with all major diagnoses leading to disease- and prematurity-related childhood deaths, as well as comparisons across the diagnostic groups, provides additional insight and understanding for healthcare professionals. The provision of specialised palliative and end-of-life care services in Switzerland, including the capacity of community healthcare services, need to be expanded to meet the specific needs of seriously ill children and their families.

Keywords: End-of-life care, Terminal care, Paediatrics, Neonatology, Child, Practice patterns, Retrospective studies

Background

Despite continued advancements in medical care and improved (expected) survival, infant and childhood deaths due to complex chronic conditions (CCC) or prematurity are inevitable [1]. Deaths during the first year of life constitute approximately 50% of disease-related infant and childhood deaths in developed countries, the causes of which include perinatal complications, prematurity, or congenital anomalies [2, 3]. Beyond the age of one year, the three most common life-limiting CCCs are neurological/neuromuscular and cardiovascular conditions (including genetic disorders), and malignancies [4, 5]. The majority of disease- and prematurity-related deaths occur in hospitals, [6, 7], and for children dying at home, hospital use in their terminal stage is high [1, 4]. Symptom burden and reliance on medical technology has been reported to be considerable [3, 8]. Circumstances and characteristics of deaths, however, are known to vary by age and medical conditions [1, 4].

Paediatric palliative care (PPC) emerged as a medical subspecialty aimed at meeting the specific needs of seriously ill children and their families. According to the World Health Organization (WHO) "palliative care is an approach that improves the quality of life of patients and their families facing the problem associated with life-threatening illness, through the prevention and relief of suffering by means of early identification and impeccable assessment and treatment of pain and other problems, physical, psychosocial and spiritual" [9]. More specifically and as part of palliative care, the term end-of-life (EOL) care refers to care when death is imminent [10]. Meeting the needs of affected children and their families requires a wide-ranging and integrative approach from a compassionate and skilled multidisciplinary team [11]. PPC and EOL care should be provided in all settings where it is required [12]; although, specialised PPC teams are mostly hospital based [13]. A thorough understanding of paediatric subspecialties and related knowledge of disease-specific aspects of paediatric EOL are needed. This understanding should go beyond the horizon of a single hospital and take into account the heterogeneous settings where care can be provided (tertiary settings, general hospitals, paediatric primary care and in the community). There is not much evidence on which to base best practice, and most existing studies focus on specific diagnostic groups or specific care settings [1, 14, 15]. It was therefore the aim of this national study to comprehensively describe, explore and compare current practices in paediatric EOL care in four distinct diagnostic groups (cardiology, neonatology, neurology and oncology) across healthcare settings including all relevant levels of healthcare providers in Switzerland.

Methods

Study design

This retrospective chart review was part of PELICAN (Paediatric End-of-LIfe-CAre Needs in Switzerland), a nationwide study "to provide comprehensive information and to understand the current practice of EOL care (i.e. in this study and similar to other studies, the last 4 weeks of life prior to death [16]) in paediatric settings in Switzerland (hospital and community care) and to explore and describe parental perspectives and the perspectives of the healthcare professionals involved" [17]. Human Research Ethics Committees from the 11 Swiss cantons in which the study took place approved the PELICAN study. Parents who had lost a child due to a cardiac, neurological or oncological condition or during the neonatal period (independent of the underlying condition) in the years 2011 and 2012 were invited to participate. Neonates < 24 h of life and patients > 18 years were excluded. Information on how, where and when recruitment took place is described in detail elsewhere [18].

Setting and data collection

Data from all eligible patients, whose parents had consented to the review of their child's medical chart, were collected in 13 hospitals, 2 institutions and 10 community-based healthcare service providers throughout Switzerland. Among the 13 hospitals, there were 5 tertiary paediatric centres, 4 dedicated children's hospitals, 3 general hospitals with paediatric units and 1 tertiary care centre with a neonatal intensive care unit. A multiprofessional PPC team was available in two tertiary paediatric centres and one dedicated children's hospital; no paediatric hospices exist in Switzerland.

Data collection was conducted mainly by the first author, who also developed the coding manual and all case report forms as well as instructing and supervising five assistants, who supported data collection [19]. The coding manual was developed within the PELICAN study group [17] and pilot tested with 10 children who were treated in 5 different hospitals and died in the year 2010. In accordance with this study's definition of EOL care as care during the last four weeks of life, data collection was restricted to the 28 days prior to the child's death. All extracted data was entered into secuTrial®, a browser-based electronic data capture system (InterActive Systems, Berlin, Germany). During the first two months of data collection, 5 % of the medical records reviewed by one of the five assistants were randomly selected and audited by KZ by performing a dual review. Any data entry discrepancies were checked for its nature of assessment error. No systemic data entry errors were detected. There were very few data entry discrepancies and those that occurred were almost always related to mixed documentation quality in the medical records that left room for interpretation, e.g., change of do-not-resuscitate (DNR) order. Emerging questions around those inconsistencies were continuously discussed among data collectors. Variable instructions in the manual were revised as needed to ensure the quality of ongoing data extraction and reduce the likelihood of inter-rater discrepancies [19].

Variables

The following data were collected for this study: (1) demographics (age, gender); (2) diagnostic information (the underlying diagnosis primarily responsible for the patient's death, gestational age for newborns only, time since diagnosis, and whether the diagnosis was made prenatally); (3) circumstances of death (place of death, occurrence of resuscitation, existence of DNR orders and whether these orders changed during the last four weeks of life, and treatment withdrawal); (4) interventions (at least once during the last four weeks of life, Yes-No: anaesthesia, e.g., surgery, imaging; ventilation; central access device; enteral feeds) and medications (number and types of medications were recorded only for the last two weeks of life to reduce the time burden related to reviewing the medical records); (5) symptoms (presence of various symptoms); (6) hospital and community healthcare utilisation (hospital days and admissions, days spent at home, number of days and hours, and types of care provided by community services). We also assessed whether the treatment approach was documented as palliative care and whether this approach changed during the last four weeks of life.

A diagnostic chapter and code from the International Statistical Classification of Diseases and Related Health Problems (ICD), 10th Revision, online version 2016 [20] was assigned to each patient, based on the exact diagnostic information extracted from the patient's last medical report. Coding was done by two independent appraisers to establish reliability and any discrepancies were discussed until there was consensus about the diagnosis. All symptoms documented in the patient's chart were recorded during data collection. The ones most frequently reported were grouped into 20 symptoms categories, based on symptoms most frequently reported in the literature [8, 14, 21]. Symptoms that affected similar areas, e.g. spasticity/dystonia for muscular impairments, or agitation/irritability for behavioural problems, were grouped.

Statistical analysis

Descriptive statistics (measures of central tendency and dispersion, frequencies and percentages) were used to explore and summarize all variables. A binary logistic model with likelihood ratio statistics was utilised for two-tailed comparisons between the diagnostic groups of variables with a binominal response (Yes – No). For count outcome variables, negative binomial regression was utilised to adjust for overdispersion [22]. For variables with a categorical response, equivalence of proportions between diagnostic groups was tested in contingency tables using the Pearson's chi-square test or Fisher's exact test when cell sizes were < 5. No measures of missing value replacement were pursued. Due to the multiple comparisons performed, we set a conservative p-value of < 0.001 to indicate statistical significance. Statistical analyses were performed using IBM© SPSS© Statistics 21 for Mac® (IBM Corp, Armonk, NY, USA).

Results

Of the 307 eligible families, 267 could be contacted and were invited to participate in the PELICAN study. Of those, 147 families (55%) consented. Two families lost twins resulting in a study sample of 149 neonates, children and adolescents (Table 1). With neonates comprising 38% of the sample, the median age at death was 0.5 years for the entire sample but substantially higher (*Mdn* = 8.4, *range* = 1.7 -17.4 years) for the oncology group. The neonates' median age was 5 days (*range* = 1 - 26) and substantially lower than age in the other diagnostic groups (Table 1). Seven ICD-10 diagnostic chapters were represented in our four groups' categorisation, with the highest variety found within the neurology group. The median time between diagnosis of the life-limiting CCC (made after birth) and death for the total sample was one month (*interquartile range [IQR]*, 0 – 6). Within the four groups, the median time between diagnosis and death was longest for the neurology group (*Mdn* = 6 months, *IQR* = 3 – 29). Diagnoses made

Table 1 Demographic and diagnostic patient characteristics

Characteristics	Total $N = 149$ (100%)	Cardiology $n = 19$ (13%)	Neonatology $n = 57$ (38%)	Neurology $n = 36$ (24%)	Oncology $n = 37$ (25%)
Age at death, *Mdn (range)*					
in months	6 (0 – 209)	6 (1 – 109)	Na	19 (1 – 207)	101 (20 – 209)
in years	0.5 (0.0 – 17.4)	0.5 (0.1 – 9.1)	Na	1.6 (0.1 – 17.2)	8.4 (1.7 – 17.4)
Gender, *n* (%)					
Female	72 (48)	10 (53)	32 (56)	15 (42)	15 (40)
Male	77 (52)	9 (47)	25 (44)	21 (58)	22 (60)
ICD-10 chapter, description, *n* (%)					
II Neoplasms	36 (24)	0 (0)	0 (0)	0 (0)	36 (97)
III Blood/immune system	1 (1)	0 (0)	0 (0)	0 (0)	1 (3)[a]
IV Endocrine, nutritional, metabolic	6 (4)	0 (0)	0 (0)	6 (16)	0 (0)
VI Nervous system	21 (14)	0 (0)	2 (4)	19 (53)	0 (0)
IX Circulatory system[b]	5 (3)	4 (21)	0 (0)	1 (3)	0 (0)
XVI Conditions originating in perinatal period	45 (30)	0 (0)	44 (77)	1 (3)	0 (0)
XVII Congenital, chromosomal	35 (24)	15 (79)	11 (19)	9 (25)	0 (0)
Gestational age (for the neonatology group only)			n = 52[c]		
24 0/7 – 27 6/7	Na	Na	17 (33)	Na	Na
28 0/7 – 31 6/7	Na	Na	8 (15)	Na	Na
32 0/7 – 36 6/7	Na	Na	9 (17)	Na	Na
37 0/7 - > 42 0/7	Na	Na	18 (35)	Na	Na
Time since diagnosis[d]					
in days, *Mdn (range)*	Na	Na	4 (1 – 26)	Na	Na
in months, *Mdn (range)*	1 (0 – 205)	7 (0 - 66)	Na	9 (0 - 205)	4 (0 - 139)
in years, *Mdn (range)*	0 (0 – 17)	0.5 (0.5 – 5.5)	Na	0.5 (0.0 – 17.0)	0.5 (0.0 – 12.0)
Diagnosis made prenatally	n = 147[c]			n = 34[c]	
Yes, *n* (%)	31 (21)	11 (58)	13 (23)	7 (21)	0 (0)

Na Not applicable, *ICD-10* International Classification of Diseases, 10th Revision
[a]Aplastic anaemia
[b]Stroke included
[c]Information was missing for some cases
[d]Calculated from date of birth, even if diagnosis was suspected prenatally

prenatally, were significantly more frequent in the cardiology group compared to the other groups ($p = < 0.001$) and not present in the oncology group. Information related to gestational age was missing for 5 neonates (8.8%) and information related to diagnoses made prenatally for 2 patients (1.3%) (Table 1).

Place and circumstances of death

Ninety-three patients (62%) died in an intensive care unit (ICU), with the highest proportion of ICU deaths occurring in the neonatology group (Table 2). Twenty-five patients (17%) died at home, with the highest proportion of home deaths occurring in the oncology group. Twenty-six patients (17%) received cardiopulmonary resuscitation (CPR) within 24 h before death, despite 15 patients (17%, $n = 147$) had a documented DNR order. A DNR order was documented in 91 patients' charts (62%). Of those, 51 patients (57%) had a change of the DNR order within the last four weeks of life. This change occurred most frequently in the neonatology group (Table 2), often within hours before the child's death. For 78 patients (84%) of the 93 who died in an ICU, death was preceded by a decision to withdraw life-sustaining interventions.

Interventions, medication and symptoms

Patients underwent several interventions, suffered from a variety of symptoms, and received a considerable amount of medication, as documented in their charts. This information is detailed in Table 3 and Fig. 1. Fifty-one patients (34%) received anaesthesia at least once

Table 2 Place and circumstances of death

	Total $N = 149$ (100%)	Cardiology $n = 19$ (13%)	Neonatology $n = 57$ (38%)	Neurology $n = 36$ (24%)	Oncology $n = 37$ (25%)	*p*-value
Place of death, *n* (%)						< 0.001[a]
PICU	63 (42)	13 (67)	27 (48)	13 (36)	10 (27)	
NICU	30 (20)	0 (0)	27 (48)	3 (8)	0 (0)	
Hospital ward / long-term institution	26 (18)	2 (11)	0 (0)	13 (36)	11 (30)	
Home	25 (17)	2 (11)	2 (3)	7 (20)	14 (38)	
Emergency department / Transport	5 (3)	2 (11)	1 (1)	0 (0)	2 (5)	
CPR[b]						
Yes, *n* (%)	26 (17)	7 (37)	6 (11)	7 (19)	6 (16)	0.097[c]
DNR order						
Yes, *n* (%)	91 (62)	11 (58)	20 (35)	33 (92)	27 (77)	< 0.001[c]
DNR order change within the last four weeks of life						
Yes, *n* (%)	51 (57)	7 (64)	18 (90)	13 (41)	13 (48)	0.002[c]
Withdrawal of life-sustaining interventions[d]	$n = 93$	$n = 13$	$n = 54$	$n = 16$	$n = 10$	
Yes, *n* (%)	78 (84)	10 (77)	49 (91)	12 (75)	7 (70)	0.203[c]

PICU Paediatric intensive care unit, *NICU* Neonatal intensive care unit, *CPR* Cardiopulmonary resuscitation, *DNR* Do not resuscitate
[a]Across the four groups, based on Fisher's exact test
[b]Within 24 h before death
[c]Across the four groups, based on likelihood ratio chi-square
[d]Only applies to patients who died in an intensive care unit

during their last four weeks of life, some patients more than once and for different interventions. The most commonly documented interventions requiring anaesthesia were surgical interventions in 28 patients (55% of the 51 patients who received anaesthesia) and diagnostic procedures, e.g. imaging in 27 patients (53%). The overall median and mean number of medications with orders for standard daily doses and as-needed orders rose from 9 (*range* = 0 - 42), 12 (*SD* = 9.20) respectively during the second-to-last week to 12 (*range* = 1 – 46), 14 (*SD* = 9.15) respectively during the last week. For 133 patients (89%) the last treatment approach was documented as palliative. The approach changed from curative to palliative during the last month in 88 patients (59%), most commonly in the neonatology group and least commonly in the oncology group (90% vs. 32%, $p = < 0.001$). Information was missing for six variables related to interventions and medication and ranged between 0.7% and 2.7% (Table 3).

Pain was the most frequently documented symptom, and occurred in 110 patients (78%, $N = 141$), with no significant differences between the diagnostic groups. One hundred and forty patients (95%, $N = 148$) received some pain medication, most commonly opioids (93%), followed by paracetamol (67%). Other common symptoms included breathing problems ($n = 107$, 72%), followed by behavioural problems such as agitation or irritability ($n = 89$, 60%). Some symptoms, such as respiratory secretion, fever, nausea/vomiting, coughing, sweating, fatigue, drowsiness, anxiety (including worry and sadness), and poor appetite, differed significantly ($p = < 0.001$) between the diagnostic groups (Figure 1). Overall, an average of 6.42 ($SD = 3.14$) symptoms were recorded per patient. Significantly fewer symptoms were reported in neonates ($M = 4.39$, $SD = 2.15$) compared to all other groups ($p = < 0.001$).

Hospital and community healthcare utilisation

Overall, our study patients stayed in the hospital for a median of six days ($IQR = 2 – 19$) during their last four weeks of life, with the highest number of hospital days for patients in the cardiology group (Table 4). Nineteen patients (13%) had no hospital days: 11 of them (58%) from the oncology group, 5 (26%) from the neurology group, 3 (16%) from the cardiology group, and none from the neonatology group. Among the 130 patients who had at least one hospital day, 62 patients (48%) had one hospital admission, 10 patients (8%), and 2 patients (1%) had 3 admissions during the last four weeks of life. Fifty-six patients (43%) had zero hospital admissions, meaning that those patients were hospitalised at the beginning of data collection and remained there until their death or discharge. Of the 57 patients in the neonatology group, 23 patients (40%) were born in a hospital with no ICU and had to be transferred to a referral tertiary hospital with an ICU. Patients from the other diagnostic groups were most commonly admitted from home (Table 4).

Table 3 Interventions and medications during the last four weeks of life

	Total $N = 149$ (100%)	Cardiology $n = 19$ (13%)	Neonatology $n = 57$ (38%)	Neurology $n = 36$ (24%)	Oncology $n = 37$ (25%)	*p*-value
Interventions requiring anaesthesia	$n = 148^a$			$n = 35^a$		
Yes, *n* (%)	51 (34)	11 (58)	21 (37)	6 (17)	13 (35)	0.021^b
Mechanical ventilation						
Yes, *n* (%)	94 (63)	14 (74)	55 (97)	15 (42)	10 (27)	$< 0.001^b$
ECMO						
Yes, *n* (%)	7 (5)	4 (21)	3 (5)	0 (0)	0 (0)	$< 0.001^b$
Presence of CAD	$n = 148^a$				$n = 36^a$	
Yes, *n* (%)	106 (72)	14 (74)	55 (97)	12 (33)	25 (69)	$< 0.001^b$
Enteral feeds via nasogastric or gastrostomy tube	$n = 148^a$			$n = 35^a$		
Yes, *n* (%)	114 (77)	17 (90)	51 (90)	33 (94)	13 (35)	$< 0.001^b$
Medication count in the last week of life[c]	$n = 146^a$			$n = 35^a$	$n = 35^a$	
Mdn, (range)	12 (1 - 46)	19 (3 - 45)	12 (1 - 34)	10 (3 - 39)	13 (4 - 46)	0.006^b
Mean, (SD)	14 (9.15)	21 (11.73)	12 (7.02)	13 (8.82)	15 (9.69)	
Pain medication	$n = 148^a$			$n = 35^a$		
Yes, *n* (%)	140 (95)	18 (95)	54 (95)	33 (94)	35 (95)	1.000^b
Anxiolytic medication	$n = 145^a$			$n = 35^a$	$n = 34^a$	
Yes, *n* (%)	84 (58)	14 (74)	27 (47)	18 (51)	25 (74)	0.032^b
Antiemetic medication	$n = 146^a$			$n = 35^a$	$n = 35^a$	
Yes, *n* (%)	25 (17)	2 (11)	0 (0)	0 (0)	23 (66)	$< 0.001^b$

ECMO Extracorporeal membrane oxygenation, *CAD* Central access device, either venous or arterial
[a]Information was missing for some cases
[b]Across the four groups, based on likelihood ratio chi-square
[c]Includes both standing daily dosages and as-needed orders

Seventy-two patients (48%) stayed at home for at least one day, with patients from the oncology group having the highest number of home days (*Mdn* = 24, *IQR* = 4 - 28), followed by patients from the neurology group (*Mdn* = 21, *IQR* = 4 - 26). Of the 72 patients who stayed at home, 36 (50%) received professional care from a community-based service. The provision of education and support to empower the family was the most commonly provided service, as documented by the care provider, and patients from the neurology group received more care hours than patients from the other groups (Table 4).

Discussion

There are several principal findings in this nationwide study examining patterns of care at EOL in four distinct diagnostic groups: patients had a variety of primary diagnoses, covering seven different ICD-10 diagnostic chapters; 62% of all patients died in ICUs, with 84% of them following a decision to withdraw life-sustaining treatment; reliance on invasive medical interventions was prevalent and patients were exposed to multiple medications; patients experienced many symptoms with an average of six symptoms per patient; finally, community-based health care services were involved in only half of the cases of the 72 patients (48%) of patients who spent time at home during their last four weeks of life.

Strengths and limitations

The study provides a wide-ranging overview of current EOL care practices in a heterogeneous real-life setting of hospitals, long-term institutions and community health-care organisations. The inclusion of patients with all major diagnoses leading to disease- and prematurity-related infant and childhood deaths, as well as comparisons across the diagnostic groups, provides additional insight and understanding for healthcare professionals. Previous studies in this field have frequently been limited to the hospital setting [1, 3] or to a specific diagnostic group [8, 14, 15]. Our study is limited by its cross-sectional, primarily descriptive design incorporating a retrospective chart review. This approach does not allow conclusions to be drawn about care quality and quality of life at the EOL. Generalisability is further limited by the way that EOL care is often delivered in Switzerland. Specialised PC/EOL care was offered in only 3 of the 13 hospitals where data were collected, and no children's hospices exist in Switzerland. The study's definition of EOL care as the last four weeks of life is

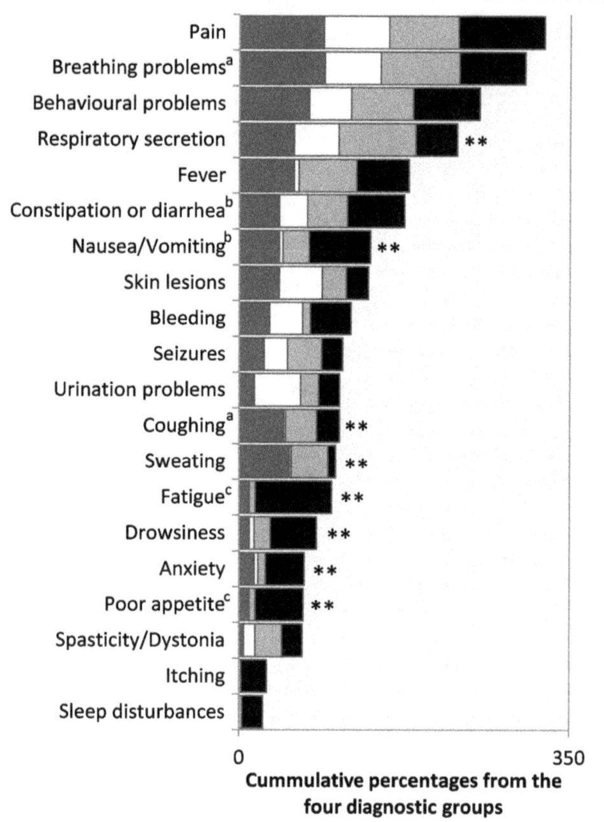

Fig. 1 Symptom prevalence and comparison between the four diagnostic groups. ** = *p*-value < 0.001 based on a negative binomial regression model.[a]Adjusted for mechanical ventilation. [b]Adjusted for enteral feeds. [c]Neonatology group excluded due to 0% of symptom presence

somehow artificial, yet was justified by the literature, experts' opinion and feasibility constraints. The study, therefore, provides insight in paediatric EOL care in a limited time frame, not necessarily covering all aspects of EOL care across a broader time period. Known reliability issues related to chart reviews were kept to a minimum by utilising established and appropriate measures, resulting in few discrepancies in the data collected. However, the mixed quality of documentation among healthcare personnel, resulting in incomplete or missing data independent of data collection quality still limits the study's reliability [19]. The comparisons between the four major diagnostic groups highlight elements that warrant discussion.

Medication and symptoms

Medication counts in our study were high, with an overall mean of 14 drugs or as-needed medication orders during the last week of life. This number is higher than the reported average of 9 drugs in a study involving 515 paediatric patients with a similar diagnostic profile receiving PPC [3]. A similar average number of 13.9 ($SD = 8.9$) of medications used in the last week of life was reported in a study of 30 children dying in an Australian hospital in 2001. Two thirds of the 30 children died in the ICU, which might have influenced the high numbers found in this study [23]. We found that the medication count increased from the second-to-last week to the last week of life. Thus, it seems that the intensity of medical treatment increases as the child nears death, a phase which is accompanied by a greater need for pharmacological interventions, especially for relieving pain, based on our clinical experience. The high number of medications in the cardiology group was often due to the frequent need for CPR and a high prevalence of surgical interventions, which are also described in other studies with cardiology patients [15, 21]. Although not perfectly comparable, symptom type and prevalence differed from the aforementioned study of 515 patients receiving PPC, in which pain was only the sixth most frequent symptom extracted from patients' charts [3]. However, pain has been reported to be the most frequent symptom in other studies with various paediatric cohorts in PC or EOL care [8, 14]. Our study adds to existing knowledge by demonstrating that symptom prevalence is dependent on the underlying CCC and that it can differ considerably.

Hospital and community healthcare utilisation

Most patients ($n = 130$) stayed at least one day in hospital during their last four weeks of life. Of those, 62 patients (48%) had at least one hospital admission and 10 patients (8%) had more than one admission. This is a lower percentage than reported in a recent North American study about trends in high-intensity EOL care among children with cancer [24]. In this population-based study with a cohort of 815 children diagnosed with cancer who died between 2000 and 2012, 143 patients (17.6%) of the patients had more than one hospital admission within 30 days of death. Compared with our oncology sub-group ($n = 37$), twenty-six patients stayed at least one day in hospital and 3 (11%) of them had more than one admission during their last four weeks of life.

Slightly less than 50% of our study's patients were at home at some point during their last four weeks of life. Naturally, this was the case for very few neonates. In light of the probably growing rate of prenatal diagnosis of a life-limiting CCC, early initiation of PPC may allow better planning and implementation of specialised care services at home [25]. Perinatal palliative care is an even younger specialty than PPC [25] and was not integrated in the three PPC programmes in Switzerland. A recent survey about the provision of services showed that perinatal palliative care programmes in the US were based in academic medical centres, regional and local hospitals, or community based hospitals [26]. Back in

Table 4 Hospital and community healthcare utilisation during the last four weeks of life

	Total $N = 149$ (100%)	Cardiology $n = 19$ (13%)	Neonatology $n = 57$ (38%)	Neurology $n = 36$ (24%)	Oncology $n = 37$ (25%)	*p*-value
Hospital days, *Mdn* (*range*)	6 (0 - 28)	20 (0 - 28)	5 (1 - 26)	7 (0 - 28)	4 (0 - 28)	0.035[a]
Care setting before hospital admission[b], *n* (%)	$n = 88$	$n = 17$	$n = 23$	$n = 26$	$n = 22$	
Home	37 (42)	11 (64)	0 (0)	16 (62)	10 (45)	NA[c]
Other hospital	35 (40)	3 (18)	23 (100)	4 (15)	5 (23)	NA[c]
Emergency department	8 (9)	3 (18)	0 (0)	4 (15)	1 (5)	NA[c]
Outpatient clinic	7 (8)	0 (0)	0 (0)	1 (4)	6 (27)	NA[c]
Long-term institution	1 (1)	0 (0)	0 (0)	1 (4)	0 (0)	NA[c]
Patients at home at least for one day, *n* (%)	72 (48)	11 (58)	3 (5)	27 (75)	31 (84)	< 0.001[a]
Days spent at home, *Mdn* (*range*)	0 (0 - 28)	8 (0 - 28)	0 (0 - 16)	21 (0 - 28)	24 (0 - 28)	0.001[a]
Care days with community care service[d],	$n = 72$	$n = 11$	$n = 3$	$n = 27$	$n = 31$	
Mdn (*range*)	1 (0 - 28)	0 (0 - 24)	1 (0 - 5)	5 (0 - 28)	0 (0 - 28)	0.001[a]
Hours of care by community care service[d]	$n = 36$	$n = 5$	$n = 2$	$n = 15$	$n = 14$	
Mdn (*range*)	34 (2 - 315)	12 (7 - 190)	6 (3 - 8)	38 (4 - 315)	23 (2 - 108)	0.111[a]
Type of community care service						
Family education/support, *n* (%)	35 (97)	5 (100)	2 (100)	14 (93)	14 (100)	NA[c]
Needs assessment, *n* (%)	31 (86)	4 (80)	1 (50)	13 (87)	13 (93)	NA[c]
Monitoring of vital signs/general condition, *n* (%)	29 (81)	5 (100)	2 (100)	13 (87)	9 (64)	NA[c]
Administration of medication, *n* (%)	25 (69)	5 (100)	0 (0)	10 (67)	10 (71)	NA[c]
Interventions related to enteral feeds, *n* (%)	22 (61)	5 (100)	1 (50)	13 (87)	3 (21)	NA[c]
Respiratory interventions, *n* (%)	18 (50)	2 (40)	0 (0)	11 (73)	5 (36)	NA[c]
Interventions related to excretion, *n* (%)	14 (39	1 (20)	0 (0)	6 (40)	7 (50)	NA[c]

NA Not applicable
[a]Across the four groups, based on likelihood ratio chi-square
[b]Representing the cumulative hospital admissions in all patients
[c]No significance testing conducted due to small numbers
[d]Consisting of nurses, most of them specialised in paediatric and/or community nursing

2013, Feudtner et al. [13] showed however, that only 54% of hospital-based PPC programmes provided prenatal consultation [13].

Only half of the patients who spent time at home received community-based healthcare services. Recent data from Germany and the US show that the coordination and provision of specialised palliative home care can alleviate caregivers' distress and burden [27], and improve both the child's [28] and the caregivers' quality of life [27]. As reported by our study, community nursing care encompasses a range of service types. The high level of coordination with the leading team in the hospital and the expertise required makes it especially challenging. Subgroup analysis of our study's at-home population targeting facilitators for and barriers to EOL care in the home setting has been performed and is published elsewhere [29].

Implications

PPC is growing internationally and the provision of consultation by a hospital-based multiprofessional PPC team seems to be the favoured model of care [13]. There is some evidence suggesting that PPC programmes providing specialised services may reduce healthcare resource utilisation by reducing hospital admissions, shortening hospital stays, and lessening aggressive care to prolong life [30]. Additionally, provision of hospital-based specialised PPC may shift and extend the care setting beyond the hospital [30]. In order to provide good quality EOL care a high level of expertise with a good understanding of the different illness trajectories, and efficient collaboration across a variety of paediatric subspecialties is required. Outcome measurement has to be introduced into practice and prospective studies are needed to evaluate meaningful family-oriented clinical outcomes, quality of care, and the impact of specialised PPC to advance clinical practice and research in the field [30, 31].

Conclusions

Swiss paediatric patients, similar to what is reported from other countries, experience high-intensity EOL care with invasive interventions, high medication counts and high symptom prevalence. Transitions between the inpatient and the home care setting were experienced by most patients outside the neonatology group. Professional home care was only utilised by half of the patients/families. The provision of specialised palliative and EOL care services, including the capacity of community healthcare services were limited. There is therefore a need for PPC services to be expanded to meet the specific needs of seriously ill children and their families in Switzerland.

Abbreviations

CCC: Complex chronic conditions; CPR: Cardiopulmonary resuscitation; DNR: Do not resuscitate; EOL: End-of-life; ICD: International Statistical Classification of Diseases and Related Health Problems; ICU: Intensive care unit; IQR: Interquartile range; PELICAN: Paediatric End-of-LIfe CAre Needs; PPC: Paediatric palliative care

Acknowledgements

We would like to thank Anouk Dorsaz, Marie-Madeleine Minder, Simone Keller, and Judith Wieland for their invaluable contribution in collecting the large amount of data. We also thank Heather Murray for her language editing. The authors wish to express their special thanks to all the members of the PELICAN Consortium who supported and facilitated the study conduction in all participating institutions: Marc Ansari; Christoph Aebi; Reta Baer; Maja Beck Popovic; Vera Bernet; Pierluigi Brazzola; Hans Ulrich Bucher; Regula Buder; Sandra Cagnazzo; Barbara Dinten; Anouk Dorsaz; Franz Elmer; Raquel Enriquez; Patricia Fahrni-Nater; Gabi Finkbeiner; Bernhard Frey; Urs Frey; Jeannette Greiner; Ralph-Ingo Hassink; Simone Keller; Oliver Kretschmar; Judith Kroell; Bernard Laubscher; Kurt Leibundgut; Reta Malaer; Andreas Meyer; Christoph Stuessi; Mathias Nelle; Thomas Neuhaus; Felix Niggli; Geneviève Perrenoud; Jean-Pierre Pfammatter; Barbara Plecko; Debora Rupf; Felix Sennhauser; Caroline Stade; Maja Steinlin; Lilian Stoffel; Karin Thomas; Christian Vonarburg; Rodo von Vigier; Bendicht Wagner; Judith Wieland; Birgit Wernz.

Funding

The research received funding from the following sponsors: The Swiss Cancer League / Swiss Cancer Research; Nursing Science Foundation, Basel, Switzerland; Federal Office of Public Health, Switzerland; Start Stipend Award, PhD Program in Health Sciences, Faculty of Medicine, University of Basel, Switzerland.

Authors' contributions

EC and EB designed the study. KZ elaborated the methodology, conducted the study, under the guidance of EC and EB, had full access to the data and performed the statistical analysis, and wrote the manuscript. KZ, KE and AS were involved in recruitment processes and data collection. All authors, including SE and NW, contributed to the interpretation of results, revised the manuscript critically and approved the final version.

Ethics approval and consent to participate

Human Research Ethics Committees from the 11 Swiss cantons in which the study took place approved the PELICAN study (leading committee: Kantonale Ethikkommission Zürich, KEK ZH Nr. 2012-0537). Parents of eligible deceased children were informed and invited to participate in the study by the former treating team, who also acted as gatekeeper as needed. Participation was entirely voluntary and written informed consent was obtained from all participants.

Competing interests

The authors declare that they have no competing interests.

Author details

[1]Department Public Health (DPH), Nursing Science, University of Basel, Bernoullistrasse 28, 4056 Basel, Switzerland. [2]Paediatric Palliative Care, University Children's Hospital Zurich, Children's Research Center CRC, Steinwiesstrasse 75, 8032 Zurich, Switzerland. [3]Department of Pediatrics, Inselspital Bern University Hospital, Bern, Switzerland. [4]Health Division, University of Applied Sciences Bern, Bern, Switzerland. [5]School of Nursing, University of Pittsburgh, 3500 Victoria Street, Pittsburgh, PA 15261, USA. [6]Institute of Higher Education and Research in Healthcare – IUFRS, University of Lausanne, Route de la Corniche 10, 1010 Lausanne, Switzerland. [7]Nurse Research Consultant, Department of Woman-Mother-Child, Lausanne University Hospital CHUV, Lausanne, Switzerland. [8]Paediatric Haematology-Oncology, University Children's Hospital UKBB, Spitalstrasse 33, 4056 Basel, Switzerland. [9]Triemli Hospital Zurich, Zurich, Switzerland.

References

1. Ananth P, Melvin P, Feudtner C, Wolfe J, Berry JG. Hospital use in the last year of life for children with life-threatening complex chronic conditions. Pediatrics. 2015;136(5):938–46. https://doi.org/10.1542/peds.2015-0260.
2. Fraser LK, Miller M, Hain R, Norman P, Aldridge J, McKinney PA, Parslow RC. Rising national prevalence of life-limiting conditions in children in England. Pediatrics. 2012;129(4):e923–9. https://doi.org/10.1542/peds.2011-2846.
3. Feudtner C, Kang TI, Hexem KR, Friedrichsdorf SJ, Osenga K, Siden H, Friebert SE, Hays RM, Dussel V, Wolfe J. Pediatric palliative care patients: a prospective multicenter cohort study. Pediatrics. 2011;127(6):1094–101. https://doi.org/10.1542/peds.2010-3225.
4. Feudtner C, Christakis DA, Zimmerman FJ, Muldoon JH, Neff JM, Koepsell TD. Characteristics of deaths occurring in children's hospitals: implications for supportive care services. Pediatrics. 2002;109(5):887–93.
5. Hain R, Devins M, Hastings R, Noyes J. Paediatric palliative care: development and pilot study of a 'Directory' of life-limiting conditions. BMC Palliat Care. 2013;12(1):43. https://doi.org/10.1186/1472-684X-12-43.
6. Fontana MS, Farrell C, Gauvin F, Lacroix J, Janvier A. Modes of death in pediatrics: differences in the ethical approach in neonatal and pediatric patients. J Pediatr. 2013;162(6):1107–11. https://doi.org/10.1016/j.jpeds.2012.12.008.
7. Feudtner C, Feinstein JA, Satchell M, Zhao H, Kang TI. Shifting place of death among children with complex chronic conditions in the United States, 1989-2003. JAMA. 2007;297(24):2725–32. doi:297/24/2725 [pii]
8. Wolfe J, Orellana L, Ullrich C, Cook EF, Kang TI, Rosenberg A, Geyer R, Feudtner C, Dussel V. Symptoms and distress in children with advanced cancer: prospective patient-reported outcomes from the PediQUEST study. J Clin Oncol. 2015;33(17):1928–35. https://doi.org/10.1200/JCO.2014.59.1222.
9. WHO Definition of Palliative Care http://www.who.int/cancer/palliative/definition/en/. 30.01.2016.
10. Wolfe J, Hinds PS, Sourkes BM. The language of pediatric palliative care. In: Wolfe J, Hinds PS, Sourkes BM, editors. Textbook of interdisciplinary pediatric palliative care. 1st ed. Philadelphia: Elsevier Saunders; 2011. p. 3–6.
11. Craig F, Abu-Saad Huijer H, Benini F, Kuttner L, Wood C, Feraris PC, Zernikow B. IMPaCCT: standards of paediatric palliative care. Schmerz. 2008; 22(4):401–8. https://doi.org/10.1007/s00482-008-0690-4.
12. Radbruch L, Payne S, EAPC Board of Directors. White paper on standards and norms for hospice and palliative care in Europe: part 2. Eur J Palliat Care. 2010;17(1):22–33.
13. Feudtner C, Womer J, Augustin R, Remke S, Wolfe J, Friebert S, Weissman D. Pediatric palliative care programs in children's hospitals: a cross-sectional national survey. Pediatrics. 2013;132(6):1063–70. https://doi.org/10.1542/peds.2013-1286.
14. Steele R, Siden H, Cadell S, Davies B, Andrews G, Feichtinger L, Singh M. Charting the territory: symptoms and functional assessment in children with progressive, non-curable conditions. Arch Dis Child. 2014;99(8):754–62. https://doi.org/10.1136/archdischild-2013-305246.
15. Morell E, Wolfe J, Scheurer M, Thiagarajan R, Morin C, Beke DM, Smoot L, Cheng H, Gauvreau K, Blume ED. Patterns of care at end of life in children with advanced heart disease. Arch Pediatr Adolesc Med. 2012;166(8):745–8. https://doi.org/10.1001/archpediatrics.2011.1829.
16. Wolfe J, Grier HE, Klar N, Levin SB, Ellenbogen JM, Salem-Schatz S, Emanuel EJ, Weeks JC. Symptoms and suffering at the end of life in children with cancer. N Engl J Med. 2000;342(5):326–33. https://doi.org/10.1056/NEJM200002033420506

17. Bergstraesser E, Zimmermann K, Eskola K, Luck P, Ramelet AS, Cignacco E. Paediatric end-of-life care needs in Switzerland: current practices, and perspectives from parents and professionals. A study protocol. J Adv Nurs. 2015;71(8):1940–7. https://doi.org/10.1111/jan.12650.
18. Zimmermann K, Bergstraesser E, Engberg S, Ramelet AS, Marfurt-Russenberger K, Von der Weid N, Grandjean C, Fahrni-Nater P, Cignacco E, Consortium P. When parents face the death of their child: a nationwide cross-sectional survey of parental perspectives on their child's end-of life care. BMC Palliat Care. 2016; 15(1):30. https://doi.org/10.1186/s12904-016-0098-3.
19. Gregory KE, Radovinsky L. Research strategies that result in optimal data collection from the patient medical record. Appl Nurs Res. 2012;25(2):108–16. https://doi.org/10.1016/j.apnr.2010.02.004.
20. ICD-10 Online: 2016. http://apps.who.int/classifications/icd10/browse/2016/en. Accessed 6 Nov 2015.
21. Blume ED, Balkin EM, Aiyagari R, Ziniel S, Beke DM, Thiagarajan R, Taylor L, Kulik T, Pituch K, Wolfe J. Parental perspectives on suffering and quality of life at end-of-life in children with advanced heart disease: an exploratory study*. Pediatr Crit Care Med. 2014;15(4):336–42. https://doi.org/10.1097/PCC.0000000000000072.
22. UCLA: Statistical Consulting Group. Data analysis examples 24.01.2016.
23. Drake R, Frost J, Collins JJ. The symptoms of dying children. J Pain Symptom Manag. 2003;26(1):594–603.
24. Kassam A, Sutradhar R, Widger K, Rapoport A, Pole JD, Nelson K, Wolfe J, Earle CC, Gupta S. Predictors of and trends in high-intensity end-of-life care among children with cancer: a population-based study using health services data. J Clin Oncol. 2017;35(2):236–42. https://doi.org/10.1200/JCO.2016.68.8283.
25. Balaguer A, Martin-Ancel A, Ortigoza-Escobar D, Escribano J, Argemi J. The model of palliative care in the perinatal setting: a review of the literature. BMC Pediatr. 2012;12:25. https://doi.org/10.1186/1471-2431-12-25.
26. Wool C, Cote-Arsenault D, Perry Black B, Denney-Koelsch E, Kim S, Kavanaugh K. Provision of Services in Perinatal Palliative Care: a multicenter survey in the United States. J Palliat Med. 2016;19(3):279–85. https://doi.org/10.1089/jpm.2015.0266.
27. Groh G, Borasio GD, Nickolay C, Bender HU, von Luttichau I, Fuhrer M. Specialized pediatric palliative home care: a prospective evaluation. J Palliat Med. 2013;16(12):1588–94. https://doi.org/10.1089/jpm.2013.0129.
28. Friedrichsdorf SJ, Postier A, Dreyfus J, Osenga K, Sencer S, Wolfe J. Improved quality of life at end of life related to home-based palliative care in children with cancer. J Palliat Med. 2015;18(2):143–50. https://doi.org/10.1089/jpm.2014.0285.
29. Eskola K, Bergstraesser E, Zimmermann K, Cignacco E. Maintaining family life balance while facing a child's imminent death-a mixed methods study. J Adv Nurs. 2017;73(10):2462–72. https://doi.org/10.1111/jan.13304.
30. Conte T, Mitton C, Trenaman LM, Chavoshi N, Siden H. Effect of pediatric palliative care programs on health care resource utilization and costs among children with life-threatening conditions: a systematic review of comparative studies. CMAJ Open. 2015;3(1):E68–75. https://doi.org/10.9778/cmajo.20140044.
31. Bausewein C, Daveson BA, Currow DC, Downing J, Deliens L, Radbruch L, Defilippi K, Lopes Ferreira P, Costantini M, Harding R, et al. EAPC white paper on outcome measurement in palliative care: improving practice, attaining outcomes and delivering quality services - recommendations from the European Association for Palliative Care (EAPC) task force on outcome measurement. Palliat Med. 2016;30(1):6–22. https://doi.org/10.1177/0269216315589898.

9

Opioid substitution treatment and heroin dependent adolescents: reductions in heroin use and treatment retention over twelve months

Bobby P. Smyth[1,2,3,5*], Khalifa Elmusharaf[2] and Walter Cullen[4]

Abstract

Background: Opioid dependence is a major health concern across the world and does also occur in adolescents. While opioid substitution treatment (OST) has been thoroughly evaluated in adult populations, very few studies have examined its use in adolescents. There are concerns that OST is underutilised in adolescents with heroin dependence. We sought to measure changes in drug use among adolescents receiving OST and also to examine treatment attrition during the first 12 months of this treatment.

Methods: We included all heroin dependent patients aged under 18.5 years commencing OST at one outpatient multidisciplinary adolescent addiction treatment service in Dublin, Ireland. Psycho-social needs were also addressed during treatment. Drug use was monitored by twice weekly urine drugs screens (UDS). Change in the proportion of UDS negative for heroin was examined using the Wilcoxon signed rank test. Attrition was explored via a Cox Regression multivariate analysis.

Results: OST was commenced by 120 patients (51% female and mean age 17.3 years). Among the 39 patients who persisted with OST until month 12, heroin abstinence was 21% (95% confidence interval [CI] = 9–36%) at month three and it was 46% (95% CI = 30–63%) at month 12. Heroin use declined significantly from baseline to month three ($p < 0.001$) and from month three to month 12 ($p = 0.01$). Use of other drugs did not change significantly. People using cocaine during month 12 were more likely to be also using heroin ($p = 0.02$). Unplanned exit occurred in 25% patients by 120 days. The independent predictors of attrition were having children, single parent family of origin, not being in an intimate relationship with another heroin user and evidence of cocaine use just before treatment entry.

Conclusions: We found that heroin dependent adolescent patients achieved significant reductions in heroin use within three months of starting OST and this improved further after a year of treatment, about half being heroin abstinent at that stage. Patient drop out from treatment remains a challenge, as it is in adults. Cocaine use before and during treatment may be a negative prognostic factor.

Keywords: Adolescents, Heroin dependence, Methadone treatment, Buprenorphine treatment, Treatment adherence

* Correspondence: smythbo@tcd.ie
[1]Department of Public Health and Primary Care, Trinity College Dublin, Dublin 2, Ireland
[2]Graduate Entry Medical School, University of Limerick, Limerick, Ireland

Background

There is global ongoing concern regarding opioid dependence. While this is primarily focused on non-prescribed use of pharmaceutical opioids in USA currently, heroin has been the main concern elsewhere, including Ireland [1, 2]. The prevalence of heroin dependence tends to fluctuate over time and is much more common in adults than adolescents [1, 3]. In Dublin, heroin use first emerged as a concern among adolescents in the 1990s, in the midst of a dramatic increase in heroin dependence among adults [3, 4].

Opioid substitution treatment (OST) is now the main first line treatment intervention for heroin dependence among adults [5]. The main medications used are methadone, a full agonist or buprenorphine, a partial agonist. There are legislative and administrative obstacles in many jurisdictions to provision of OST to adolescents [1]. The limited evidence base for this treatment in this younger age range is also an issue which may be contributing to wariness by clinicians to prescribe [2, 6]. A recent study in USA found that just 2.4% of adolescents attending treatment for heroin use received medication [1].

There are no clinical trials examining outcome of OST beyond three months in people aged under 18 years old [6]. There are a small number of 'open label' longer term studies. The largest study has involved just 153 patients and was conducted over 40 years ago [7]. However, it provided no information on cessation of heroin use among those who remained on methadone treatment (MT), and the dose of methadone was limited to just 20mgs so its implications for modern practice are very unclear. Although the primary goal of OST is to assist the patient in reducing their heroin use, the other adolescent studies also fail to provide any firm information on this issue. The absence of scientific information on the rates of ongoing heroin use by adolescents on OST acts as an obstacle to provision of this treatment [2].

The DARP study of adolescents in USA in the 1970s did report a progressive decline in heroin use over the first year of MT but it did not provide any specific information on the actual rates of heroin use during treatment [8]. More recently, the NIDA multisite buprenorphine/naloxone treatment (BT) trial examined treatment of youth over a three month period, although only 12 participants were under eighteen years-old. At week eight, 77% of those retained on BT provided an opiate negative urine drug screen [9]. Abstinence from heroin at the end of that trial was associated with greater baseline medical and psychiatric problems, a history of recent injecting and evidence of early cessation of heroin use during BT [10].

Adolescents entering addiction treatment typically present with polysubstance use and this is also the case for those with primary dependence upon heroin [11–13]. An adolescent's motivation to address use of one substance such as heroin may not generalise to other substances [13]. Although there is evidence that adults on OST can also achieve significant reductions in use of other drugs, there is no such evidence for OST programs for adolescents [14]. The DARP study from the USA in the 1970s reported evidence of increased use of cannabis and alcohol among youth on OST at follow up [8].

Drop out from OST has been examined by a small number of studies in this age range. Studies of MT indicate that 25% of patients drop out within approximately four months [7, 8, 15]. Bell & Mutch found that the drop out from BT was significantly greater than from MT [16]. Other studies of BT in this age range also indicate frequent early drop out from treatment, with typically a quarter of patients exiting within 4 to 8 weeks [17–19].

Given this paucity of outcome studies of OST in adolescent heroin dependence, we sought to address a number of questions which are of importance to clinicians and patients in order to make informed decisions. What proportion of adolescents ceases heroin use while on OST? Does abstinence increase incrementally or simply stabilise beyond three months on OST? What is the rate of drop out? Are there any baseline or treatment characteristics which are associated with either abstinence or drop out?

Methods

Setting, assessment and treatment

This study was based at the Young Persons' Programme (YPP) within the National Drug Treatment Centre (NDTC) in Dublin, Ireland. The approach to assessment and treatment of heroin dependent adolescents at this service is summarised below but has been described in detail elsewhere [20, 21]. Although published a number of years after the establishment of the YPP, the approach to treatment is consistent with the UK guidance on pharmacological management of substance dependence among young people [22].

Assessment typically involved three clinic visits to meet different members of the multi-disciplinary team, a supervised urine drug screen (UDS) being obtained at each visit. In addition to assessing for heroin dependence using ICD-10 criteria, co-existing psychological, developmental, social and physical needs were identified.

The main pillars of treatment involved OST (methadone or buprenorphine), counselling and in some cases, family therapy. Induction onto a stable dose of methadone typically occurred over a period of about two weeks while buprenorphine induction took 2–3 days [23]. If patients continued to use heroin or resumed use after a period of abstinence, an increase in medication was considered. Use of other substances was also addressed during treatment. Where the initial opioid agonist medication was associated with a poor treatment response, the patient was offered the option of switching to the alternative.

Patients provided two supervised UDS per week for on-site drug toxicology testing during treatment. These samples were screened for opiates, EDDP (a methadone metabolite), cocaine, benzodiazepines and alcohol. They were intermittently screened for amphetamines and cannabis. The provision of 'take-away' doses of medication was utilised as a contingent reinforcer of drug abstinence, as evidenced by urine toxicology.

Patients were also provided with treatment of co-morbid medical or psychiatric problems [21]. They were actively supported in addressing co-existing housing, vocational and criminal justice related needs as part of their care plan.

The overarching goal of the service was to reduce the harm which young people were experiencing related to their drug use. It held an aspiration, but not an insistence, that patients progress towards complete abstinence via gradual OST dose reduction and ultimate cessation of this medication. This ultimately occurs in about one in every four cases [20]. Where dose tapering occurred, it was generally conducted slowly on an outpatient basis over a period of about three months, negotiated with the individual patient.

Patients

The inclusion criteria were:- heroin dependence, aged under 18.5 years and commenced OST. The cohort under study included patients who commenced treatment between May 2000 and June 2016. Patients with a primary diagnosis of dependence on prescription opioids were excluded, as such patients have been rarely encountered in Ireland.

Data collection

The study was approved by the Research Ethics Committee of the NDTC. Baseline descriptive characteristics were obtained from the patients' initial structured assessment, this being adapted from the Maudsley Addiction Profile [24]. We recorded information on patient treatment participation at three, six and twelve months. If a patient was not attending the service on these dates, we noted the date of and reason for exit.

Those who were referred to and commenced on another OST program were categorised as "transfers for ongoing treatment". This typically involved transfer to an adult OST program, this option being available to patients after their 18th birthday. However, most opted to persist with treatment on the YPP beyond this age [20]. Patients were categorised as exiting via "dose taper" if they adhered to the prescribed dose reduction regime and showed urinalysis evidence of heroin abstinence at discharge from the treatment program. Patients who ended treatment because they were incarcerated were categorised as exiting due to "prison". Finally, patients who simply stopped attending, relocated without arranging alternative treatment or left treatment prematurely against medical advice were all categorised as being "drop outs". Patients were generally not deemed to have dropped out of their index treatment episode unless that had failed to attend for four weeks. If they were deemed a drop out, then the date of last attendance for medication was recorded as the date of discharge. Although many patients re-entered treatment after dropping out or following a relapse to heroin use after a successfully completed dose taper, only their first or index treatment episode was included for the purposes of this study. The pattern of transitions out of and back into treatment have been described in a separate study [20]. If a patient switched from BT to MT or vice versa, but continued in treatment, this was not viewed as a treatment exit.

To examine changes in drug use, five periods during the first year of treatment contact were examined for each patient. The results of all urine drug screens (UDS) provided by each patient during each period was collated. The periods in question were (a) pre treatment assessment phase which was typically 7 to 10 days in duration and involved provision of 2–4 UDS, (b) induction phase which comprised the remaining days in that first month of patient contact after commencing OST, (c) third entire month of treatment, (d) sixth entire month of treatment and (e) twelfth entire month of treatment. During phases (b) to (e), patients were typically providing two UDS per week. For each patient, a dichotomous outcome variable to indicate abstinence/use was created for each of the phases they were being treated (a) to (e). They were deemed to be using heroin if any one UDS sample tested positive for opiates during that phase. If all UDS were opiate negative, they were deemed heroin abstinent. Similarly, a single positive for cocaine in a month resulted in that month being deemed one of cocaine use.

Statistics

In order to conduct an exploratory analysis, we used Pearson chi square test to examine association between categorical covariates and dichotomous outcome variables of interest, except in instances where a predicted cell value was less than five, where Fisher's Exact test was utilised. Odds ratios and their 95% confidence intervals were calculated to indicate the direction and magnitude of associations. Continuous variables were converted into categorical variables, by choosing the median value as the point of split, apart from age where we used 18th birthday as the cut-off.

When reporting the proportion of patients who were heroin abstinent, we also calculated the 95% confidence intervals of those rates using the exact confidence limits for binomial proportions. McNemar's paired proportions test with continuity correction was employed to determine whether OST was associated with changes in the binary category of drug use. We sought to confirm that heroin abstinence in month three was greater than baseline, and that abstinence at months six and twelve were greater than month three. We also examined changes in the proportion of samples which tested negative for heroin using the related samples Wilcoxon signed rank test. For each period, we calculated this proportion by dividing the number of negative tests by the total number of UDS obtained. All of these analyses were confined to the subgroup of patients who persisted with OST for a full year.

To examine drop out and factors associated with same, the Kaplan-Meier test was conducted. The event of interest was unplanned exit from treatment via drop out or imprisonment. The time to treatment exit, in days, was recorded for each patient who left their index treatment episode during the first year, whether by unplanned exit or via planned exit (following completion of dose taper or via transfer to another OST service). For patients who persisted with OST, the number of days entered was 365 days. The Log Rank was used to test for the equality of the survival distributions within each covariate. To facilitate interpretation of these differences, the estimated number of days to drop out by 25% is reported. In order to explore independent predictors of unplanned exit, we then conducted a multivariate analysis using Cox Regression. Covariates were selected for entry into the final equation using the forward and backward selection technique. All analyses were conducted using IBM SPSS Statistics, version 21.

Results

Description of participants

There were 120 eligible patients who commenced OST. One patient with primary methadone dependence was excluded and there were no presentations with primary prescription opioid dependence. The patient characteristics are provided in Table 1. The mean age was 17.3 years (range 14–18 years). There were 13 (11%) who had not yet reached their 16th birthday. Eighty-eight per cent were using heroin daily at treatment entry. Thirty-nine patients persisted with treatment to month 12 and their profile is also outlined in Table 1. Twenty-nine (24%) left following completion of dose taper and nine (8%) were transferred elsewhere for ongoing OST. There were 43 unplanned treatment exits, with 36 (30%) dropping out and 7 (6%) going to prison. There were no deaths during treatment.

Cessation of heroin use and other drugs

Table 2 presents the results of urine drug screens from the subgroup of patients who persisted with OST for at least 12 months. This table indicates the proportion demonstrating abstinence from each drug at each time period examined. During the third month of treatment 8 (21% [95% confidence interval (CI) = 9–36%]) were abstinent from heroin. Six (15% [95%CI = 6–31%]) were abstinent from heroin, cocaine and benzodiazepines. At month 12, there were 18 (46% [95%CI = 30–63%]) abstinent from heroin, of whom nine (23% [95%CI = 11–39%]) were also abstinent from cocaine and benzodiazepines.

Changes in drug use over time

Table 2 also indicates that heroin abstinence increased significantly from baseline to three months, from baseline to twelve months and from third month to twelfth month. Rates of use of other substances did not change significantly from baseline. When looking beyond heroin abstinence to examine changes in the proportions of negative urine screens, it also emerged that there were significant reductions in heroin use between baseline and month 3 and from month 3 to month 12. However, there was no significant change in heroin use between months 3 and 6. When comparing the proportions of heroin negative urine screens between months 3 and 12, we found that eight (21%) patients deteriorated, six (15%) were unchanged and 25 (64%) improved.

Correlates of heroin abstinence

There were very few pre-treatment characteristics significantly associated with heroin abstinence at month 12. Full results of this analysis are presented in Additional file 1: Table S1 in an on-line supplement. None of the patients who had a previous psychiatric admission were abstinent ($p = 0.02$). Abstinence was not significantly associated with higher medication dose ($p = 0.88$). All of the patients who were using cocaine during month 12 were also using heroin ($p = 0.02$). Early reductions in heroin use, as evidenced by provision of at least one heroin negative sample during induction tended to be associated with reduced likelihood of heroin abstinence at month 12 ($p = 0.07$).

We repeated the analysis, with imputed positive heroin results for the 43 patients who had an unplanned discharge. This indicated that heroin abstinence was significantly associated with being in an intimate/sexual relationship with another heroin user (OR 3.4 [95%CI 1. 1–10.0], $p = 0.02$). No other baseline characteristic was significantly associated with abstinence in that analysis with imputed results.

Persistence with OST

Information on attrition during treatment is reported in Table 3. Overall, the estimated length of time to 25% leaving treatment in an unplanned manner was 120 (Standard Error 41) days. The table only presents results of the covariates where the Log Rank test indicated a p value of less than 0.2, although all covariates in Table 1 were explored. There was no significant difference

Table 1 Characteristics of 120 adolescents commencing opioid substitution treatment, and subgroup who persisted in treatment until month 12

	Total Group	Missing data	In treatment until month 12			
	N (%)[c]		*N* (%)[d]	OR	95% CI OR	*P* value
Number in Treatment	120		39 (33)			
Socio-demographic characteristics						
Female	61 (51)		25 (41)	2.0	(0.9–4.4)	0.07
Aged under 18.0 years	104 (87)		35 (34)	1.5	(0.5–5.1)	0.49
Left school under 15 years	51 (46)	8	18 (35)	1.0	(0.5–2.3)	0.92
Not in employment, education or training	81 (70)	4	29 (36)	1.7	(0.7–4.1)	0.24
Two parent family support	59 (50)	1	27 (46)	3.8	(1.6–8.6)	0.001
Has a child	6 (5)		0 (0)	n/a		0.18[a]
Has been in care	38 (32)	2	10 (26)	0.7	(0.3–1.6)	0.35
Sibling Heroin Use	45 (39)	4	17 (38)	1.4	(0.6–3.0)	0.45
Parental heroin Use	25 (22)	4	6 (24)	0.6	(0.2–1.5)	0.25
Partner uses heroin	47 (39)	1	18 (38)	1.5	(0.7–3.3)	0.30
Homeless or hostel in past month	34 (28)		11 (32)	0.9	(0.4–2.2)	0.89
Previous criminal convictions	46 (41)	8	14 (30)	0.9	(0.4–2.0)	0.80
Ever incarcerated	31 (27)	6	8 (26)	0.8	(0.3–1.9)	0.55
Psychiatric History						
Ever assessed by a psychiatrist	62 (53)	2	22 (36)	1.4	(0.6–2.9)	0.44
Past Inpatient psychiatric admission	10 (9)	4	6 (60)	3.2	(0.8–12)	0.09[a]
Past DSH	36 (31)	5	12 (33)	1.1	(0.5–2.5)	0.86
Substance Use						
Lifetime Drug Use						
Non-prescribed benzodiazepines	107 (90)	1	36 (34)	1.0	(0.3–3.6)	1.0[a]
Non-prescribed methadone	90 (78)	5	30 (33)	0.8	(0.3–1.9)	0.54
Cocaine use	76 (68)	8	30 (40)	2.7	(1.1–7.0)	0.04
Injected	53 (45)	2	17 (32)	1.0	(0.5–2.2)	0.99
Commenced heroin under 15 years of age	43 (36)	2	20 (47)	2.6	(1.2–5.7)	0.02
Regular heroin use for more than 12 months	73 (64)	6	26 (36)	1.2	(0.5–2.7)	0.67
Past Month Drug Use						
Non-prescribed benzodiazepines	71 (60)	1	26 (37)	1.4	(0.6–3.1)	0.40
Non-prescribed methadone	71 (60)	1	27 (38)	1.7	(0.7–3.7)	0.22
Cocaine	31 (26)	2	10 (32)	1.0	(0.4–2.3)	0.91
Cannabis	80 (73)	11	27 (34)	1.3	(0.5–3.4)	0.54
Amphetamine	9 (9)	19	4 (44)	1.9	(0.5–7.7)	0.45[a]
Alcohol	46 (45)	18	17 (37)	1.2	(0.5–2.8)	0.61
Injecting	35 (29)	1	13 (37)	1.5	(0.7–3.4)	0.34
Using more than 3 'bags' heroin per day	60 (53)	7	18 (30)	0.9	(0.4–2.0)	0.81
Pre-treatment UDS[b] positives						
Benzodiazepines	71 (59)		26 (37)	1.6	(0.7–3.6)	0.25
Methadone	67 (56)		20 (30)	0.8	(0.4–1.6)	0.49
Cocaine	13 (11)		3 (23)	0.6	(0.2–2.3)	0.54[a]
Cannabis	47 (47)	20	13 (28)	0.7	(0.3–1.6)	0.38

Table 1 Characteristics of 120 adolescents commencing opioid substitution treatment, and subgroup who persisted in treatment until month 12 *(Continued)*

	Total Group	Missing data	In treatment until month 12			
	N (%)[c]		*N* (%)[d]	OR	95% CI OR	*P* value
Early Treatment						
Suboxone Commenced	32 (27)		7 (22)	0.5	(0.2–1.3)	0.13
At least one heroin negative UDS during induction	50 (46)	12	14 (28)	0.6	(0.3–1.4)	0.28

[a]*P* value calculated using Fishers Exact Test Statistic as estimated value in cell was less than 5
[b]UDS = Urine drug screen
[c]This column indicates the proportion (%) of the total group showing that characteristic (e.g. 51% of total group are female)
[d]This column indicates the proportion (%) of the subgroup with the characteristic who are still in treatment at month 12 (e.g. 25/61 [41%] of the females were still in treatment at month 12)

between those commenced on Buprenorphine or methadone (log rank test statistic 1.04, $p = 0.31$). To further assist understanding of the analysis and the pattern of drop out, an example is provided in Fig. 1, which contrasts patients who showed UDS evidence of cocaine use during assessment against those without such cocaine use.

The Cox regression analysis (see Table 3) indicated that patients who had no children, grew up in families with two parents, were in an intimate relationship with another heroin user and were abstinent from cocaine in pre-treatment drug screens demonstrated significantly lower rates of unplanned exit from treatment.

Of the 20 people commenced on buprenorphine who persisted with treatment for three months, six (30%) had switched to methadone at that point. Only one person (2%) had switched from methadone to buprenorphine by month three. Seven people who commenced buprenorphine remained in treatment for 12 months, by which time six has switched to methadone. Only two of the 32 commenced on methadone had switched to buprenorphine by month 12.

Discussion

Reductions in heroin use and incremental change

Heroin use is associated with a vast array of risks [2, 5, 25]. A key goal of OST is to assist patients in reducing, and ideally stopping, their use of heroin [25]. Our study indicates that this treatment delivers substantial reductions in heroin use among adolescents. Almost half of these young patients who persisted with OST for a year demonstrated complete cessation of heroin use during their twelfth month of treatment. Previous studies of OST in adolescent heroin dependence have largely ignored the issue of abstinence during treatment. In a slightly older cohort, Kellogg et al. reported that patients who persisted with OST were heroin abstinent every other month on average, although urine drug screens were conducted inconsistently which increases the possibility that occasional use was not detected in that study [15].

The rate of heroin abstinence in month twelve constituted a significant improvement compared to the third month of treatment, at which point one in five demonstrated abstinence. This is consistent with one other study in adolescents and also with research on adult

Table 2 Evidence of drug use from urine drug screens (UDS), at baseline and during treatment, among 39 patients who persisted with treatment for 12 months

	Month 1		Month 3	Month 6	Month 12	Baseline vs Month 3	Baseline vs Month 12	Month 3 vs Month 6	Month 3 vs Month 12
	Pre-treatment baseline	Induction phase[b]							
Median number of UDS conducted (range)	3 (2–4)	4 (0–7)	7 (2–10)	7 (1–9)	8 (1–11)	Related samples Wilcoxon signed rank test *p* value			
Median % of UDS heroin negative (interquartile range)	0 (0–0)	0 (0–33)	50 (0–89)	40 (0–100)	87 (33–100)	< 0.001	< 0.001	0.86	0.01
All UDS negative during period						*p* value from McNemar test			
Heroin	1 (3)	4 (11)	8 (21)	12 (31)	18 (46)	0.04	< 0.001	0.34	0.04
Benzodiazepine	13 (33)	18 (50)	15 (38)	18 (46)	15 (38)	0.77	0.79	0.45	1.0
Cannabis[a]	19/32 (59)	18/28 (64)	20/37 (54)	16/33 (48)	14/36 (39)	0.69	0.11	1.0	0.29
Cocaine	36 (92)	36 (100)	32 (82)	31 (79)	33 (85)	0.22	0.45	1.0	1.0
Heroin, benzos & cocaine	0 (0)	1 (3)	6 (15)	8 (21)	9 (23)	n/a	n/a	0.63	0.55

[a]Urine drug screens were randomly tested for cannabis, which caused information on use to be missing for some patients during each period
[b]Three patients did not have any urine screens during induction
n/a not applicable

Table 3 Unplanned treatment exit among 120 heroin dependent adolescents during the first year on opioid substitution treatment (OST)

	Univariate analysis[a]				Multivariate cox regression		
	Estimated 25% drop out		Log rank statistic	*P* value	Hazard ratio (HR)	(95% CI of HR)	*P* value
	Days	(SE)					
Overall	120	(41)					
Socio-demographic characteristics							
Sex							
Female	75	(9)					
Male	225	(55)	2.36	0.13			
Age							
Under 18 years	120	(45)					
Aged 18 years	62	(69)	0.14	0.70			
Early school leaver							
Left Education under age 15	75	(18)					
Left school after 15th birthday	197	(69)	1.83	0.18			
Family of origin							
Has two parents	270				1.0		
Single parent/other relative/adopted	75	(19)	8.56	0.003	3.5	(1.7–6.9)	0.001
Own children							
Has a child	72	(61)			5.3	(1.9–14.8)	0.001
No children	123	(40)	5.11	0.02	1.0		
History of being in social care							
Has been in care	75	(28)					
Never in social care	155	(41)	3.52	0.06			
Parental heroin use							
No heroin use by parents	186	(66)					
A parent has heroin problems	72	(52)	2.91	0.09			
Heroin use by partner							
Partner has used heroin	270	(89)			1.0		
No partner/No heroin use by partner	86	(19)	3.53	0.06	2.1	(1.1–4.3)	0.03
Accommodation in past month							
Homeless or hostel	69	(25)					
Stable accommodation	176	(54)	2.40	0.12			
Deliberate self harm (DSH)							
Has a history of DSH	75	(28)			1.8	(1.0–3.3)	0.07
No history of past DSH	176	(67)	2.21	0.14	1.0		
Pre-treatment Drug Use							
Lifetime Cocaine							
Use	103	(29)					
No use	176	(69)	2.99	0.08			
Past month non-prescribed methadone use							
Self reported Use	197	(29)					
No self reported use	73	(23)	3.42	0.07			

Table 3 Unplanned treatment exit among 120 heroin dependent adolescents during the first year on opioid substitution treatment (OST) *(Continued)*

	Univariate analysis[a]				Multivariate cox regression		
	Estimated 25% drop out		Log rank statistic	*P* value	Hazard ratio (HR)	(95% CI of HR)	*P* value
	Days	(SE)					
Cocaine							
Positive baseline urine drug screen	50	(15)			3.2	(1.4–7.4)	0.006
All baseline urine drug screens negative	176	(55)	3.97	< 0.05	1.0		
Quantity of heroin use per day							
Using 3 'bags' or more per day	69	(19)					
Using less than 3 'bags' day	225	(40)	5.77	0.02			
Dose of OST at month three[b]							
Dose >50mgs methadone (or equivalent)	239	(24)					
Dose <= 50mgs methadone (or equivalent)	> 365		2.90	0.09			

[a]Kaplan Meier Survival analysis. The model estimate of the number of days to unplanned discharge by 25% of patients with that characteristic is reported, for comparison
[b]includes the 72 people being prescribed OST after 90 days, with methadone equivalent dose for those on buprenorphine being multiplied by 5 (i.e. if on 12mgs of buprenorphine, assigned value of 60mgs in methadone equivalents)

patients showing that longer treatment with OST builds incremental improvements in outcome [8, 14, 15, 26]. In their NIDA clinical trial, Woody et al. found a rapid return to heroin use once patients were tapered off their three months of buprenorphine treatment [9].

The confirmation that adolescents on OST can achieve substantial reductions in heroin use, with many doing so very early in treatment, should act as source of optimism for clinicians. It suggests that it is realistic for staff and treatment services to have a high expectation of reduced heroin use early in treatment and to be confident that many patients will achieve periods of sustained abstinence during treatment.

We found no indication of a relationship between medication dose and heroin abstinence. There was no upper ceiling dose used in this service and our finding may indicate that dose was appropriately titrated against clinical need. There is research to indicate increased heroin use at lower OST doses in both adolescents and adults [18, 27]. In contrast, Kellogg et al. detected greater heroin use among young adults on higher methadone doses [15].

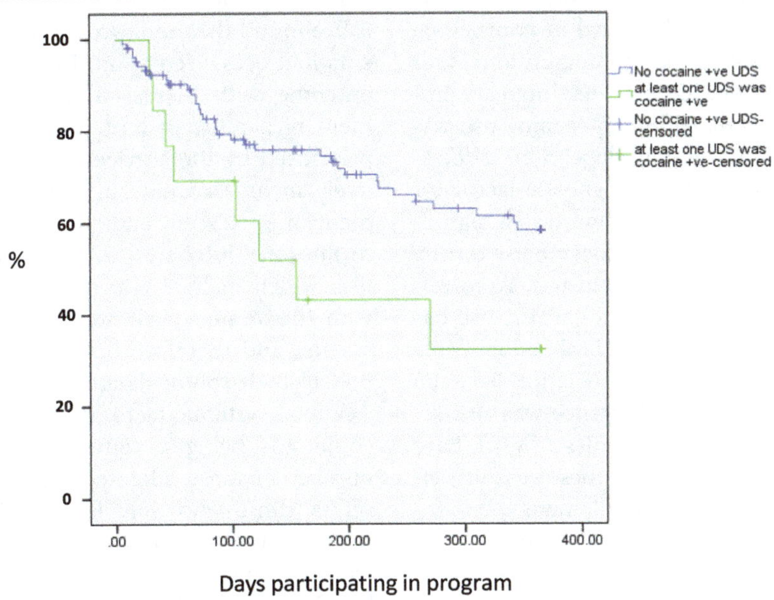

Fig. 1 Unplanned treatment exit by 120 adolescents on OST; impact of cocaine use at treatment entry

Treatment retention

The second main focus of this study was treatment retention. We found that one in four patients had an unplanned treatment exit by 120 days. Retention rates were similar in DARP in the 1970s and in the more recent study by Kellogg et al. [8, 15]. Those two studies examined methadone treatment. A number of studies examining use of buprenorphine in other settings report much higher rates of attrition among adolescent patients [16–18]. In contrast to Bell & Mutch, we found no significant difference between the two opioid agonist medications, although many patients in our study did switch from buprenorphine to methadone during treatment [16]. One factor which complicates comparisons of retention rates across all of these studies relates to the variable criteria used to define 'drop out'. In our study, patients who recommenced regular attendance after a period of up to four weeks non-attendance were viewed as still being in their index treatment episode. Other studies have viewed patients as having dropped out with much shorter periods of non-attendance.

Use of other substances

Unfortunately, half of those who were heroin abstinent demonstrated some ongoing use of benzodiazepines. Overall, the rates of abstinence from drugs other than heroin did not increase significantly from pre-treatment levels. Studies of OST in adults suggest that they can achieve reductions in use of other drugs [14, 26]. However, previous research on younger cohorts has also failed to demonstrate reductions in use of other drugs and the DARP study found some evidence of increased use of cannabis and alcohol at follow-up [8, 15].

At this service, efforts were made to address cocaine use. Where use occurred it was discussed in counselling sessions and also during key working interventions. Our failure to successfully reduce cocaine use appears important for this patient group. Although cocaine use was not extensive among these heroin dependent adolescents, it seems to act as a negative prognostic factor for those who use it. Cocaine use at baseline was a significant predictor of treatment drop out. Cocaine use during OST was correlated with ongoing heroin use. A correlation between persistent heroin use and cocaine use has also been demonstrated by others in both adolescents and adults [15, 27, 28]. The adverse association between cocaine use and poorer treatment adherence was also reported by Kellogg et al. [15]. Adult studies of OST have made similar observations [29, 30]. For these reasons, efforts have been made in Ireland to implement interventions targeting cocaine use among adults attending OST. The results have been quite disappointing to date, with poor uptake of counselling treatments being a key obstacle [31]. With polydrug using adolescents, it has been shown in Ireland and elsewhere that their motivation to address their main drug may be very different to their motivation to address substances which they perceive as quite secondary [13]. In spite of these challenges, services working with heroin dependent adolescents should have protocols in place to assess and respond to use of cocaine and other substances.

Association of systemic factors with outcome

Other potential prognostic factors were identified in the exploratory analysis, many of which suggested the importance of the family and social support system around the adolescent. Some characteristics of family systems may provide support to an adolescent who is facing a severe drug use disorder while other family types may add to the strain on an adolescent who is already coping poorly [32, 33]. Our finding of increased abstinence when analysis included imputed data, and of better treatment retention, in those with a heroin using sexual partner was unexpected. The general view in addiction treatment is that increased social ties with other drug users brings poorer outcome [33]. Interestingly, in a separate study examining outcome after inpatient detoxification of heroin dependent adults in Ireland, it also emerged that being in a relationship with another heroin user was associated with better outcome [34]. Although these findings are counter-intuitive, the issue may warrant further exploration by other researchers. We have previously reported that female patients are much more likely to be in an intimate relationship with another heroin user [13]. Typically partners enter treatment at the same time. It seems possible that a shared goal and a shared understanding of the challenges faced by a partner may support rather than undermine recovery [35].

We found that adolescents from families with two parents had better retention. Crome et al. also found better outcome with increased family support [36]. Involvement of parents in both assessment and treatment was prioritised by the service [21]. Efforts were made to actively include parents in the care plan. Family involvement in adolescent addiction treatment has been shown to improve outcomes [37]. It may be the case that families which include two parents are better able to cope with the strain which addiction places upon the family system, and therefore better positioned to provide support to their son or daughter [32].

A final systemic factor which was correlated with outcome was being a young parent. While only a small number of these adolescent patients had a child themselves, those who were faced with this additional strain on their personal resources were less likely to persist with treatment. Drop out occurred in spite of the efforts by the service to support these young parents via provision of crèche facilities on site. Others have highlighted the particular challenges faced by single parents with addiction issues, and some services have developed targeted programs of support such as the Parents under Pressure intervention [38].

Those who had a previous psychiatric admission appeared less likely to be abstinent. Crome et al. also reported poorer outcome in those with a psychiatric history [36]. However, Subramaniam et al. found that greater baseline psychiatric problems was associated with better outcome in the NIDA clinical trial of buprenorphine [10]. Our previous research has indicated that there are improvements in mental health symptoms among the adolescents attending OST at this service and lower depressive symptoms correlate with reduced heroin use [21].

Strengths and limitations

The strengths of this study include the sample size which is quite large relative to other studies of OST in this age range. However, the sample size is still relatively small for statistical purposes, with limited power. In view of the large number of statistical tests conducted in this study, and the decision not to alter the p value via a Bonferoni correction, this raises the possibility that some significant findings may also constitute type 1 statistical errors.

The treatment intervention was delivered at a single site making it easier for clinicians elsewhere to determine how applicable our findings may be to their own treatment setting. The monitoring of drug use by twice weekly supervised UDS constitutes a very thorough level of evaluation of drug use and we can be reasonably confident that the patients whom we determined to be abstinent are truly abstinent. A limitation can arise from assessing change via very regular urine screens. For example, a patient could change from injecting heroin four times a day at treatment entry to smoking heroin just twice a week. While this constitutes a very positive achievement from a harm reduction perspective, all UDS would be likely to remain opiate positive and our results would indicate no change in such a scenario.

Conclusions

This study adds to the currently limited evidence base for OST in adolescents who are heroin dependent. The positive outcomes appear broadly similar to those achieved in adults, among whom there is widespread acceptance of this treatment. One of the lingering doubts about OST in adolescents since the DARP study relates to the limited success in achieving reductions in use of other drugs [8]. In spite of our efforts to address this use, we also found that levels of use of other substances remained stubbornly elevated. This does not negate the fact that the reductions in heroin use were substantial. Importantly, abstinence increased significantly from month three to one year, with half of the patient group on OST having ceased heroin use during their full twelfth month of treatment. It seems difficult to predict which patients are going to persist with this treatment and to have better outcomes. However, use of cocaine, both prior to and during treatment, appears to be a negative prognostic factor. With adolescent patients it appears to be particularly important to be mindful of potential systemic factors which may either support or undermine treatment success.

Overall, the efforts currently being made to ensure greater provision of OST to adolescents by groups such as the American Academy of Pediatrics appear appropriate and timely [2]. Also, where treatment is commenced, we echo the view of Woody et al. that "clinicians should be in no hurry to stop an effective medication simply because the patient is young" [9].

Abbreviations

BT: Buprenorphine treatment; CI: Confidence interval; DARP: Drug abuse reporting program; EDDP: 5-ethylidene-1,5-dimethyl-3, 3-diphenylpyrrolidine; MT: Methadone treatment; NDTC: National Drug Treatment Centre; NIDA: National Institute of Drug Abuse; OST: Opioid substitution treatment; UDS: Urine drugs screens; YPP: Young Persons' Programme

Acknowledgements

The authors are grateful to the staff of the YPP for their assistance in collating the data, in particular to Robbie Dolan and Martin Meagher. We are also grateful to the staff in the laboratory at the NDTC where all urine drug screens were analysed.

Authors' contributions

BPS conducted the analysis and lead on the drafting of the manuscript. KE & WC also contributed to the drafting of the manuscript. BPS, KE & WC were involved in interpretation of the data. BPS, KE & WC read and approved the final manuscript. BPS, KE & WC have agreed to be accountable for all aspects of the work.

Ethics approval and consent to participate

The study received ethical approval from the research ethics committee of the National Drug Treatment Centre, and this committee agreed that consent from individual patients was not required for this study. Only routinely gathered patient information was obtained. Patient specific information was not made available to anyone external to the clinical service where they were treated. This approach to consent is consistent with national data protection guidelines (see https://www.dataprotection.ie/documents/guidance/Health_research.pdf).

Competing interests

BPS has received lecture fees from Pfizer, Shire and Eli Lilly. BPS was a co-PI in a RCT examining buprenorphine induction which recruited patients from the NDTC. That RCT was funded by Schering-Plough (now Merck), a distributor of buprenorphine worldwide. BPS was the lead clinician at the treatment service (the YPP) where this study was conducted. BPS has no other competing interest. Neither KE nor WC has any competing interest.

Author details

[1]Department of Public Health and Primary Care, Trinity College Dublin, Dublin 2, Ireland. [2]Graduate Entry Medical School, University of Limerick, Limerick, Ireland. [3]National Drug Treatment Centre, 30/31 Pearse St, Dublin 2, Ireland. [4]Academic General Practice, School of Medicine, University College Dublin, Belfield, Dublin 4, Ireland. [5]HSE Addiction Service, Bridge House, Cherry Orchard Hospital, Dublin 10, Ireland.

References

1. Feder KA, Krawczyk N, Saloner B. Medication-assisted treatment for adolescents in specialty treatment for opioid use disorder. J Adoles Health. 2017;60:747–50. https://doi.org/10.1016/j.jadohealth.2016.12.023.
2. Levy S, Ryan SA, Gonzalez PK, Patrick SW, Quigley J, Siqueira L, et al. Medication-assisted treatment of adolescents with opioid use disorders. Pediatrics. 2016;138:e20161893. https://doi.org/10.1542/peds.2016-1893.
3. Smyth BP, O'Brien M. Children attending addiction treatment services in Dublin, 1990–1999. Eur Addiction Res. 2004;10:68–74. https://doi.org/10.1159/000076116.
4. Gervin M, Hughes R, Bamford L, Smyth BP, Keenan E. Heroin smoking by "chasing the dragon" in young opiate users in Ireland: stability and associations with use to "come down" off "ecstasy". J Subst Abus Treat. 2001;20(4):297–300.
5. Marsch L. The efficacy of methadone maintenance interventions in reducing illicit opiate use, HIV risk behavior and criminality: a meta-analysis. Addiction. 1998;93:515–32.
6. Minozzi S, Amato L, Bellisario C, Davoli M. Maintenance treatments for opiate -dependent adolescents . Cochrane Database of Systematic Reviews 2014, Issue 6. Art. No.: CD007210. https://doi.org/10.1002/14651858.CD007210.pub3.
7. Millman RB, Khuri ET, Nyswander ME. Therapeutic detoxification of adolescent heroin addicts. Ann N Y Acad Sci. 1978;311:153–64.
8. Sells SB, Simpson DD. Evaluation of treatment outcome for youths in the drug abuse reporting program (DARP): a follow-up study. In: Beschner GM, Friedman AA, editors. Youth drug abuse: problems, issues and treatment. Lanham, MD: Lexington Books; 1979. p. 571–622.
9. Woody GE, Poole SA, Subramaniam G, Dugosh K, Bogenschutz M, Abbott P, et al. Extended vs short-term buprenorphine-naloxone for treatment of opioid-addicted youth: a randomized trial. JAMA. 2008;300:2003–11. https://doi.org/10.1001/jama.2008.574.
10. Subramaniam GA, Warden D, Minhajuddin A, Fishman MJ, Stitzer ML, Adinoff B, et al. Predictors of abstinence: National Institute of drug abuse multisite buprenorphine/naloxone treatment trial in opioid-dependent youth. J Am Acad Child & Adoles Psychiatry. 2011;50:1120–8. https://doi.org/10.1016/j.jaac.2011.07.010.
11. Gilvarry E. Substance abuse in young people. J Child Psychol & Psychiatry. 2000;41:55–80.
12. Smyth BP, James P, Cullen W, Darker C. So prohibition can work? Changes in use of novel psychoactive substances among adolescents attending a drug and alcohol treatment service following a legislative ban Int J Drugs Policy. 2015;26:887–9. https://doi.org/10.1016/j.drugpo.2015.05.021.
13. Smyth BP, Kelly A, Cullen W, Darker C. Outcome for adolescents abusing alcohol and cannabis following outpatient treatment: how many 'reliably improve'? Irish Med J. 2015;108:137–9.
14. Gossop M, Marsden J, Stewart D, Kidd T. The National Treatment Outcome Research Study (NTORS): 4–5 year follow-up results. Addiction. 2003;98:291–303.
15. Kellogg S, Melia D, Khuri E, Lin A, Ho A, Kreek MJ. Adolescent and young adult heroin patients: drug use and success in methadone maintenance treatment. J Addict Disease. 2006;25:15–25. https://doi.org/10.1300/J069v25n03_03.
16. Bell J, Mutch C. Treatment retention in adolescent patients treated with methadone or buprenorphine for opioid dependence: a file review. Drug Alcohol Rev. 2006;25:167–71. https://doi.org/10.1080/09595230500537670.
17. Matson SC, Hobson G, Abdel-Rasoul M, Bonny AE. A retrospective study of retention of opioid-dependent adolescents and young adults in an outpatient buprenorphine/naloxone clinic. J Addict Med. 2014:8176–82. https://doi.org/10.1097/ADM.0000000000000035.
18. Mutlu C, Demirci AC, Yalcin O, Kilicoglu AG, Topal M, Karacetin G. One-year follow-up of heroin-dependent adolescents treated with Buprenorfine/naloxone for the first time in a substance treatment unit. J Subst Abus Treat. 2016;67:1–8. https://doi.org/10.1016/j.jsat.2016.04.002.
19. Warden D, Subramaniam GA, Carmody T, Woody GE, Minhajuddin A, Poole SA, et al. Predictors of attrition with buprenorphine/naloxone treatment in opioid dependent youth. Addict Behaviors. 2012;37:1046–53. https://doi.org/10.1016/j.addbeh.2012.04.011.
20. Smyth BP, Fagan J, Kernan K. Outcome of heroin-dependent adolescents presenting for opiate substitution treatment. J Subst Abus Treat. 2012;42:35–44. https://doi.org/10.1016/j.jsat.2011.07.007.
21. Smyth BP, Ducray K, Cullen W. Changes in psychological well-being among heroin-dependent adolescents during psychologically supported opiate substitution treatment. Early Interv Psychiatry. 2016; https://doi.org/10.1111/eip.12318.
22. Department of Health. Guidance for the pharmacological management of substance misuse among young people. London: Department of Health, 2009. http://webarchive.nationalarchives.gov.uk/20130124051653/http://www.dh.gov.uk/prod_consum_dh/groups/dh_digitalassets/documents/digitalasset/dh_106429.pdf (accessed 5 Jan 2018).
23. Amass L, Pukeleviciene V, Subata E, Almeida AR, Pieri MC, D'egidio P, Stankova Z, Costa A, Smyth BP, Sakoman S, Wei Y. A prospective, randomized, multicenter acceptability and safety study of direct buprenorphine/naloxone induction in heroin-dependent individuals. Addiction. 2012 Jan 1;107(1):142–51. https://doi.org/10.1111/j.1360-0443.2011.03577.x.
24. Marsden J, Gossop M, Stewart D, et al. The Maudsley addiction profile (MAP): a brief instrument for assessing treatment outcome. Addiction. 1998;93:1857–67.
25. Smyth BP, Keenan E, O'Connor JJ. Evaluation of the impact of Dublin's expanded harm reduction programme on prevalence of hepatitis C among short-term injecting drug users. J Epid Comm Health. 1999;53(7):434.
26. Teesson M, Mills K, Ross J, Darke S, Williamson A, Havard A. The impact of treatment on 3 years' outcome for heroin dependence: findings from the Australian treatment outcome study (ATOS). Addiction. 2008;103(1):80–8. https://doi.org/10.1111/j.1360-0443.2007.02029.x.
27. Kamal F, Flavin S, Campbell F, Behan C, Fagan J, Smyth R. Factors affecting the outcome of methadone maintenance treatment in opiate dependence. Irish Med J. 2007;100:393–7.
28. Williamson A, Darke S, Ross J, Teesson M. The effect of persistence of cocaine use on 12-month outcomes for the treatment of heroin dependence. Drug Alcohol Depend. 2006;81:293–300. https://doi.org/10.1016/j.drugalcdep.2005.08.010.
29. DeMaria PA, Sterling R, Weinstein SP. The effect of stimulant and sedative use on treatment outcome of patients admitted to methadone maintenance treatment. Am J Addict. 2000;9:145–53.
30. Levine AR, Lundahl LH, Ledgerwood DM, Lisiesko M, Rhodes GL, Greenwald MK. J gender-specific predictors of retention and opioid abstinence during methadone maintenance treatment. Subst Abuse Treat. 2015;54:37–43. https://doi.org/10.1016/j.jsat.2015.01.009.
31. Darker C, Sweeney B, El Hassan H, Kelly AS, O'Connor S, Smyth B, Barry J. Non-attendance at counselling therapy in cocaine-using methadone-maintained patients: lessons learnt from an abandoned randomised controlled trial. Irish J Med Sci. 2012;181(4):483–9. https://doi.org/10.1007/s11845-011-0803-4.
32. Orford J, Copello A, Velleman R, Templeton L. Family members affected by a close relative's addiction: the stress-strain-coping-support model. Drugs: education, prevention and policy. 2010;17(S1):36–43. https://doi.org/10.3109/09687637.2010.514801.

33. Goehl L, Nunes E, Quitkin F, Hilton I. Social networks and methadone treatment outcome: the costs and benefits of social ties. Am J Drug Alcohol Abuse. 1993;19:251–62.
34. Smyth BP, Barry J, Keenan E, Ducray K. Lapse and relapse following inpatient treatment of opiate dependence. Irish Med J. 2010;103:176–9.
35. Ruff S, McCOMB JL, Coker CJ, Sprenkle DH. Behavioral couples therapy for the treatment of substance abuse: a substantive and methodological review of O'Farrell, Fals-Stewart, and Colleagues' program of research. Fam Process. 2010;49(4):439–56. https://doi.org/10.1111/j.1545-5300.2010.01333.x.
36. Crome IB, Christian J, Green C. The development of a unique designated community drug service for adolescents: policy prevention education implication. Drugs: Educ, Prevent Policy. 2000;7:87–108.
37. James P, Kearns C, Campbell A, Smyth BP. Adolescents and substance use: the handbook for professionals working with young people. Oxford: Radcliffe Publishing; 2013. p. 100–9.
38. Dawe S, Harnett PH, Rendalls V, Staiger P. Improving family functioning and child outcome in methadone maintained families: the parents under pressure programme. Drug Alc Review. 2003;22(3):299–307. https://doi.org/10.1080/0959523031000154445.

10

Stabilization of the obesity epidemic and increasing thinness in children in Caribbean Bonaire

Joana Kist-van Holthe[1*], Tirza Blom[1], Laura Melchers[1], Alcira Janga-Jansen[2], Tahirih van Kanten[2], Marian Luinstra-Passchier[2], Teatske Altenburg[1], Remy HiraSing[1] and Mai Chinapaw[1]

Abstract

Background: In 2008, the prevalence of overweight and obesity among children in Bonaire was twice as high as the prevalence in northern Europe but comparable to that of other Caribbean islands and the United States. The aim of this study was to examine change in the body mass index status of children in Bonaire and report children's energy balance-related behaviours (EBRB) in 2015.

Methods: Two school-based cross sectional surveys of children age 4-14 years were conducted in 2008 and 2015. Height (m) and weight (kg) were measured, body mass index (BMI) calculated and children's BMI categorised according to the International Obesity Task Force criteria. In 2015, children age 10-14 years completed a questionnaire on EBRB and responses were compared between non-overweight/obese children and overweight/obese children.

Results: In total 2117 children age 4-14 years participated (92.4% response rate). The prevalence of thinness significantly increased between 2008 and 2015 (adjusted OR 1.5 95% CI: 1.2-1.8). There were no other significant differences in children's weight status between survey years. One quarter of children (25.4%) were overweight/obese in 2015. There were no significant differences in EBRB between non-overweight/obese and overweight/obese children in 2015. Few children met recommendations for EBRB.

Conclusions: The prevalence of overweight/obesity in children in Bonaire did not significantly change between 2008 and 2015 and remained high. However, the prevalence of thinness has significantly increased. Interventions to improve children's current EBRB are required.

Keywords: Obesity, Children, Overweight, Thinness, Caribbean, Lifestyle, Diet, Physical activity, Sedentary behavior

Background

The prevalence of childhood overweight and obesity has rapidly increased worldwide in recent decades [1]. Children are developing obesity at a younger age, and the degree of obesity among children is increasing. More importantly, overweight and obesity "track" into adulthood, implicating a 2-15 times higher chance of becoming an obese adult when being obese during childhood [2]. Overweight and obesity can lead to important health issues, e.g., type 2 diabetes, cardiovascular disease, fatty liver disease, psychological problems and musculoskeletal disorders [3, 4]. In Bonaire, an island in the Caribbean and part of the Netherlands, 35% of the adult population in 2013 was overweight, 25% was obese, and 8 % had type 2 diabetes [5, 6].

In 2008, we first studied the prevalence of overweight and obesity in children in Bonaire. At that time, 14.3% of the boys (aged 4-14 years) and 18.6% of the girls were overweight, and 9.8% of the boys and 13.0% of the girls were obese [7]. The prevalence of overweight is approximately twice as high as that in countries in northern Europe but is comparable to that of other islands in the Caribbean and the United States [7]. Thinness was observed in 10.4% of boys and 8.5% of girls.

* Correspondence: j.kist@vumc.nl
[1]Department of Public and Occupational Health, Amsterdam Public Health Research Institute, VU Medical Center, Amsterdam, the Netherlands

The aim of this study was to obtain an update on the body mass index (BMI) status of children in Bonaire. In addition, we studied energy balance-related behaviors to obtain clues for the tailored prevention of obesity.

Methods

General

All schools in Bonaire (nine elementary schools and one high school) were asked to participate in a cross-sectional study from March to May 2015. Because attending school is mandatory up to the age of 16 years, the study population comprised all school-attending children. No incentives were given. One small elementary school ($n = 103$ children) declined to participate for unknown reasons. Weight and height were measured in all 4- to 14-year-old children, and children 10-14 years of age were asked to complete a questionnaire pertaining to energy balance-related behaviors. The same study design was used as that in a previous study in children in Bonaire in 2008 [7]. The VU University Medical Ethical Committee has revised the study protocol and concluded that the study does not fall within the scope of the Medical Research Involving Human Subjects Act. Parental permission for participation in the study was given by means of passive informed consent. All parents received a letter informing them of the study and that they could opt out by filling in a form and sending it back to the school.

Anthropometric measurements

Two trained assistants performed the anthropometric measurements at the schools. Body weight was measured to the nearest 0.1 kg using a digital scale (Seca 877®, Hamburg, Germany). Because children were weighed in summer clothes without shoes, the following correction for clothing was performed: – 300 g for children 4-6 years; – 600 g for children 7-9 years; – 800 g for those aged 10-11 years; and – 1000 g for children ≥12 years. Height was measured to the nearest 0.1 cm without shoes using a microtoise (Seca 206®, Hamburg, Germany). BMI was calculated as weight (kg) /height (m^2) and classified as thinness, normal weight, overweight, obesity and morbid obesity according to the cut points of the International Obesity Task Force [8].

Energy balance-related behavior questionnaire

Children ≥10 years of age were asked to complete a questionnaire during class pertaining to energy balance-related behaviors based on a previously validated questionnaire among European children 10-12 years of age [9]. The questionnaire was adapted to the Caribbean situation so that the children could easily understand the questions (Additional file 1, energy balance-related questionnaire), e. g., by giving examples of frequently used (brand) names of sweetened drinks and local vegetables. The questionnaire was translated into Papiamento and Dutch. The results were compared to recommendations for children for fruit (≥ 2 pieces per day) and vegetable intake (≥ 150-200 g per day equal to 3-4 ladles per day) [10], physical activity (≥ 1 h per day of moderate- to vigorous-intensity physical activity) [11], television / media time (maximum 2 h per day) [12] and sleep [13, 14]. The recommended sleep duration for children 10 years of age is ≥10.5 h; for 11- and 12-year-olds, the recommendation is ≥10 h, and for 13- and 14-year-olds, the recommendation is ≥9.5 h [13, 14].

Statistics

Analyses were performed with SPSS 22.0 (IBM®, New York, USA). Differences in BMI status (thinness, overweight, obesity and morbid obesity) in 2015 compared to 2008 were tested with logistic regression. Analyses were adjusted for age, gender and clustering of data within schools. In addition, we checked whether differences in BMI status between 2008 and 2015 differed by gender and age group by including an interaction term. As gender and age group were no effect modifiers only the overall Odds ratios are presented.

The difference in energy balance-related behaviors between non-overweight and overweight children was tested with the Pearson Chi-squared test (categorical variables), t-test (continuous variables with normal distribution) and the Mann-Whitney test (continuous variables with skewed distribution). Because of the large number of tests, a p-value < 0.01 was considered statistically significant.

Results

BMI status

A total of 2117 of 2291 (92.4%) 4- to 14-year-old children (1070 (50.5%) boys) in Bonaire participated in the study. Anthropometric measurements were not performed in 174 children (7.6%) because these children were not at school on the day of the measurements or because the parents did not want their child to participate in the study. Table 1 presents the prevalence (%) of the body mass index (BMI) status of children in Bonaire in 2008 and 2015. The prevalence of thinness, normal weight, overweight, obesity and morbid obesity in children was 13.7, 61.0, 15.5, 6.4 and 3.5%, respectively. In 2015, the prevalence of thinness was higher in 4-11 than 12-14 year olds (15.1 versus 9.7%), while the prevalence of overweight and obesity were higher in 12-14 than 4-11 year olds (19.6 versus 14% and 7.7 versus 5.9%, respectively). BMI status was similar in boys and girls (Fig. 1). The prevalence of thinness in primary school children in Bonaire was significantly higher in 2015 than in 2008 AOR 1.5 (95%CI: 1.2-1.8). The prevalence of overweight, obesity or morbid obesity was similar in 2015 and 2008 AOR 1.1 (95% CI: 0.9-1.3), 1.0 (95% CI:0.7-1.2) and 1.0 (95% CI: 0.7-1.4), respectively.

Table 1 Prevalence (%) of the body mass index (BMI) status of children in Bonaire in 2008 and 2015

		Boys		Girls		All	
Age group	BMI status	2008	2015	2008	2015	2008	2015
		%	%	%	%	%	%
4-11 years	Thinness	11.4	16.3	9.6	13.8	10.5	15.1
	Normal weight	66.8	62.2	59.7	60.8	63.4	61.5
	Overweight	12.4	12.5	18.2	15.6	15.2	14.0
	Obesity	5.8	5.5	7.6	6.3	6.7	5.9
	Morbid obesity	3.6	3.5	4.8	3.5	4.2	3.5
	Total	100	100	100	100	100	100
		N = 678	N = 793	N = 643	N = 768	N = 1330	N = 1561
12-14 years	Thinness	8.0	8.3	6.1	11.1	7.0	9.7
	Normal weight	61.8	63.2	60.4	55.9	61.1	59.5
	Overweight	19.5	18.8	19.5	20.4	19.5	19.6
	Obesity	7.3	7.9	10.9	7.5	9.2	7.7
	Morbid obesity	3.4	1.8	3.1	5.0	3.2	3.4
	Total	100	100	100	100	100	100
		N = 262	N = 277	N = 293	N = 279	N = 555	N = 556
Total		100 N = 949	100 N = 1070	100 N = 936	100 N = 1047	100 N = 1885	100 N = 2117

Energy balance-related behavior questionnaire

A total of 768 (75%) of 1029 10- to 14-year-old children in Bonaire completed the questionnaire. The response rate varied per question from 583 (57%) to 768 (75%). The percentage of missing questionnaires included children who were not at school on the day of the survey (7.9%). Table 2 denotes the results of the questionnaire pertaining to energy balance-related behaviors. There were no significant differences between non-overweight and overweight children in self-reported dietary patterns, physical activity, screen time or sleep duration. A large number of the children in Bonaire did not fulfill the recommendations for a healthy lifestyle; for example, only 50% of the children attained the recommended daily intake of vegetables, and only 37% met the recommendations for fruit intake.

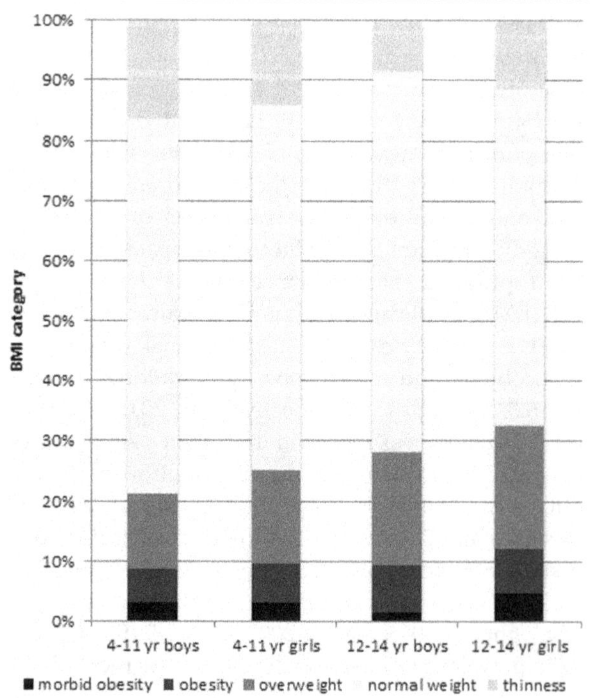

Fig. 1 Body mass index (BMI) categories in 4- to 11 and 12- 14-year-old boys and girls in in 2015 in Bonaire

Discussion

Although the prevalence of overweight and obesity in children in Bonaire in 2015 was high, it was similar to that of 2008. This is a promising development. Two recent large-scale studies on childhood obesity, with data from the United States, China, Australia, New Zealand and Europe, demonstrated a similar stabilization in the prevalence of overweight and obesity [15, 16]. To the best of our knowledge, this is the first study examining the prevalence of overweight and obesity over time in Caribbean children.

Remarkably, thinness was noted in nearly 14% of the children. This is more than two times the prevalence of thinness in Puerto Rico (5.7%) [17]. Equally, using the International Obesity Task Force definition of thinness in 5- to 14-year-old children in Guadeloupe, Martinique, French Guiana and French Polynesia, thinness varied from 12.7 to 19.4% in girls and from 4.8 to 13.3% in boys [18]. Our study was not designed to provide clues as to why the prevalence of thinness – especially that in young children

Table 2 Energy balance-related behaviors among 10- to 14-year-old children (N = 768) in 2015 in Bonaire

Energy balance-related behaviors (Percentage complying with recommendations)	overweight or obese children $N = 247$	non-overweight children $N = 521$	*p*-value
Nutrition			
Ate breakfast this morning	71.7	75.4	0.26
Eats two or more pieces of fresh fruit/day	37.4	37.4	0.97
Eats two or more portions of vegetables/day	50.2	50.3	0.97
Drinks one or less sweetened drinks/week	17.9	15.0	0.28
Physical activity/screen behavior			
Participates one or more times / week in organized sports	82.8	75.7	0.03
Participates in one or more hours of physical activity on a school day	68.0	67.8	0.94
Watches two or more hours of television on a school day	73.1	72.8	0.93
Uses the computer for two or more hours on a school day	62.8	65.9	0.39
Uses active transportation to school	21.1	23.8	0.40
Sleep duration			
10-year-old children, 10.5 h or more	94.4	88.6	0.33
11- & 12-year-old children, 10 h or more	73.8	66.1	0.17
13- & 14-year-old children, 9.5 h or more	88.2	86.0	0.65
Mean (SD) sleep duration (h)	8.7 (1.37)	8.7 (1.36)	0.98

The response rate per question varied from 583 (57%) to 768 (75%). Fruit and vegetable consumption, physical activity, television and computer time pertain to the previous day and breakfast to the morning of the survey; active transportation to school includes walking or biking. In view of the many parameters tested, $P < 0.01$ is considered significant

(4 and 5 years of age) - in Bonaire is high and has increased since 2008.

There were no significant differences between non-overweight and overweight children in Bonaire in terms of self-reported dietary patterns, physical activity, screen time or sleep duration. However, a large number of the children in Bonaire did not fulfill the recommendations for a healthy lifestyle. Only 50% of children attained the recommended daily intake for vegetables (≥ 2 portions), and 37% met the recommendations for fruit (≥ 2 pieces). High prices of fresh fruit and vegetables may play a role. Nearly all fresh fruits and vegetables are imported into Bonaire. However, compared with 10-12-year-old European children, the percentage of children in Bonaire complying with the recommendations was similar for fruit (European children 15 to 34%) and higher for vegetables (European children 15 to 32%) [19]. Approximately 25% of the children in Bonaire skipped breakfast, which resembles data from 10- to 12-year-old children in Europe, where skipping breakfast at least once a week varied from 14% (Spain) to 51% (Slovenia) [20]. In the same study, children slept (parent-reported) a mean of 9.2 h a night, varying from 8.7 h in Greek boys to 9.7 h in Belgian girls [20]. Compared with children in Europe, sleep duration in children in Bonaire was relatively short (8.7 h).

Two-thirds of children in Bonaire reported to engage in the recommended ≥1 h of moderate-to-vigorous physical activity per day. This percentage is higher than found in a large cross-sectional survey of almost 220,000 youths (11–15 years) from 42 participating countries of the 2013–2014 Health Behaviour in School-Aged Children Study. The percentage of study participants that reported to engage in moderate-to-vigorous physical activity for 60 or more minutes per day ranged from 8 to 47% for boys and from 5 to 34% for girls [21]. More than one-quarter of the children in Bonaire watched more than the advised maximum of 2 hours of television on a school day. This is less than the proportion of 10-12-year-old European children, of whom approximately 38% reported to watch more than 2 hours of television per day [22].

The strength of this study is the high response rate: nearly all (92.4%) 4- to 14-year-old children in Bonaire participated in the study. In addition, all anthropometric measurements were performed by the same trained research assistants. Furthermore, the same study design was used in the previous study in Bonaire (2008) by the same research group, thereby justifying comparison of the anthropometric data [7]. However, the content and delivery of the questionnaire in 2015 differed from that in 2008, impeding the comparison of energy balance-related behavior.

There are some weaknesses in the study. As some children who seemed overweight were not allowed to participate in the study by their parents, the prevalence of overweight and obesity may be slightly underestimated. However, the same phenomenon applied in our previous study in 2008 [7]. A limitation of the study is that psychometric testing was not done after adaptation of the questionnaire to the local situation in Bonaire. However, the adaptation only included providing cultural appropriate examples of fruits, vegetables and drinks.

Another weakness is that approximately one-quarter of the questions from the questionnaire were not completed. Furthermore, one can debate as to how correct children are in estimating the quantity of their food and drink intake, as well as their physical activity, screen- and sleep time [23–25]. To try and obtain as many reliable answers as possible, the questionnaire asked to recall intake at a certain recent moment in time (e.g., fruit and vegetable intake the day before or breakfast consumption the morning of the questionnaire). However, a three-day prospective food frequency diet may have given a more reliable overview of dietary intake. Additionally, it is possible that children gave socially acceptable answers; this may especially apply to overweight and obese children [26].

Conclusions

The prevalence of overweight and obesity among children in Bonaire remains high. However, it is a promising development that, compared with 2008, the prevalence of overweight and obesity in children has stabilized. Conversely, the prevalence of thinness, especially in the youngest children, was high. More studies are needed to clarify the cause of thinness among (young) children in Bonaire.

Self-reported energy balance-related behaviors were not significantly different between non-overweight and overweight children. However, a large number of children in Bonaire did not fulfill the recommendations for a healthy lifestyle. This knowledge can be used as a basis for governmental health policy measures in schools (e.g., providing healthy food choices and free water in school canteens, stimulating active transport and physical activity options during recess and after school) and in the community as a whole (e.g., promoting affordable locally grown fruit and vegetables, access to affordable sport participation, and safe neighborhoods and roads).

Acknowledgements
We would like to thank all children, schoolteachers and principals for their participation in the study.

Funding
The study was supported by the Department of Public Health of Bonaire. Alcira Janga-Jansen MD, Tahirih van Kanten MSc and Marian Luinstra-Passchier MD from the Department of Public Health of Bonaire were involved in the design of the study and critically reviewed the manuscript.

Authors' contributions
JKvH, AJJ, TvK, MLP, RH and MC designed the study; TB and LM carried out the study; JKvH, TB and LM wrote the manuscript; JKvH, TA and MC analysed the data; TvK, MLP, AJJ, TA, RH and MC critically reviewed the manuscript. All authors have read and approved the final manuscript.

Competing interests
The authors declare that they have no competing interests.

Author details
[1]Department of Public and Occupational Health, Amsterdam Public Health Research Institute, VU Medical Center, Amsterdam, the Netherlands. [2]Department of Public Health, Openbaar Lichaam Bonaire, Bonaire, the Netherlands.

References

1. Ng M, Fleming T, Robinson M, et al. Global, regional, and national prevalence of overweight and obesity in children and adults during 1980-2013: a systematic analysis for the global burden of disease study 2013. Lancet. 2014;384:766–81.
2. Singh AS, Mulder C, Twisk JW, van Mechelen W, Chinapaw MJ. Tracking of childhood overweight into adulthood: a systematic review of the literature. Obes Rev. 2008;9:474–88.
3. Ludwig DS. Childhood obesity–the shape of things to come. N Engl J Med. 2007;357:2325–7.
4. van Emmerik NM, Renders CM, van de Veer M, et al. High cardiovascular risk in severely obese young children and adolescents. Arch Dis Child. 2012;97:818–21.
5. Central Bureau for Statistics. Overweight and Obesity in Dutch Caribbean. Retrieved 27-2-0014. Accessed 1-8-2015. http://www.cbs.nl/nl-NL/menu/themas/dossiers/nederland-regionaal/publicaties/artikelen/archief/2014/2014-27feb-gezondheid-leefstijl-cn-2013-art.htm.
6. Central Bureau for Statistics. Diabetes. 2015. Accessed 1-8-2015. http://statline.cbs.nl/Statweb/publication/?DM=SLNL&PA=82291ned&D1=2-4&D2=0-2&D3=a&D4=0&D5=l&VW=T.
7. Schwiebbe L, van Rest J, Verhagen E, Visser RW, Kist-van Holthe JE, Hirasing RA. Childhood obesity in the Caribbean. West Indian Med J. 2011;60:442–5.
8. Cole TJ, Lobstein T. Extended international (IOTF) body mass index cut-offs for thinness, overweight and obesity. Pediatr Obes. 2012;7:284–94.
9. Singh AS, Vik FN, Chinapaw MJ, et al. Test-retest reliability and construct validity of the ENERGY-child questionnaire on energy balance-related behaviours and their potential determinants: the ENERGY-project. Int J Behav Nutr Phys Act. 2011;8:136.
10. Netherlands Nutrition Centre. Accessed 1-8-2015. http://www.voedingscentrum.nl/nl/schijf-van-vijf/eet-veel-groente-fruit-en-brood.aspx.
11. Netherlands Center for Sports and Physical Excercise. Recommendations for Healthy Physical Excercise. Accessed 1-8-2015. http://www.nisb.nl/weten/normen.html.
12. American Academy of Pediatrics. Children, adolescents, and television. Pediatrics. 2001;107:423–6.
13. Spruyt K. Sleep. Tielt: Lannoo; 2008. ISBN 9789020978483.
14. Paruthi S, Brooks LJ, D'Ambrosio C, et al. Recommended amount of sleep for pediatric populations: a consensus statement of the American Academy of sleep medicine. J Clin Sleep Med. 2016;12(6):785–6.
15. Ogden CL, Carroll MD, Kit BK, Flegal KM. Prevalence of childhood and adult obesity in the United States, 2011-2012. JAMA. 2014;311:806 14.
16. Olds T, Maher C, Zumin S, et al. Evidence that the prevalence of childhood overweight is plateauing: data from nine countries. Int J Pediatr Obes. 2011;6:342–60.
17. Rivera-Soto WT, Rodriguez-Figueroa L, Calderon G. Prevalence of childhood obesity in a representative sample of elementary school children in Puerto Rico by socio-demographic characteristics, 2008. P R Health Sci J. 2010;29:357–63.
18. Daigre JL, Atallah A, Boissin JL, et al. The prevalence of overweight and obesity, and distribution of waist circumference, in adults and children in the French overseas territories: the PODIUM survey. Diabetes Metab. 2012;38:404–11.
19. Lynch C, Kristjansdottir AG, Te Velde SJ, et al. Fruit and vegetable consumption in a sample of 11-year-old children in ten European countries–the PRO GREENS cross-sectional survey. Public Health Nutr. 2014;17:2436–44.
20. Brug J, van Stralen MM, Te Velde SJ, et al. Differences in weight status and energy-balance related behaviors among schoolchildren across Europe: the ENERGY-project. PLoS One. 2012;7:e34742.

21. Inchley J, Currie D, Young T et al. Growing up unequal: gender and socioeconomic differences in young peoples' s health and well-being. Health Behaviour in School-aged Children (HBSC) study. International report form the 2013-2014 study. World Health Organization. http://www.euro.who.int/__data/assets/pdf_file/0003/303438/HSBC-No.7-Growing-up-unequal-Full-Report.pdf.
22. Te Velde SJ, De Bourdeaudhuij I, Thorsdottir I, et al. Patterns in sedentary and exercise behaviors and associations with overweight in 9-14-year-old boys and girls–a cross-sectional study. BMC Public Health. 2007;7:16.
23. Bryant MJ, Lucove JC, Evenson KR, Marshall S. Measurement of television viewing in children and adolescents: a systematic review. Obes Rev. 2007;8(3):197–209.
24. Livingstone MB, Robson PJ, Wallace JM. Issues in dietary intake assessment of children and adolescents. Br J Nutr. 2004;92(Suppl 2):S213–22.
25. Slootmaker SM, Schuit AJ, Chinapaw MJ, Seidell JC, van Mechelen W. Disagreement in physical activity assessed by accelerometer and self-report in subgroups of age, gender, education and weight status. Int J Behav Nutr Phys Act. 2009;6:17.
26. Jayawardene W, Lohrmann D, YoussefAgha A. Discrepant body mass index: behaviors associated with height and weight misreporting among US adolescents from the National Youth Physical Activity and nutrition study. Child Obes. 2014;10:225–33.

11

Knowledge, attitudes and misconceptions of Italian healthcare professionals regarding fever management in children

Elena Chiappini[1*], Antonina Marta Cangelosi[1], Paolo Becherucci[2], Monica Pierattelli[2], Luisa Galli[1] and Maurizio de Martino[1]

Abstract

Background: Fever phobia is still a major issue in paediatrics. We report knowledge of a sample of Italian paediatricians performed six years after the release of the Italian guidelines for the management of fever in children (IFG).

Methods: A questionnaire, developed following the IFG recommendations and previously administered to 300 paediatricians in 2012, was proposed to all the paediatricians attending the 2015 National Congress of Practice Paediatrics, held in Florence, Italy. Changes in answers over time were analyzed.

Results: 70.2% (562/800) paediatricians returned the questionnaire. The recommended site and device for body temperature measurement in children > 1 year was correctly chosen by 89.3% of participants (vs. 80.7% of 2012 participants; $P < 0.001$), but with children aged less than 1 year the correct answer was selected only by the 50.3% (vs. 39.3% of 2012 participants: $P < 0.001$).
Use of physical methods was still incorrectly recommended by 51.6% of paediatricians (vs. 63.6% in 2012; $P < 0.001$). Use of antipyretics according to discomfort was adopted only by 38.2% of participants, while 12.2% of them recommended alternate use of antipyretics. These proportions were substantially stable since 2012 (45 and 11% respectively), rectal administration of antipyretics only in case of vomiting was correctly recommended by 86.8% of paediatricians vs. 74.7% in 2012 ($P < 0.001$).

Conclusion: Improvements in some pediatricians' misconceptions were observed over time. However, some incorrect habits persist. Further studies are needed to better understand the "weak points" of the communication between Scientific Societies and paediatricians in order to impact everyday clinical practice.

Keywords: Fever, Children, Antipyretics, Thermometer, Paracetamol, Ibuprofen

Background

Since the 1980's, when Barton Schmitt coined the term "fever phobia" [1], several studies have been published in this regard, reporting its presence both among healthcare professionals and parents/tutors, in Western countries as well as in limited resource settings [2, 3]. Despite the dissemination of several international guidelines [4, 5], poor knowledge about the correct use of antipyretics still persists among paediatricians. The results of the most recent surveys performed in Italy and in other European countries show improvements, but also the potential for further optimization [2, 6]. The present study investigated changes in knowledge/misconceptions over time by surveying a large sample of paediatricians, comparing results with those obtained in a previous similar national survey [6].

Methods

Study design

A survey was conducted including paediatricians attending the National Congress of Practice Paediatrics, held in Florence in November 2015. All the paediatricians

* Correspondence: elena.chiappini@unifi.it
[1]Department of Health Sciences, Anna Meyer Children's University Hospital, University of Florence, Viale Pieraccini, 24, 50100 Florence, Italy

Table 1 Temperature monitoring site/method used by paediatricians participating in the 2012 and 2015 surveys and type of thermometer recommended

	2012 n (%; 95% CI) *n* = 300	2015 n (%; 95% CI) *n* = 562	*P*
Children < 1 year of age			
Axillary*	118 (39.3; 33.8–44.9)	283 (50.4; 46.2–54.5)	0.001
Rectal	124 (41.3; 35.8–46.9)	192 (34.2; 30.2–38.1)	0.020
Groin crease	38 (12.7; 8.9–16.4)	71 (12.6; 9.9–15.4)	0.980
Oral	0 (0.0; 0.0–0.0)	1 (0.2; 0.0–0.5)	0.950
Auricular	18 (6.1; 3.3–8.7)	7 (1.2; 0.3–2.2)	< 0.0001
Forehead	2 (0.6; 0.0–1.6)	8 (1.4; 0.4–2.4)	< 0.0001
Children > 1 year of age			
Axillary*	242 (80.7; 76.2–85.1)	502 (89.3; 86.8–91.9)	0.0003
Rectal	9 (3.0; 1.1–4.9)	20 (3.6; 2.0–5.1)	0.660
Groin crease	15 (5.0; 2.5–7.5)	24 (4.3; 2.6–5.9)	0.630
Oral	2 (0.7; 0.0–1.6)	1 (0.2; 0.0–0.5)	0.240
Auricular	29 (9.6; 6.3–13.0)	6 (1.1; 0.2–1.9)	< 0.0001
Forehead	3 (1.0; 0.0–2.1)	10 (1.8; 0.7–2.9)	0.370
Type of recommended thermometer			
Digital*	203 (67.7; 62.4–73.0)	385 (68.5; 64.7–72.3)	0.430
Auricular	15 (5.0; 2.5–7.5)	9 (1.6; 0.6–2.6)	0.003
Other**	32 (10.6; 7.2–14.2)	168 (29.8; 26.1–33.7)	< 0.0001

Note: * right answer according to the Guidelines of the Italian Paediatric Society
**mercury, skin infrared, plastic streap placed forehead, dummy-pacifier style thermometers

Table 2 Use of physical methods and antipyretics among paediatricians participating in the 2012 and 2015 surveys

First choice drug			
	2012 n (%)	2015 n (%)	*P*
Paracetamol*	295 (98.3; 96.1–99.3)	546 (97.1; 95.4–98.4)	0.656
Ibuprofen*	4 (1.3; 0.5–3.4)	12 (2.1;1.2–3.7)	0.40
Other	1 (0.3; 0.0–1.8)	4 (0.7; 0.3–1.8)	0.48
Second choice drug			
Paracetamol*	19 (6.3; 4.1–9.7;)	61 (10.8; 8.5–13.7)	0.03
Ibuprofen*	276 (92.0; 88.4–94.6)	495 (88.1; 85.1–90-5)	0.04
Acetylsalicilic acid	2 (0.7; 0.2–2.4)	0 (0.0; 0.0–0.0)	0.12
Other	3 (1.0;0.3–2.9)	6 (1.1; 0.5–2.3)	0.92
Choice of administration of paracetamol			
Oral	249 (83.0; 78.3–86-8)	517 (92.0; 89.4–94.0)	< 0.0001
Rectal	51 (17.0;13.2–21.7)	45 (8.0;6.0–10.5)	< 0.0001
Alternating use			
Yes	34 (11.3; 8.2–15.4)	69 (12.3; 9.8–15.2)	0.40
Use of physical methods			
Together with antipyretic drug	29 (9.7; 6.8–13.5)	36 (6.4; 4.7–8.7)	0.08
Before the antipyretic drug	9 (3.0; 1.6–5.6)	14 (2.3; 14.5–41.4)	0.66
If fever persists	153 (51.0; 45.4–56.6)	242 (43.1; 39.0–47.2)	0.15
Never*	109 (36.3; 31.3–41.9)	270 (48.0; 43.9–52.2)	< 0.0001

Note:* right answer according to the Guidelines of the Italian Paediatric Society recommendation

attending the conference received an anonymous, standardized and self-administered paper-based questionnaire. They were requested to participate to the survey by returning the filled questionnaire to the conference registration desk. Results were entered into an electronic database, analyzed and compared with those obtained from a previous similar survey, performed in 2012, at the 12th National Congress of the Italian Society of Paediatric Infectious Diseases and based on the same questionnaire (Appendix 1) [6].

Questionnaire

The questionnaire was developed on the basis of previous similar surveys [6, 7], and in consideration of the IFG recommendations [4]. The questionnaire consisted in multiple choice questions, as previously described [6]. Briefly, the main topics included: methods and devices recommended for the measurement of body temperature, knowledge regarding the use of physical methods and antipyretics.

Statistical analysis

The results were expressed as absolute numbers, percentages and 95% confidence intervals (95% CIs) were calculated. The χ^2 or the Fischer's exact test (2 grades of freedom) were used in order to calculate differences among responses between the years 2012 and 2015. SPSS software package was used and p value < 0.05 was considered as statistically significant.

The study was not commercially sponsored.

Results

The questionnaire was returned by 562/800 (70.%) of participants; the majority (91.9%; 517/562) were primary care paediatricians; 16 (2.8%) were hospital paediatricians, and 29 (5.1%) residents/other; 393 (69.9%) participants declared to be aware of IFG.

Methods for body temperature measurement

In children under one year of age, axillary site was correctly chosen by an increased number of paediatricians over time: 50.3% in 2015 vs. 39.3% in 2012 ($p < 0.0001$). However, the rectal measurement, which was discouraged by the IFG because considered invasive, was still commonly adopted: the proportion of participants who recommended rectal measurement in children under one year of age was 41.3% in 2012 and 34.2% in 2015 ($p = 0.002$) (Table 1).

In children > 1 year of age, a correct answer indicating axilla as the preferred site for temperature measurement was provided by 89.3% of paediatricians vs 80.7% in the 2012 survey ($p = 0.0003$).

Considering the type of thermometer recommended, the digital one was the most widely recommended (68.5%); while the use of auricular thermometer decreased overtime and was only 1.6% in 2015 vs 5.0% in 2012 ($P = 0.003$) (Table 1).

Use of physical methods and antipyretics

Wet bandages, ice bags and other physical methods (discouraged by IFG) were never recommended by 48.0% of paediatricians in 2015, with a significant increase from the

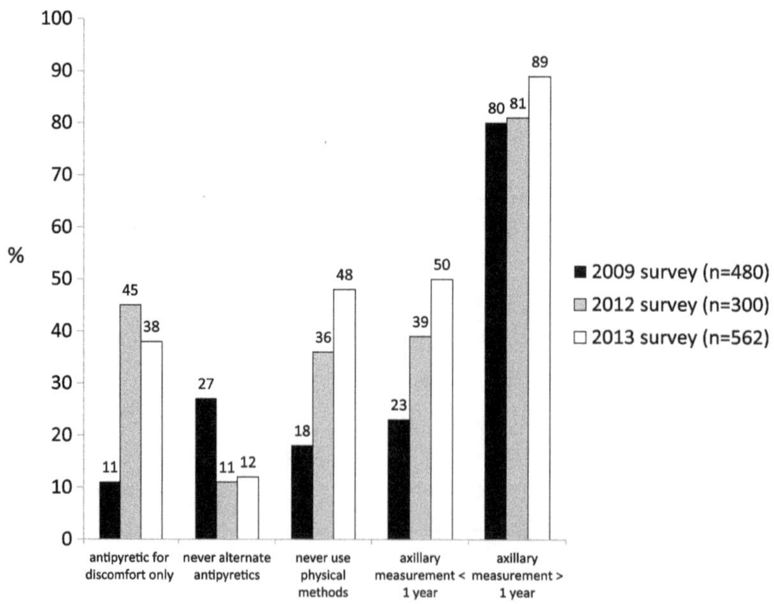

Fig. 1 Change in Italian paediatricians' knowledge over time

results reported in the 2012 survey (36.4%; $P < 0.0001$) (Table 2).

The use of antipyretics according to the presence of discomfort, and not for a specific cut-off of body temperature, was recommended only by 38.2% of paediatricians (vs. 45.3% in 2012).

Paracetamol was confirmed as the first choice antipyretic drug for 97% of paediatricians (Table 2).

None of the participants recommended acetylsalicylic acid but, unfortunately, a small proportion of paediatricians recommended other drugs, besides paracetamol and ibuprofen (including steroids and metamizole) with an antipyretic purpose (Table 2).

Rectal administration only in case of vomiting was correctly recommended by 86.8% of paediatricians in 2015 vs. 74.7% in 2012 ($P < 0.0001$).

The alternate use of paracetamol and ibuprofen was recommended by 12.2% of paediatricians in 2015, similarly to 2012 (Table 2; Fig. 1).

Discussion

In the present study, changes in knowledge and misconceptions among paediatricians over time were evaluated. Considering also results from our 2009 survey, which included 480 Italian paediatricians [7], progressive improvements in the amount of correct answers were observed (Fig. 1). However, several incorrect habits, including use of physical methods, use of antipyretics not focused on the presence of discomfort, alternate use of antipyretics, and rectal misuse of these drugs are still common.

Several previous studies investigated misconceptions of paediatricians concerning the management of fever in children. Italian pediatricians' knowledge seems to be in line, or slightly better, than those reported in other European countries in recent years. As an example, the use of physical methods was recommended by 77% of paediatricians in Switzerland [8] and 74% of them [9] in France; this proportion is higher than observed in our study (about 50%). Alternate use of antipyretics was recommended by 65% of Swiss paediatricians [8] but only by 11% of our participants.

The reasons behind the persistence of fever phobia over time have been previously explored [2]. The lack of a strict definition of the child's discomfort is one major obstacle. Moreover, the evaluation of the child's discomfort is usually subjectively assessed by one caregiver, and it is influenced by his/her fever-phobia level, in a sort of "vicious circle" [2]. Another issue is the quality of educational material provided by the Scientific Societies that has been found to be often unclear [10]. Finally, paediatricians should improve their ability to communicate with caregivers, not only in terms of time spent for the parents' education, but also in efforts toward an empathetical and trustful connection with the caregiver [11].

Our study has several limitations. Our results may not be generalized to all paediatricians in Italy, since those included represent approximatively 7% of the entire population of the Italian paediatricians [6]. The two surveys were conducted during two different Conferences. Therefore, the two populations of paediatricians may differ in some characteristics. Personal data (i.e. age and residence) of participants were not collected. Hence our results do not provide information regarding possible differences according to the geographical provenience, age, or other variables. Moreover, adjustment for potential confounders was not possible. It is well-known that self-reported behaviors can be misleading, since some participants might not complete the survey as carefully as they would do in real settings [6]. Participants could be more interested in

Table 3 Main recommendations by the Italian fever guidelines [4]

- ✓ Rectal measurement should not be used routinely in children aged < 5 years because it is invasive and causes discomfort (evidence level III; strength of recommendation D).
- ✓ Oral measurement of body temperature should be avoided in children (evidence level III; strength of recommendation D).
- ✓ Axillary measurement using a digital thermometer is recommended in children aged < 4 weeks (evidence level III; strength of recommendation B).
- ✓ In the hospital or ambulatory care setting, axillary measurement using a digital thermometer or tympanic measurement using an infrared thermometer is recommended in children aged ≥4 weeks (evidence level II; strength of recommendation B).
- ✓ For measurements taken at home by parents/caregivers, axillary measurement using a digital thermometer is recommended in all children (evidence level II; strength of recommendation B).
- ✓ Use of a tympanic infrared thermometer is not recommended, as this mode of measurement is prone to operator-related error.
- ✓ Use of antipyretics in children is recommended only when the fever is associated with evident discomfort (eg, prolonged crying, irritability, reduced activity, reduced appetite, disturbed sleep) (evidence level I; strength of recommendation B).
- ✓ Use of physical methods to reduce fever is not recommended (evidence level I; strength of recommendation E).
- ✓ Paracetamol and ibuprofen are the only antipyretic drugs recommended for use in children (evidence level I; strength of recommendation A).
- ✓ Use of acetylsalicylic acid in children is not recommended because of the risk of Reye's syndrome (evidence level III; strength of recommendation E).
- ✓ Because of their poor benefit– risk ratio, steroids should not be used as antipyretics in children (evidence level III; strength of recommendation E).
- ✓ Combined or alternating use of ibuprofen and paracetamol is not recommended (evidence level VI; strength of recommendation D).
- ✓ Rectal administration of antipyretics should be considered only in the presence of vomiting or other conditions that prevent oral administration (evidence level I; strength of recommendation A).

fever management than non-responding paediatricians. On the other hand, we were able to administer the same questionnaire to large samples of Italian pediatricians, from 2009 to 2015, exploring changes in the adherence to the guideline's recommendations over time and which messages should be strengthened (Table 3).

Conclusion

Our study highlights improvements in the management of the febrile child in Italy, but also detected the persistence of some incorrect habits. Several key messages of the IFG must be further stressed. In particular, the recommendation regarding the use of antipyretics according to the child's discomfort seems to be adopted only by a minority of paediatricians. Similarly, recent literature reports suggest that improvements in educational interventions are needed in many European countries [2]. Our results may be of help for targeting educational interventions and adherence to practices recommended by the IFG. Further studies are needed in order to understand "weak points" of the communication between Scientific Societies and pediatricians, as well as between paediatricians and caregivers.

Appendix

Questionnaire

1. Where should body temperature be measured in children under one year?

a) the armpit
b) the rectum
c) groin crease
d) the mouth
e) the ear
f) on the forehead

2. Where should the body temperature be measured in children over one year?

a) the armpit
b) the rectum
c) groin crease
d) the mouth
e) the ear
f) on the forehead

3. What kind of thermometer do you suggest to measure temperature?

a) mercury-in-glass
b) electronic
c) auricular
d) skin infrared
e) plastic strip placed on forehead
f) "dummy"
g) I don't suggest any particular thermometer

4. Above what temperature do you administer antipyretics?

a) < 37 °C
b) 37.5 °C
c) 38 °C
d) 38.5 °C
e) 39 °C
f) not exist a temperature cut off, depend on patient malaise

5. Which antipyretic drugs do you usually suggest to use?

a) acetaminophen
b) ibuprofen
c) aspirin
d) other (metamizole, betamethasone)

6. When the temperature is not going down quickly, do you believe it is useful to associate two or more antipyretic drugs?

a) yes
b) no

7. Do you suggest to use physical methods as sponging or ice pack to reduce a child's body temperature?

a) yes, with the antipyretic drug
b) yes, before the antipyretic drug
c) only if the temperature is not going down after the antipyretic drug
d) no, never

8. When do you suggest to administer antipyretic drug rectally?

a) it's more useful
b) it's more practical
c) because parents prefer this way
d) only in the presence of vomiting

Abbreviation

IFG: Italian Fever Guideline

Authors' contributions

EC conceived the study, participated in the design and coordination, and drafted the manuscript. MC and LG performed the statistical analyses and drafted the manuscript. PB, MP and MdM participated in study design and helped to draft and review the manuscript. All authors read and approved the final manuscript.

Competing interests
The authors declare that they have no competing interests.

Author details
[1]Department of Health Sciences, Anna Meyer Children's University Hospital, University of Florence, Viale Pieraccini, 24, 50100 Florence, Italy. [2]Primary Care Paediatrician, Florence, Italy.

References

1. Schmitt BD. Fever phobia: misconceptions of parents about fevers. Am J Dis Child. 1980;134:176–81.
2. Crocetti M, Moghbeli N, Serwint J. Fever phobia revisited: have parental misconceptions about fever changed in 20 years? Paediatrics. 2001;107:1241–6.
3. Bertille N, Purssell E, Corrard F, Chiappini E, Chalumeau M. Fever phobia 35 years later: did we fail? Acta Paediatr. 2016;105:9–10.
4. Chiappini E, Venturini E, Remaschi G, Principi N, Longhi R, Tovo PA, Becherucci P, Bonsignori F, Esposito S, Festini F, Galli L, Lucchesi B, Mugelli A, Marseglia GL, de Martino M. Italian pediatric society panel for the Management of Fever in children. 2016 update of the Italian pediatric society guidelines for Management of Fever in children. J Pediatr. 2017;180:177–83.
5. Fields E, Chard J, Murphy MS, Richardson M, Guideline Development Group and Technical Team. Assessment and initial management of feverish illness in children younger than 5 years: summary of updated NICE guidance. BMJ. 2013;f286:346.
6. Chiappini E, D'Elios S, Mazzantini R, Becherucci P, Pierattelli M, Galli L, de Martino M. Adherence among Italian paediatricians to the Italian guidelines for the management of fever in children: a cross sectional survey. BMC Paediatr. 2013;13:210.
7. Chiappini E, Parretti A, Becherucci P, Pierattelli M, Bonsignori F, Galli L, de Martino M. Parental and medical knowledge and management of fever in Italian pre-school children. BMC Paediatr. 2012;12:97.
8. Lava SA, Simonetti GD, Ramelli GP, Tschumi S, Bianchetti MG. Symptomatic management of fever by Swiss board-certified paediatricians: results from a cross-sectional, web-based survey. Clin Ther. 2012;34:250–6.
9. Bertille N, Pons G, Khoshnood B, Fournier-Charrière EA. National Survey of healthcare Professionals' practices in France. PLoS One. 2015;10(11):e0143230.
10. Freda MC. The readability of American Academy of Pediatrics patient education brochures. J Pediatr Health Care. 2005;19:151–6.
11. Sahm LJ, Kelly M, McCarthy S, O'Sullivan R, Shiely F, Romsing J. Knowledge, attitudes and beliefs of parents regarding fever in children: a Danish interview study. Acta Paediatr. 2016;105:69–73.

12

Transcutaneous bilirubin estimation in extremely low birth weight infants receiving phototherapy

Vidit Bhargava[1*], Daniel Tawfik[1], Bruce Niebuhr[2] and Sunil K. Jain[3]

Abstract

Background: Measurement of transcutaneous bilirubin (TcB) is a quick, reliable and painless method to guide management of hyperbilirubinemia. Studies in term and late preterm infants have found that TcB measurements from covered areas (TcB-C) during phototherapy (PHT) co-relate well with serum bilirubin levels. Limited data exists in extremely low birth weight (ELBW) infants.

Methods: In this prospective observational study, an opaque patch was placed on the back of an ELBW infant prior to initiation of PHT. TcB-C and TcB-E (TcB from exposed area) levels were measured at birth and at 24-h intervals for 5 days. Total serum bilirubin (TSB) levels were also measured within 30 min of obtaining TcB levels. A Wilcoxon signed rank test was used for data analysis. A mixed effect model was used to adjust for repeated measurements over time. The p value < 0.05 was considered significant.

Results: A total of 19 infants were enrolled in the study, with a mean gestational age of 26 ± 2 weeks and mean weight 827 ± 127 g. The difference between TcB-C and TSB was 2.68 ± 2.41 mg/dl (mean ± SD, $p < 0.001$). In contrast, the difference between TcB-E and TSB was − 0.51 ± 1.74 mg/dl ($p = 0.02$). TcB-C consistently overestimates TSB, while TcB-E consistently underestimates TSB.

Conclusions: During PHT exposure, TcB-C does not correlate with TSB values in ELBW infants. TcB-C levels cannot be used as a surrogate for TSB measurement in ELBW infants.

Keywords: Hyperbilirubinemia, ELBW, Kernicterus, Transcutaneous bilirubinometry

Background

Hyperbilirubinemia is seen in almost two-thirds of term and more than two-thirds of all preterm infants [1]. The incidence of kernicterus has dramatically decreased since the onset of regular screening and aggressive management with phototherapy (PHT). In one post-mortem series of premature infants, kernicterus was found to be virtually non-existent [2]. The USA Kernicterus Registry reported 125 infants ≥35 weeks estimated gestational age with kernicterus/acute bilirubin encephalopathy between 1992 to 2004. No specific serum bilirubin values coincided with onset of kernicterus in these infants [3]. Hence, while the incidence has substantially decreased, a considerable disease burden still exists in term and preterm infants with hyperbilirubinemia. The American Academy of Pediatrics Subcommittee on Hyperbilirubinemia recommends that every infant be screened for hyperbilirubinemia by TSB or TcB at 24 h of life and with subsequent measurements guided by the bilirubin level at 24 h of life and the presence of other risk factors [4]. A recent NICHD Neonatal Research Network study focused exclusively on the management of hyperbilirubinemia in ELBW infants demonstrated that aggressive management of hyperbilirubinemia with

* Correspondence: viditbhumi@yahoo.com
[1]Department of Pediatrics, Division of Pediatric Critical Care, Lucile Salter Packard Children's Hospital, 770 Welch Road, Suite 435, Palo Alto, CA 94304, USA

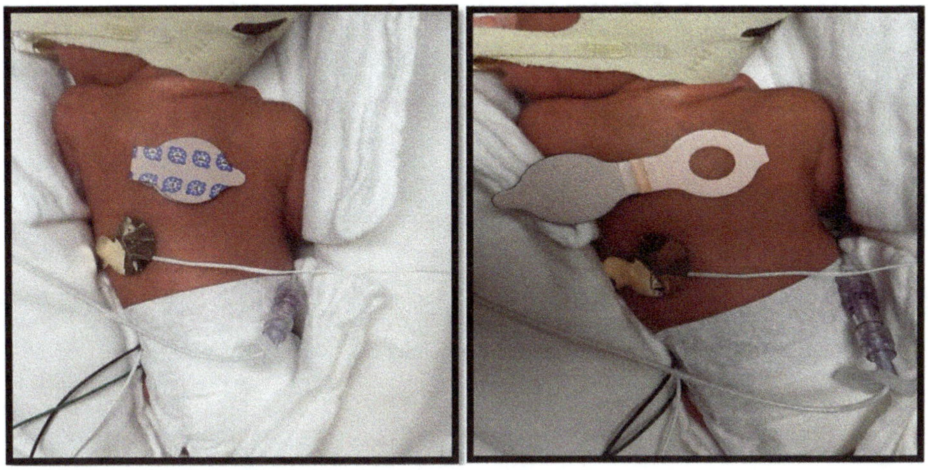

Fig. 1 Demonstrating photo-opaque patch placement in an ELBW neonate

PHT demonstrated significant benefits in neurodevelopmental outcomes [5].

Transcutaneous bilirubinometry is a quick, painless and reliable alternative to serum bilirubin measurements in the management of hyperbilirubinemia [6]. Following PHT, TcB measurements are considered unreliable, as PHT causes bleaching of the skin [7]. We and others have identified a moderate correlation between TcB measurements taken from skin covered by an opaque patch and TSB levels in term and late preterm infants following phototherapy [8, 9]; however, there is little data on the reliability of TcB-C in ELBW infants. We aim to investigate if TcB-C following PHT exposure is a suitable surrogate for TSB in ELBW infants.

Methods

A prospective observational study was performed in NICU at University of Texas Medical Branch (UTMB) at Galveston after approval from the local institutional review board (IRB). Subjects were enrolled in the study from January 2014 to June 2016. The study population consisted of ELBW infants born at UTMB receiving phototherapy for hyperbilirubinemia. ELBW infants were defined as infants with a birth weight of less than 1000 g. Following IRB approval, subjects were enrolled in the study with parental assent. The requirement for written consent was waved by the IRB at our institution. In our NICU, all ELBW infants get prophylactic PHT for first 5 days. All ELBW infants were eligible for the study. Infants with congenital viral infections, conjugated hyperbilirubinemia, sepsis, major congenital malformations, ABO/Rh incompatibility or gastrointestinal illness were excluded from the study.

Table 1 Patient demographics

Sample size	19
Males	13 (68%)
Females	6 (32%)
Gestational age (in weeks)	26 ± 2
Birth weight (in grams)	827 ± 127 g
Race	19 (100%)
Caucasian	6 (31.6%)
African-American	3 (15.8%)
Hispanic	8 (42.1%)
Other	2 (10.5%)

Prior to starting PHT, an opaque patch was placed on the back of the infant. (Fig. 1) The forehead could not be used to place the patch as most of these infants required CPAP. After placing the opaque patch, PHT was started by using a Giraffe Blue Lite PT system (GE Healthcare, Chicago, IL) and continued for 5 days. TcB-C, TcB-E and TSB levels were obtained at birth and every 24 h for 5 days by trained NICU nurses. TcB-C was obtained from the skin covered by the opaque patch. TcB-E was obtained from a site not covered by the patch but adjacent to it. TcB measurements were obtained using the Respironics™ BiliCheck noninvasive bilirubin meter. Clinical data was collected from the electronic medical record (EMR) and included gestational age, birth weight, sex, ethnicity, blood group, maternal blood group, and ABO/Rh incompatibility, if any.

Serum bilirubin levels (TSB) were used as the gold standard. The required sample size for each method was calculated using a power analysis. The power analysis indicated that 32 subjects (16 in each group) were needed to have 80% power for detecting a medium-sized effect (± 0.5 mg/dl) with $p < 0.05$ for statistical significance. A Wilcoxon signed rank test was used to compare the means of the absolute difference between transcutaneous and serum bilirubin measurements for each patient at each time point (24, 48, 72 and 96 h).

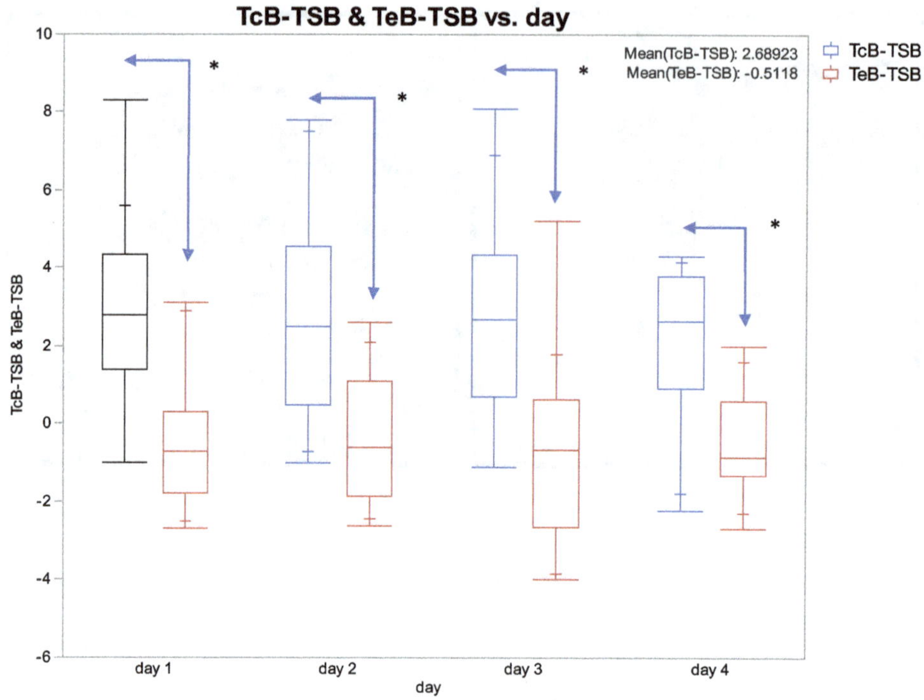

* (P < 0.05)

Fig. 2 Graph depicting the difference between TcB-C or TcB-E and TSB on various days

The absolute difference between transcutaneous and serum bilirubin measurements for each patient is shown on a Bland-Altman plot for easy visualization. Analysis was performed using a mixed effect model to account for repeated measures over time. All analysis was done using JMP® Pro software.

Results

Twenty subjects were initially enrolled in the study. One subject was excluded from the study due to neonatal demise at day 2 of life. The mean birth weight was 827 ± 127 g, and the mean estimated gestational age was 26 ±2 weeks. Caucasians, Hispanics and African-Americans constituted the majority of study group participants. Patient demographics are shown in Table 1. Differences between TcB-C or TcB-E and TSB are shown in Fig. 2.

A Wilcoxon signed rank test was used to compare the TcB-C or TcB-E to TSB. The mean of difference between TcB-C and TSB was 2.68 ± 2.41 mg/dl ($p < 0.001$, IQR 1.1–4.2) mg/dl. In contrast, the mean of difference between TcB-E and TSB was − 0.51 ± 1.74 mg/dl ($p = 0.02$, IQR -1.77 – 0.47, shown in Table 2 and Fig. 3) The absolute differences between the TcB-C or TcB-E and TSB for each patient were like the trends seen in the Wilcoxon signed rank test and are depicted as Bland Altman plots for easy visualization (Fig. 4). TcB-C overestimated serum bilirubin levels for most patients with a difference of 2.71 ± 0.49 mg/dl ($p < 0.001$), while TcB-E underestimated serum bilirubin levels with a difference of − 0.51 ± 0.26 mg/dl ($p = 0.07$).

Similar results were obtained following adjustment of the bilirubin estimation for repeated measures over time. There was no effect of randomization of the day of bilirubin estimation on the overall results. The TcB-C continued to overestimate the TSB ($p < 0.001$), while TcB-E continued to underestimate the TSB ($p < 0.001$). However, when the bilirubin estimation was randomized for each patient the overall model improved by 18.9% and this difference was found to be significant ($p = 0.02$).

Thus, TcB-C overestimates the estimation of bilirubin compared to serum bilirubin, while TcB-E underestimates the estimation of bilirubin compared to serum bilirubin. Hence, TcB-C and TcB-E may not be used as surrogates for bilirubin estimation in ELBW infants receiving phototherapy.

Discussion

We evaluated the role of TcB estimation in ELBW infants who were receiving PHT. We found TcB-C did not

Table 2 Serum (TSB) and transcutaneous bilirubin measurements (TcB-C/TcB-E)

	Mean	SD	IQ range (25–75%)	SEM	*P* value
TcB-C – TSB	2.68	2.41	1.1–4.2	0.29	< 0.001
TcB-E – TSB	−0.51	1.74	−1.77 – 0.47	0.21	0.02

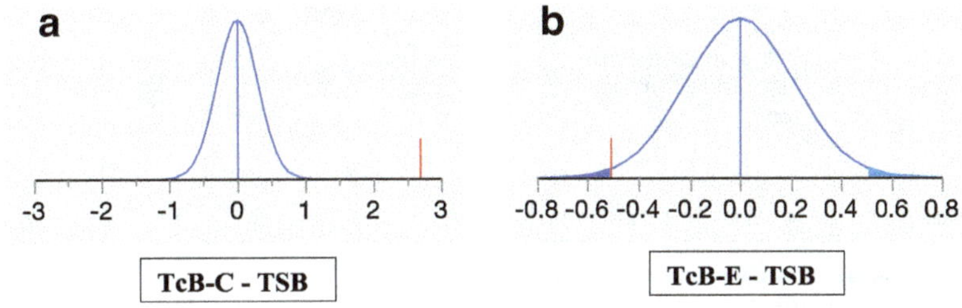

Fig. 3 **a** The probability density function and the mean of difference between the TcB-C and TSB. **b** The probability density function and the mean of difference between the TcB-E and TSB. The vertical bar represents the mean compared to the normal distribution

correlate well with TSB levels in ELBW infants and, in fact, were often higher than TSB. Within 24 h of PHT exposure, TSB values decreased significantly compared to the TcB-C values and thereafter the values decline gradually. Skin exposure to PHT converts unconjugated bilirubin into its water-soluble isomer by photoisomerisation. There is a continuous and bidirectional movement of bilirubin isomers between the blood and the skin leading to skin bleaching [10]. During PHT exposure, TcB drops due to skin bleaching. But if a part of the skin is covered by a photo-opaque patch bleaching will be minimal. The lateral movement of bilirubin from exposed to the covered areas of skin is also minimal, thus accounting for the higher bilirubin levels in the covered areas of skin [11]. This finding in our study is similar to

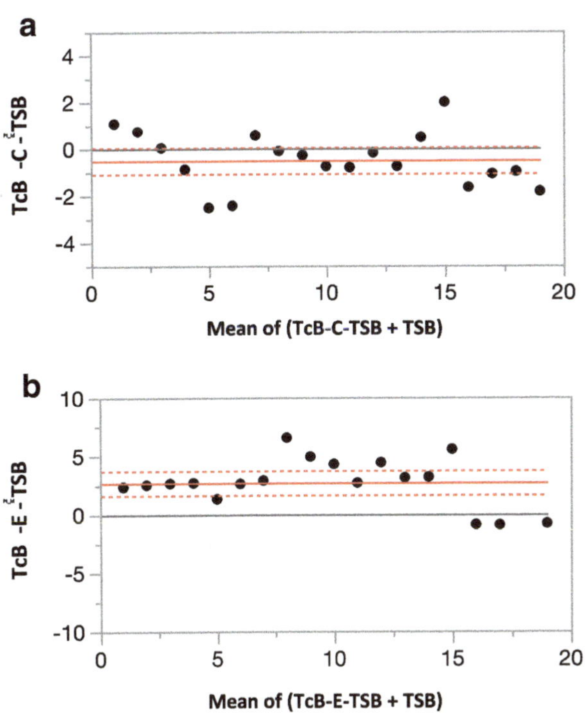

Fig. 4 **a** A Bland Altman plot depicting the difference between TcB-C and TSB for each patient. **b** A Bland Altman plot depicting the difference between TcB-E and TSB for each patient

that reported by by Ozkan, et al., who noted that TcB-C was slower to decline compared to TSB and TcB-E values. In their study, TcB-E levels declined rapidly in the first 6 h after starting PHT, while the decline in TcB-C was not noticed until 12 h after starting PHT. Serum bilirubin values were noted to decline gradually during the study period.

In studies performed in term and preterm infants, the TcB-C levels were found to be comparable with serum bilirubin levels [8]. This was likely due to a gradual decline in TSB levels, permitting equilibration of TcB-C with TSB. However, in our study TSB levels were significantly lower than TcB C levels. This significant decline in TSB in ELBW infants is likely multifactorial in nature. First, bilirubin clearance depends on a multiple factors including wavelength of light used for PHT, irradiance of light, skin surface area exposed to PHT, and rates at which bilirubin is removed from skin and blood [12]. Stratum corneum in ELBW is immature [13], allowing rapid clearance of bilirubin from exposed areas of the skin (bleaching effect) leading to a significant decline in TcB-E levels. Second, since bilirubin levels in the skin rapidly decline following initiation of phototherapy, equilibration between the skin and serum leads to a rapid decline in serum bilirubin levels.

Our study has a few limitations. The sample size of the study population was small and the study was not adequately powered to reliably predict secondary outcomes such as the correlation between TSB and TcB-E values. We measured serum bilirubin at 24-h intervals which may have affected the micro trends in bilirubin levels via different methods during the first 24 h. More frequent bilirubin sampling may be helpful in delineating dermal bilirubin kinetics in ELBW infants.

Conclusions

We suggest that TcB-C is not be a helpful surrogate for TSB in ELBW infants receiving PHT. Studies in larger cohorts may be needed to further substantiate these findings. In the future, we suggest measuring TcB and TSB at shorter intervals and in larger cohorts to evaluate the dermal bilirubin kinetics.

Abbreviations
NICU: Neonatal intensive care unit; PHT: Phototherapy; TcB-C: Transcutaneous bilirubin estimation from covered areas of skin; TcB-E: Transcutaneous bilirubin estimation from exposed areas of skin; TSB: Total serum bilirubin; UTMB: University of Texas Medical Branch, Galveston

Acknowledgments
The authors would like to acknowledge and thank the NICU transport nurses at UTMB for their sincere dedication and contribution in data collection for the study. A special mention to Cheryl Napuli RN, Christie Talbert RN and Regina Garrison RN for their help in completing the study.

Authors' contributions
VB was involved in patient enrollment, data collection, data interpretation and writing the manuscript. BN was involved in the statistical analysis and review of the manuscript. SKJ was involved in the study design, and obtaining approval for the study. He was also involved in data interpretation and review of the manuscript. DT was involved in the statistical analysis and review of the manuscript. He was also involved in reviewing the revision of the manuscript. All authors read and approved the final manuscript.

Competing interests
The authors declare that they have no competing interests.

Author details
[1]Department of Pediatrics, Division of Pediatric Critical Care, Lucile Salter Packard Children's Hospital, 770 Welch Road, Suite 435, Palo Alto, CA 94304, USA. [2]Department of Pediatrics, University of Texas Medical Branch, Galveston, TX, USA. [3]Department of Pediatrics, Division of Neonatology, University of Texas Medical Branch, Galveston, TX, USA.

References
1. Woodgate P, Jardine LA. Neonatal jaundice: phototherapy. BMJ Clin Evid. 2015;2015
2. Pearlman MA, Gartner LM, Lee K, Morecki R, Horoupian DS. Absence of kernicterus in low-birth weight infants from 1971 through 1976: comparison with findings in 1966 and 1967. Pediatrics. 1978;62(4):460–4.
3. Johnson L, Bhutani VK, Karp K, Sivieri EM, Shapiro SM. Clinical report from the pilot USA kernicterus registry (1992 to 2004). J Perinatol. 2009;29(Suppl 1):S25–45.
4. Hyperbilirubinemia AAoPSo. Management of hyperbilirubinemia in the newborn infant 35 or more weeks of gestation. Pediatrics. 2004;114(1):297–316.
5. Morris BH, Oh W, Tyson JE, Stevenson DK, Phelps DL, O'Shea TM, McDavid GE, Perritt RL, Van Meurs KP, Vohr BR, et al. Aggressive vs. conservative phototherapy for infants with extremely low birth weight. N Engl J Med. 2008;359(18):1885–96.
6. Bajpai PC, Agarwal SS, Kapoor CL, Krishna Murti CR. Skin as the site of photoconversion of bilirubin in hyperbilirubinaemia of the new born. Indian J Med Res. 1976;64(8):1214–9.
7. Tan KL, Dong F. Transcutaneous bilirubinometry during and after phototherapy. Acta Paediatr. 2003;92(3):327–31.
8. Fonseca R, Kyralessa R, Malloy M, Richardson J, Jain SK. Covered skin transcutaneous bilirubin estimation is comparable with serum bilirubin during and after phototherapy. J Perinatol. 2012;32(2):129–31.
9. Nagar G, Vandermeer B, Campbell S, Kumar M. Effect of phototherapy on the reliability of transcutaneous bilirubin devices in term and near-term infants: a systematic review and meta-analysis. Neonatology. 2016;109(3):203–12.
10. Ozkan H, Oren H, Duman N, Duman M. Dermal bilirubin kinetics during phototherapy in term neonates. Acta Paediatr. 2003;92(5):577–81.
11. Hegyi T, Hiatt IM, Indyk L. Transcutaneous bilirubinometry. I. Correlations in term infants. J Pediatr. 1981;98(3):454–7.
12. Hegyi T, Hiatt IM, Gertner IM, Zanni R, Tolentino T. Transcutaneous bilirubinometry II. Dermal bilirubin kinetics during phototherapy. Pediatr Res. 1983;17(11):888–91.
13. Kanti V, Bonzel A, Stroux A, Proquitté H, Bührer C, Blume-Peytavi U, Bartels NG. Postnatal maturation of skin barrier function in premature infants. Skin Pharmacol Physiol. 2014;27(5):234–41.

13

An outbreak of Coxsackievirus A6–associated hand, foot, and mouth disease in a kindergarten in Beijing in 2015

Jie Li[1,2†], Rong Zhu[1†], Da Huo[2], Yiwei Du[2], Yuxiang Yan[1], Zhichao Liang[2], Yanxia Luo[1], Yang Yang[2], Lei Jia[2], Lijuan Chen[2], Quanyi Wang[2*] and Yan He[1*]

Abstract

Background: Coxsackievirus A6 (CVA6) is one of the major agents to cause hand, foot and mouth disease (HFMD) outbreaks globally. The objective of this study is to investigate the epidemiologic and clinical manifestations of CVA6 outbreak, and thus guide the diagnosis and treatment of the disease, as well as disease prevention.

Methods: An HFMD outbreak in a kindergarten was reported to Shijingshan District Center for Disease Control and Prevention (SCDC) on November 2, 2015 in Beijing, China. Epidemiological investigation was conducted. We performed a nine-week follow-up study to collect and analyze the clinical manifestations of HFMD cases.

Results: The outbreak yield 56 (15.7%) clinical diagnosed HFMD cases out of 357 registered children in the kindergarten with the mean age of 3.5 years old. This outbreak lasted for three days and ceased after initiating infectious disease controlling procedures, including periodical suspension of the kindergarten activities, environmental disinfection, and family health education. Fifty-one cases were followed for nine weeks. The positive rate of clinical manifestations of rash, fever, desquamation, pigmentation and onychomadesis were 100.0%, 84.3%, 68.6%, 17.6% and 43.1%, respectively. Children developed desquamation within the first 4 weeks after disease onset and developed onychomadesis between the 3th and 8th week after disease onset. Children with desquamation had 9.3 (95%CI: 1.836–47.437) times higher odds of developing onychomadesis compared to those without this manifestation. Ten out of 14 collected samples were CVA6 positive, and five positive samples shared a high degree of similarity in the VP1 nucleotide and amino acid sequences (99.9–100.0% and 100%).

Conclusion: This HFMD outbreak was caused by CVA6, featured with delayed symptoms. Emerging CVA6-associated HFMD and its delayed symptoms should be paid more attention to reduce outbreaks and provide more information to doctors and parents.

Keywords: Hand foot and mouth disease, Disease outbreak, Coxsackievirus A6, Onychomadesis

Background

Hand, foot and mouth disease (HFMD) is an infectious disease characterized by clinical symptoms of vesicular rashes and stomatitis of the oral mucosa affecting patients' hands, feet and occasionally the buttocks. The most susceptible patient population of HFMD is children less than 5 years old. HFMD is caused by viruses belonging to the species Enterovirus A or B, genus Enterovirus, family Picornaviridae, among which, human enterovirus 71 (EV-A71) and Coxsackievirus A16 (CVA16) were the most prevalent pathogens in previous publications [1–3]. Only EV-A71 is almost exclusively associated with severe disease.

From 2012 onward, Coxsackievirus A6 (CVA6) has been reported as an emerging pathogen of the HFMD epidemic globally. In 2013, the etiological surveillance system in Beijing and other cities in China identified a

* Correspondence: bjcdcxm@126.com; heyanlb2014@163.com
†Jie Li and Rong Zhu contributed equally to this work.
[2]Institute for Infectious Disease and Endemic Disease Control, Beijing Center for Disease Prevention and Control, No.16, Hepingli Middle Street, Beijing 100013, People's Republic of China
[1]Department of Epidemiology and Biostatistics, School of Public Health, Capital Medical University, No. 10 Xitoutiao, You'anmen Wai, Fengtai District, Beijing 100069, People's Republic of China

sudden rise of CVA6 positive rate, which turned out to be one of the predominant pathogens of HFMD [4–7]. Since then, CVA6 has spread across mainland China and drawn serious public health attention.

In 2015, there were in total six HFMD outbreaks occurred in the kindergartens in Beijing. The number of cases ranged from 11 to 14 among the five of them, and remaining one had 56 cases. This outbreak occurred in a kindergarten in Shijingshan district in Beijing. There were 357 children and 51 school staffs in this kindergarten. The children were divided and assigned to 11 classes (average class size was 32). Daily extra-curricular activities were held, in which children from different classes attended lessons together. We performed a further investigation on this large-scale HFMD outbreak in this kindergarten and found that it was caused by CVA6 infection.

In this study, we aimed to collect and summarize epidemiological and clinical evidence of CVA6 infected HFMD, and thus to support and guide the diagnosis, treatment, prevention and control of the disease.

Methods

Case definition and outbreak definition

A clinical case of HFMD was defined as presenting with oral ulcers and maculopapular or vesicular rash distributed over the hands, feet and buttocks, with or without fever. Cases were classified as severe if they presented any cardiopulmonary complications (pulmonary edema, pulmonary hemorrhage, or cardiorespiratory failure) or neurological complications (aseptic meningitis, encephalitis, encephalomyelitis, acute flaccid paralysis, or autonomic nervous system dysregulation) [8].

According to the "Protocol of control practice for the clustered cases and outbreaks of hand foot and mouth disease" issued by the National Health and Family Planning Commission of China in 2012 [9], an HFMD outbreak was defined as ≥10 cases of HFMD occurring in a kindergarten or school within a week. Once an outbreak is reported from a kindergarten or a school, the health practitioners from local CDC will have a risk assessment on the situation, upon which a school suspension decision will be made. In order to confirm the disease causing agent of the outbreak, at least five samples are required to be collected and analyzed.

Sample and data collection

Once the district CDC got a report of HFMD outbreak, the epidemiological investigation was conducted immediately. Demographic information (ID, birth date, gender), clinical symptoms (fever, rash, sore throat, desquamation, onychomadesis), and epidemiological data (onset date of HFMD, the date of visiting a hospital, onset date of delayed symptoms, clinical diagnostic result and laboratory test result) and throat swab samples were collected by CDC staffs on the same day of the field investigation with prior written informed consent. The teacher in charge of each classroom was responsible for reporting any new case to the doctors of community healthcare centers who would pay the sick children a home visit, collected information with prior written informed consent, and reported to the local CDC afterwards. Parents or guardians of the sick children were followed up twice by telephone to collect information about the delayed symptoms, such as onychomadesis, desquamation and chromatosis, at 4th and 9th weeks after the onset of HFMD.

Sample processing mode, nucleotide extraction and virus identification

The specimens were vortexed for 1 min and centrifuged at 4000×g for 20 min before nucleotide extraction. Total nucleotide extraction was performed with MagNA Pure LC Total Nucleic Acid Isolation Kit-Large Volume (ROCHE, Co, USA) by a Roche MagNA Pure LC 2.0 nucleic extraction system (ROCHE, Co, USA) according to the manufacturer's instructions. EV, EV-A71 and CVA16 were identified using real-time RT-PCR Kit (DAAN Gene, Guangzhou, China) [10]. Samples of non-EV-A71 and non-CVA16 were further identified by detecting the VP1 region according to previously described method [11]. Complete nucleotide sequences of VP1 genes were amplified using previously described specific primers [12]. Polymerase Chain Reaction (PCR) products of complete VP1 genes were purified and sequenced using ABI PRISM310 Genetic Analyzer.

Phylogenetic analysis of CVA6

To further study the homology of sequences from viruses in this outbreak, sequence analysis of VP1 was carried out using Molecular Evolutionary Genetics Analysis Version 6.0 (MEGA6). The phylogenetic tree was constructed by Maximum likelihood method with bootstrapping of 1000 replicates. A total of 5 CVA6 isolates representing this outbreak were aligned and compared with the corresponding region of CVA6 isolates from HFMD casess through 2009 to 2015 in Beijing.

Statistical analysis

Statistical analysis was conducted using SPSS17.0 software (IBM SPSS Inc., Chicago, IL, USA). Continuous variables in asymmetric distribution were described using the median with 25th and 75th percentiles. Frequencies and proportions were used for categorical variables. Comparisons of proportions were performed using the Chi-square test. A two-tailed p value of less than 0.05 (2-sided significance testing) was considered to be statistically significant.

Ethics statement

This study was in compliance with the Helsinki Declaration and was approved by the Human Research Ethics Committee of Beijing CDC. The approval number of the local ethics committee was 201,809. Sample collection in this study was agreed by the patient's guardian with prior written informed consent.

Results

In 2015, a total of six outbreaks of HFMD occurred in Beijing kindergartens (Table 1). Four out of six outbreaks were caused by CVA6. The remaining two outbreaks were caused by EV71 and CVA16. Among the six outbreaks, the largest one was caused by CVA6, in which 56 cases were identified.

Epidemiological investigation

This outbreak occurred in a kindergarten in Shijingshan district and was reported on November 2, 2015. In response, Shijingshan district CDC (SCDC) initiated an epidemiological investigation immediately.

From October 26th to November 5th, a total of 56 clinically diagnosed cases from 10 classes were reported. The attack rate was 15.7% (56/357). From October 27th to 30th, 16 children from different classes were reported with fever or rash on body. During the following weekend (October 31 and November 1), this outbreak attained the peak and a total of 22 cases were obtained. From November 2nd to 5th, another 17 cases were reported (Fig. 1).

There were 357 children and a health-care doctor in this kindergarten. Every morning, school doctor did regular body checks for each child to see if they present any fever, skin rashes or herpangina. Once a symptom is found, the parents or guardians would be notified to take their children for further medical examination. During the noon break, the same regular body checks would be performed again. The first case in this outbreak appeared on October 26, 2015 a 5-year-old girl who had low-grade fever with no rash on her hands or feet. She felt ill in the afternoon and was taken home by her mother and rested at home for following days. On October 29, her mother found generalized vesicular rashes distributed over her hands and feet and took her to a hospital, where she was diagnosed with HFMD. Her parents did not recall or report exposure to any HFMD cases before diagnosis.

Outbreak control measures

Infection-control measures, including case isolation, contact medical observation, environmental disinfection, suspension of the kindergarten, and health education, were immediately implemented. All the children diagnosed with HFMD were isolated at home for at least 10 days until recovered. Kids could return to kindergarten only if the community health care center proved that they have completely recovered. Classrooms, indoor playground, bathrooms, kitchens and recreation facilities were cleaned and disinfected thoroughly. Based on the fact that children from 10 out of the 11 classes were infected (according to the clinical diagnosis) and HFMD was prone to spread rapidly, the kindergarten was advised to take a periodical suspension for 10 days. The health practitioners from local CDC and health care centers did health education for children and their parents, as well as the kindergarten staffs.

Epidemiological characteristics, clinical manifestations and laboratory test result

During this outbreak, to obtain more detailed information about the prognosis and the delayed symptoms such as desquamation and onychomadesis, we contacted all the HFMD patients in this the outbreak. Five parents of the patients refused, thus, 51(91.1%) volunteered to enroll in this study and were successfully followed up at 4th and 9th week after illness onset. Among the 51 patients, 26 (51.0%) were girls, and the median age was 44 months (IQR 41.0–51.0). Six out of 51 cases (11.8%) had a history of HFMD disease.

All the cases sought for medical treatment and were clinically diagnosed as mild HFMD in seven hospitals and fully recovered without any complications. Epidemiology and clinical presentations of HFMD cases in this study were shown in Table 2. The most common clinical manifestation was skin rash (51/51, 100.0%), followed by fever (43/51, 84.3%). A total of 35 children (68.6%, 35/51)

Table 1 Epidemiology characteristics of six HFMD outbreaks in Beijing in 2015

ID	District	Classification	Number of Cases	Attack rate (%)	[a]Age (year)	Male/Female	Date	Agent
1	Fangshan	Kindergarten	14	17.7	3.0(2.0, 3.0)	2.5:1	Apr	CVA16
2	Mentougou	Kindergarten	16	6.5	4.0(4.0, 5.0)	1.3:1	Jun	CVA6
3	Fangshan	Kindergarten	22	12.0	3.0(3.0, 3.0)	1.8:1	Jul	EV-A71
4	Fengtai	Kindergarten	11	2.1	5.0(5.0, 5.0)	0.8:1	Jul	CVA6
5	Chaoyang	Kindergarten	14	4.0	4.0(4.0, 4.3)	0.8:1	Sep	CVA6
6	Shijingshan	Kindergarten	56	15.7	3.4(3.7, 4.3)	0.9:1	Oct	CVA6

[a]Presented as the median (p25, p75)

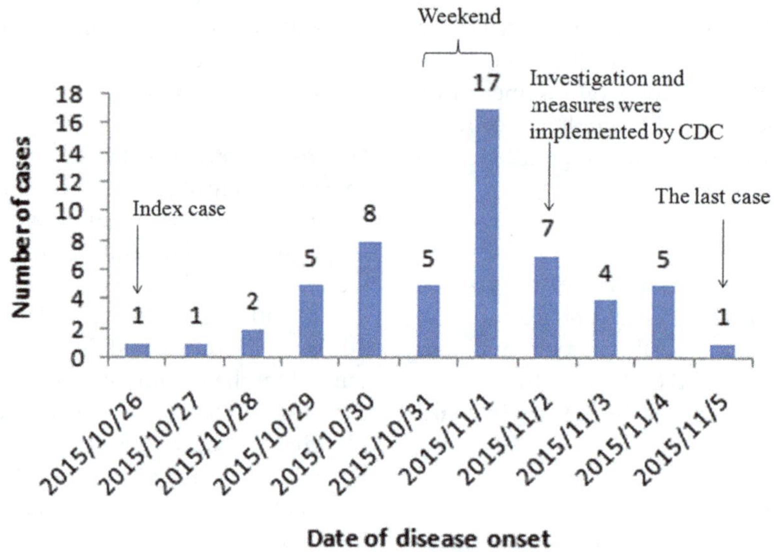

Fig. 1 Number of children with HFMD in the outbreak by date of disease onset ($n = 56$)

developed desquamation within the 1st and the 4rd week after disease onset. Of the 51 patients, 22 (43.1%) experienced onychomadesis between the 3rd and 8th week after disease onset (Additional file 1). The most common location of onychomadesis on the hands and feet were the thumbs (17/51, 33.3%) and halluces (8/51, 15.7%), respectively. In total, 68 finger nails from 22 kids and 17 ft nails from 8 children were found with onychomadesis. Twelve (54.5%, 12/22) cases showed the symptom of onychomadesis on symmetrical location. Among the 51 patients, two (3.9%) lost all their fingernails.

Laboratory results were available among 26 cases which were collected by staffs from the health care community center during home visit. The median WBC count, median CRP value, median lymphocyte count and median lymphocyte percentage of cases were $9.2*10^9$/L (6.8–10.8), 9.4 mg/L (8.0–13.5), $3.1*10^9$/L (2.3–4.0) and 36.0% (24.6–52.4), respectively. The WBC counts of 26.9% (7/26), CRP of 37.5% (6/16) and lymphocyte count of 47.6% (10/21) were above the upper limit of the normal range.

Given that onychomadesis was described as a late complication of HFMD and the role of CVA6 in causing onychomadesis was unclear, we attempted to examine factors associated with the manifestations [13, 14]. As shown in Table 3, age, sex, fever, body temperature, pigmentation and median duration from onset to initial diagnosis were not significantly associated with children's onychomadesis status ($P > 0.05$). Cases with the symptom of desquamation have 9.3 times higher odds (OR = 9.3, 95% CI, 1.836–47.437) of experiencing onychomadesis comparing with those cases without desquamation.

Pathogen detection and phylogenetic analysis

During the outbreak, parents of 14 cases (including the parents of the index case) agreed to provide samples for pathogen detection. A total of 14 throat samples from patients were analyzed, and 10 (71.4%) samples (including the sample from the index case) were CVA6 positive. Another three samples, including a swab throat from the health-care teacher and two samples from the tableware and the toilet, were CVA6 negative. Among five out of ten CVA6 positive samples, the VP1 sequences were successfully amplified. The similarity in the nucleotide and amino acid sequences among them was 99.9–100.0% and 100%, respectively. We analyzed the VP1 of CVA6 viruses from this outbreak (MG488204, MG488205, MG488206, MG488207, and MG488208) and from previous cases during 2009–2015 in Beijing. All the CVA6 strains were classified into five major groups (A-E) (Fig. 2). CVA6 isolates in Beijing from 2009 to 2012 were classified as group D. CVA6 isolates from 2013 to 2015 were classified as group E. The nucleotide identity for CVA6 strains in this study and from 2009 to 2012, 2013–2014 and 2015 in Beijing was 87.7–89.2%, 97.8–99.3% and 94.2–98.3%, respectively. CVA6 strains (including the CVA6 strain from the index case) from the outbreak in this study were all classified as group E.

Discussion

According to the etiology surveillance system of Beijing, in 2009, 2011, 2012, and 2014, CVA16 was identified as the main pathogen of HFMD, while in 2010, EV-A71 was the major pathogen. However, in 2013 and 2015, CVA6 surpassed CVA16 and EV-A71 to become the

Table 2 Epidemiology and clinical presentations of HFMD cases in this study

Characteristics	N (%)
Sex	
Male	25(49.0)
Female	26(51.0)
[a]Age(months)	44(41.0-51.0)
Fever	43(84.3)
[a]Duration(day)	1.5(1.0-2.0)
[a]The highest temperature(°C)	38.7(38.4–39.2)
≥ 39 °C	12(23.5)
Rash	
Hand	48(94.1)
Foot	37(72.5)
Oral cavity	32(62.7)
Perioral area	19(37.3)
Buttock	16(31.4)
Extremity	6(11.8)
Trunk	5(9.8)
Bullous eruption	2(3.9)
Pigmentation	9(17.6)
Desquamation	35(68.6)
Onychomadesis	22(43.1)
Hands	21(41.2)
Thumb	17(33.3)
Forefinger	10(19.6)
Middle finger	8(15.8)
Ring fingers	5(9.8)
Little finger	3(5.9)
Feet	8(15.7)
The big toe	8(15.7)
The second toe	1(2.0)
The third toe	1(2.0)
[a]Median duration from onset to diagnosis(day)	1(0.0–3.0)
Laboratory test	
[a]WBC (10^9/L)	9.2(6.8–10.8)
[a]CRP (mg/L)	9.4(8.0–13.5)
[a]Lymphocyte count(10^9/L)	3.1(2.3–4.0)
[a]Lymphocyte percentage (%)	36.0(24.6–52.4)

WBC, white blood cell; CRP, C-reactive protein
[a]Presented as the median (p25, p75)

Table 3 Factors associated with onychomadesis

	Onychomadesis		OR(95%CI)	P^a
	Yes (%)	No (%)		
Age(month)(n = 51)				
36–47	16(72.7)	15(51.7)	0.402(0.123–1.318)	0.128
48–72	6(27.3)	14(48.3)		
Sex (n = 51)				
Female	9(40.9)	17(58.6)	2.046(0.664–6.311)	0.210
Male	13(59.1)	12(41.4)		
Median duration from onset to initial diagnosis(days)				
≤ 2	16(72.7)	16(55.2)	0.462(0.140–1.517)	0.199
> 2	6(27.3)	13(44.8)		
Fever(n = 51)				
No	5(22.7)	3(10.3)	0.392(0.083–1.860)	0.228
Yes	17(77.3)	26(89.7)		
Temperature(n = 43)				
37.3 ≤ T < 39 °C	13(76.5)	14(53.8)	0.359(0.092–1.399)	0.133
T ≥ 39 °C	4(23.5)	12(46.2)		
Desquamation(n = 51)				
Yes	20(90.9)	15(51.7)	**9.3 (1.836–47.437)**	**0.003**
No	2(9.1)	14(48.3)		
Pigmentation(n = 51)				
No	16(72.7)	26(89.7)	3.250(0.711–14.851)	0.150
Yes	6(27.3)	3(10.3)		

[a]$P < 0.05$ from the x^2 test was considered to be significant
The bold values means significant difference was obtained between compared groups

predominant pathogen of HFMD [15]. In our study, CVA6 virus was identified as the dominant causative agent, which is consistent with the epidemic background of HFMD in Beijing during 2015.

Considering the fact that the average incubation period of HFMD ranges from 3 to 7 days [16], and it might begin to shed enterovirus prior to symptom onset, we speculated that the index case or someone else was the source of infection in this kindergarten [17].

Kindergartens are a highly susceptible location for HFMD outbreaks because large groups of children with close contact could create an excellent incubation site for HFMD. Children are easily infected and more likely easily to spread this disease [18]. In this outbreak, HFMD rapidly spread across 10 of the 11 classes within 11 days. It ceased after the HFMD control measures were implemented by SCDC. We speculated that at least two factors contributed to this rapid transmission. First, the interaction among children from different classes could accelerate the spread of the agent. Second, according to our previous study, some children can transmit the virus prior to symptom onset [17], and infected patients can excrete the virus for a long time. Given the highly infectious characteristics of HFMD, we strongly suggested that cases should be isolated and that thorough environmental disinfection be performed immediately once a case appeared.

As is known, EV-A71 vaccines are available in mainland China, and the protective efficacies are higher than

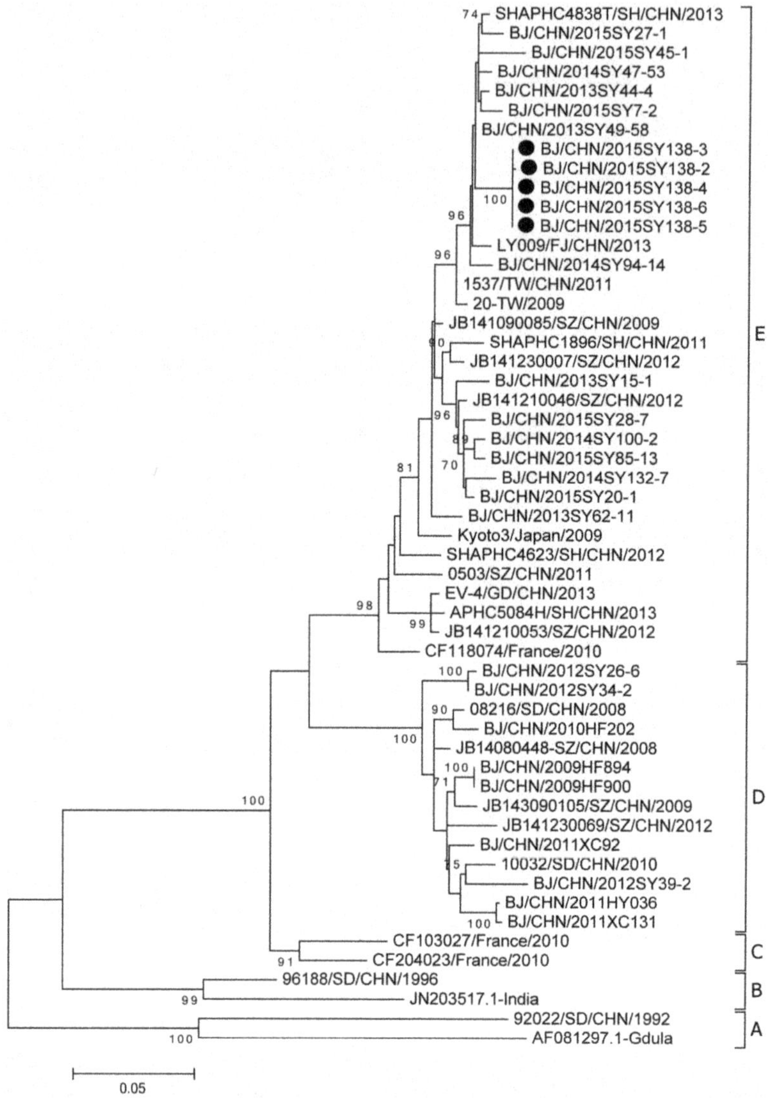

Fig. 2 Phylogenetic dendrogram based on the alignment of the complete VP1 gene sequence of CVA6 (915 bp). CVA6 strains isolated from this outbreak were indicated by a solid dot

90% against EV-A71-associated HFMD [19]. However, these vaccines cannot protect people from suffering from HFMD caused by CVA6 [20]. In the absence of any effective vaccine or antiviral therapy, primary prevention is the most effective measure to prevent the outbreak of CVA6-associated HFMD.

A previous study has reported that different genetic background strains may cause different clinical manifestations of HFMD [21]. Confirmed by the VP1 gene sequencing, our results suggested that this outbreak was caused by the same CVA6. In this study, five out of ten CVA6-positive HFMD cases developed onychomadesis. Based on the results of this study, we proposed that the difference in clinical presentations might be correlated with the host background apart from the causative pathogen. Moreover, we found that patients with symptoms of desquamation had a 9.3-time chance of experiencing onychomadesis comparing with cases without desquamation. Combining the fact that desquamation in most cases appeared earlier than onychomadesis, we suggest that desquamation might be used as an indicator of developing onychomadesis. Based on the current situation that parents and even some physicians know little about HFMD related onychomadesis, misdiagnosis could happen. We hope that this study can provide evidence for the early treatment of HFMD and help address the concerns of the parents.

There are several limitations. First, we did not assess the effectiveness of individual control measure. Second, the data collection was telephone-based and recall bias might exist. Third, due to limited knowledge about the late symptoms of HFMD, the appearance of desquamation, onychomadesis or pigmentation might be underestimated.

Conclusion

In summary, the 2015 Beijing HFMD outbreak was caused by CVA6, featured with delayed symptoms. Health care providers and parents need to pay more attention and raise awareness towards the CVA6-HFMD to be able to better control and prevent future disease outbreak.

Abbreviations

CDC: Center for Disease Control and Prevention; CRP: C-reactive protein; CVA16: Coxsackievirus A16; CVA6: Coxsackievirus A6; EV-A71: Human enterovirus 71; HFMD: Hand, foot and mouth disease; WBC: White blood cell

Acknowledgments

We thank those participants in this study who provided samples and clinical data. We also thank the staffs who work in the SCDC and local health care centers for collecting epidemiological information and samples during the execution of this study.

Funding

This work was supported by grants of key projects in the National Science & Technology Pillar Program (2015BAI09B01). This work was also supported by the grant from Beijing Natural Science Foundation to YH (7132027) and the grant from Beijing Natural Science Foundation to JL (7164240).

Authors' contributions

JL and RZ carried out the experimental design, participated in the experiment and drafted the manuscript. They contributed equally to this study and share first authorship. DH, YD and YY participated in the experimental design, performed the data analysis, and reviewed the manuscript. LZ, YL and YY participated in the experiment and reviewed the manuscript. LJ and LC participated in the clinical data collection, analysis, and reviewed the manuscript. QW and YH contributed to the experimental design and coordination with District Centers for Disease Control and Prevention and provided a final review of this manuscript. All authors read and approved the final manuscript.

Competing interests

The authors declare that they have no competing interests.

References

1. Ooi MH, Wong SC, Lewthwaite P, Cardosa MJ, Solomon T. Clinical features, diagnosis, and management of enterovirus 71. Lancet Neurol J. 2010;9:1097–105.
2. Abzug MJ. The enteroviruses: problems in need of treatments. J Inf Secur. 2014;68(Suppl 1):S108–14.
3. He Y, Zou L, Chong MK, Men R, Xu W, Yang H, et al. Genetic evolution of human enterovirus A71 subgenotype C4 in Shenzhen, China, 1998-2013. J Inf Secur. 2016;72:731–7.
4. Hongyan G, Chengjie M, Qiaozhi Y, Wenhao H, Juan L, Lin P, et al. Hand, foot and mouth disease caused by coxsackievirus A6, Beijing, 2013. Pediatr Infect Dis. 2014;33:1302–3.
5. Tan X, Li L, Zhang B, Jorba J, Su X, Ji T, et al. Molecular epidemiology of coxsackievirus A6 associated with outbreaks of hand, foot, and mouth disease in Tianjin, China, in 2013. Arch Virol. 2015;160:1097–104.
6. Hu YQ, Xie GC, Li DD, Pang LL, Xie J, Wang P, et al. Prevalence of Coxsackievirus A6 and enterovirus 71 in hand, foot and mouth disease in Nanjing, China in 2013. Pediatr Infect Dis J. 2015;34:951–7.
7. Han JF, Xu S, Zhang Y, Zhu SY, Wu DL, Yang XD, et al. Hand, foot, and mouth disease outbreak caused by coxsackievirus A6, China, 2013. J Inf Secur. 2014;69:303–5.
8. Xing W, Liao Q, Viboud C, Zhang J, Sun J, et al. Hand, foot, and mouth disease in China, 2008-12: an epidemiological study. Lancet Infect Dis. 2014;14:308–18.
9. The national health and Family Planning Commission. (2012) Protocol of control practice for the clustered cases and outbreaks of hand foot and mouth disease. http://www.chinacdc.cn/jkzt/crb/szkb/jszl_2275/201206/t20120629_63852.htm. Accessed 1 June 2012.
10. Ministry of Health of the People's Republic of China. Protocol of sample collection and laboratory tests for HFMD cases. http://www.chinacdc.cn/jkzt/crb/szkb/jszl_2275/200906/t20090612_24707.htm. Accessed 2009.
11. Nix WA, Oberste MS, Pallansch MA. Sensitive, seminested PCR amplification of VP1 sequences for direct identification of all enterovirus serotypes from original clinical specimens. J Clin Microbiol. 2006;44:2698–704.
12. Sinclair C, Gaunt E, Simmonds P, Broomfield D, Nwafor N, et al. Atypical hand, foot, and mouth disease associated with coxsackievirus A6 infection, Edinburgh, United Kingdom, January to February 2014. Euro Surveill. 2014;19:20745.
13. Jacobsen L, Zimmerman S, Lohr J. Nail findings in hand-foot-and-mouth disease. Pediatr Infect Dis J. 2015;34:449–50.
14. Apalla Z, Sotiriou E, Pikou O, Lefaki I, Lallas A, Lazaridou E, et al. Onychomadesis after hand-foot-and-mouth disease outbreak in northern Greece: case series and brief review of the literature. Int J Dermatol. 2015;54:1039–44.
15. Li J, Sun Y, Du Y, Yan Y, Huo D, Liu Y, et al. Characterization of Coxsackievirus A6- and enterovirus 71-associated hand foot and mouth disease in Beijing, China, from 2013 to 2015. Front Microbiol. 2016;7:391.
16. Wong SS, Yip CC, Lau SK, Yuen KY. Human enterovirus 71 and hand, foot and mouth disease. Epidemiol Infect. 2010;138:1071–89.
17. Li J, Lin C, Qu M, Li X, Gao Z, et al. Excretion of enterovirus 71 in persons infected with hand, foot and mouth disease. Virol J. 2013;10:31.
18. Kar BR, Dwibedi B, Kar SK. An outbreak of hand, foot and mouth disease in Bhubaneswar, Odisha. Indian Pediatr. 2013;50:139–42.
19. Chen YJ, Meng FY, Mao Q, Li JX, Wang H, Liang ZL, et al. Clinical evaluation for batch consistency of an inactivated enterovirus 71 vaccine in a large-scale phase 3 clinical trial. Hum Vaccin Immunother. 2014;10:1366–72.
20. Liu CC, Chow YH, Chong P, Klein M. Prospect and challenges for the development of multivalent vaccines against hand, foot and mouth diseases. Vaccine. 2014;32:6177–82.
21. Chen YJ, Chang SC, Tsao KC, Shih SR, Yang SL, Lin TY, et al. Comparative genomic analysis of coxsackievirus A6 strains of different clinical disease entities. PLoS One. 2012;7:e52432.

14

Clinical profile of comorbidity of rare diseases in a Tunisian patient: a case report associating incontinentia pigmenti and Noonan syndrome

Nehla Ghedira[1,2*], Arnaud Lagarde[2,4], Karim Ben Ameur[3,1], Sahar Elouej[2,6], Rania Sakka[1,3], Emna Kerkeni[1], Fatma-Zohra Chioukh[3,1], Sylviane Olschwang[2,4,5], Jean-Pierre Desvignes[2], Sonia Abdelhak[6], Valerie Delague[2], Nicolas Lévy[2,4], Kamel Monastiri[3,1] and Annachiara De Sandre-Giovannoli[2,4]

Abstract

Background: Noonan syndrome (NS) is an autosomal dominant multisystem disorder caused by the dysregulation of several genes belonging to the RAS Mitogen Activated Protein Kinase (MAPK) signaling pathway. Incontinentia Pigmenti (IP) is an X-linked, dominantly inherited multisystem disorder.

Case presentation: This study is the first report of the coexistence of Noonan (NS) and Incontinentia Pigmenti (IP) syndromes in the same patient. We report on the clinical phenotype and molecular characterization of this patient. The patient was examined by a pluridisciplinary staff of clinicians and geneticist. The clinical diagnosis of NS and IP was confirmed by molecular investigations. The newborn girl came to our clinics due to flagrant dysmorphia and dermatological manifestations. The clinical observations led to characterize the Incontinentia Pigmenti traits and a suspicion of a Noonan syndrome association. Molecular diagnosis was performed by Haloplex resequencing of 29 genes associated with RASopathies and confirmed the NS diagnosis. The common recurrent intragenic deletion mutation in *IKBKG* gene causing the IP was detected with an improved PCR protocol.

Conclusion: This is the first report in the literature of comorbidity of NS and IP, two rare multisystem syndromes.

Keywords: Noonan syndrome, RAS-MAPK pathway, RAF1, Dysmorphism, Incontinentia Pigmenti, X-linked disorder, Comorbidity, Next generation sequencing

Background

Noonan syndrome (NS, OMIM 163950) is one of the most frequent genetic disorders in children with an autosomal dominant pattern of inheritance [1, 2]. This multisystem disease is variably expressed with an estimated prevalence of 1 in 1000–2500 live births [1, 3].

The clinical diagnosis of NS is established on the basis of distinctive features according to different criteria developed by Van Der Burgt and *al* [4] in 1994. Constant clinical traits characterizing this syndrome include: dysmorphic facial features, variable developmental delay with constant short stature, congenital heart defects and chest wall anomaly often consisting of pectus carinatum or/and pectus excavatum [5–7]. NS has also a distinct constellation of ectodermal manifestations that depends on the mutated gene including short and curly hair, loose anagen hair, absent eye-brows, erythema, and granular cell tumors, abnormal pigmented lesions (multiple pigmented naevi, "café au lait" spots and freckles. Keratosis pilaris can also occurs [8–11].

NS has a heterogeneous genetic background that involves genes encoding proteins with roles in the RAS MAPK pathway [5, 12–14]. Gain of function mutations in the *PTPN11* gene (OMIM 176876) are found in 40–50% of NS patients [10, 15, 16]. Other mutations in

* Correspondence: gnehla@yahoo.fr
[1]Research Unit 01/UR/08-14, Faculty of Medicine of Monastir, University of Monastir, Avenue Avicenne, 5019 Monastir, Tunisia
[2]Aix Marseille University, INSERM, GMGF, Marseille, France

several genes of the cascade are less frequent: e.g. in *SOS1* (OMIM 182530, about 11% of cases), *RAF1* (OMIM 164760, about 5% of cases), *SHOC2* (OMIM 602775, about 2% of cases), *KRAS* (OMIM 190070, about 1.5% of cases), *NRAS* (OMIM 164790, about 0.2% of cases), *CBL* (OMIM 165360), *RIT1* (OMIM 609591) and recently, with the emergence of NGS technologies in the molecular characterization of rare diseases, other genes have been implicated such as *RRAS* (OMIM 165090), *RASA2* (OMIM 601589), *SOS2* (OMIM 601247) and *LZTR1* (OMIM 600774) [5, 17–19]. Nevertheless, about 30% of NS cases remain without molecular confirmation.

Familial Incontinentia Pigmenti (IP, OMIM 308300) is a rare X-linked dominant genodermatosis that affects ectodermal tissues and is usually prenatally lethal in males [20, 21]. However, some affected males have been reported, either presenting with X-chromosome somatic mosaicism or a concomitant diagnosis of Klinefelter syndrome [22]. In total, 900 to 1200 individuals with IP have been reported in the literature.

More than 80% of IP patients have a recurrent genomic large-scale deletion of exons 4–10 of the *NEMO* gene (*IKBKG*, OMIM 300248), which encodes a regulatory component of the IKB Kinase complex, leading to loss of NF-KB activation and increased apoptosis. Although hypomorphic mutations and CNVs have been reported, the architecture of the NEMO/IKBKG locus seems to facilitate genome instability generating the high frequency of de novo rearrangements observed in IP patients [20, 23, 24].

Case presentation

The patient was a one- month- old baby girl referred to our center for a congenital heart defect. The baby was born at full term (40-week s gestation). Pregnancy, as well as the perinatal period, were unremarkable. The baby had facial dysmorphism with broad forehead, hypertelorism, down-slanting palpebral fissures, a high arched palate, bifid uvula and low set posteriorly rotated ears, long philtrum and epicanthal folds (Fig. 1a, b). Echocardiography showed pulmonic stenosis. During the first week of life, the baby developed Incontinentia Pigmenti, a typical skin rush that started with papules, vesicles and pustules on an erythematous base, followed by plaques and warty papules linearly arranged over erythematous lesions, then a linear brownish pigmentation involving the trunk and the extremities developed by the age of 1 month. All these skin lesions were distributed along the lines of Blaschko (Fig. 1c-f). No dental or eye anomalies were observed. She had congenital stridor, delayed neurological development and growth retardation (weight was 4000 g at 2 months, < P3). These findings were consistent with Noonan syndrome associated with Incontinentia Pigmenti based on "Incontinentia Pigmenti diagnostic criteria update" by Minicand *al* [25]. The phenotypes of the two syndromes evolved with the age of the patient (Fig. 1g-j).

Methods

The clinical data were compiled by clinical geneticists and pediatricians (R. S, K.BA, K.M, and FZ.C). The patient's parents signed written informed consent to consultation and molecular studies for both diagnostic and research purposes and also for publication of the patient's pictures. Along this, parents give also their consent for participation in genetic testing in addition to their child. This work complies with the declaration of Helsinki (https://www.wma.net/policies-post/wma-declaration-of-helsinki-ethical-principles-for-medical-research-involving-human-subjects/) and with the ethical guidelines of the institutions involved. Genomic DNA of the patient and her parents was manually extracted from peripheral blood collected in EDTA tubes according to standard salting out methods and purified by QIAmp CDN kit (Qiagen). DNA quality and quantity were measured on Nanodrop Spectrophotometer (Thermo Scientific) and by Qubit ds S Assay on Qubit 2.0 Fluorometer (Thermo Fisher Scientific).

NGS analysis

A panel of 29 genes was designed using the online Sure Design software (Agilent Technologies). A predesigned Haloplex Noonan panel containing the genes *PTPN11, SOS1, RAF1, KRAS, BRAF, NRAS, HRAS, MAP2K1, MAP2K2, SHOC2, CBL, SPRED1* and *NF1* was used, to which were added other genes involved in RASopathies (the list of all analyzed genes can be provided on request). The size of the final target region was 232.387kpb with 570 amplicons and the mean sequence coverage was 93.73 at 20× priori 99.41% coverage of the target region. The preparation of the libraries was performed using the Haloplex target enrichment system dedicated to Ion Torrent PGM. Massively parallel sequencing was performed on an Ion Torrent PGM (Thermo Fisher Scientific).

Raw data generated by the PGM sequencer were processed by Torrent Suite Software v.4 and aligned using TMAPv.3. Sequence variants were identified using the Variant Caller tool from the Ion Torrent package using default "germline low stringency" parameters (min_cov_each_strand: 0, min_variant_score: 10, min_allele_freq: 0.1, snp_min_coverage: 6 snp and indel; strand_bias: 0.98 snp and 0.85 indel) then prioritized using the in-house software Varaft (http://varaft.eu) that includes Annovar [26] and UMP-Predictor [27] . Variants not previously reported in healthy controls and classified as pathogenic were evaluated for sequencing depth and

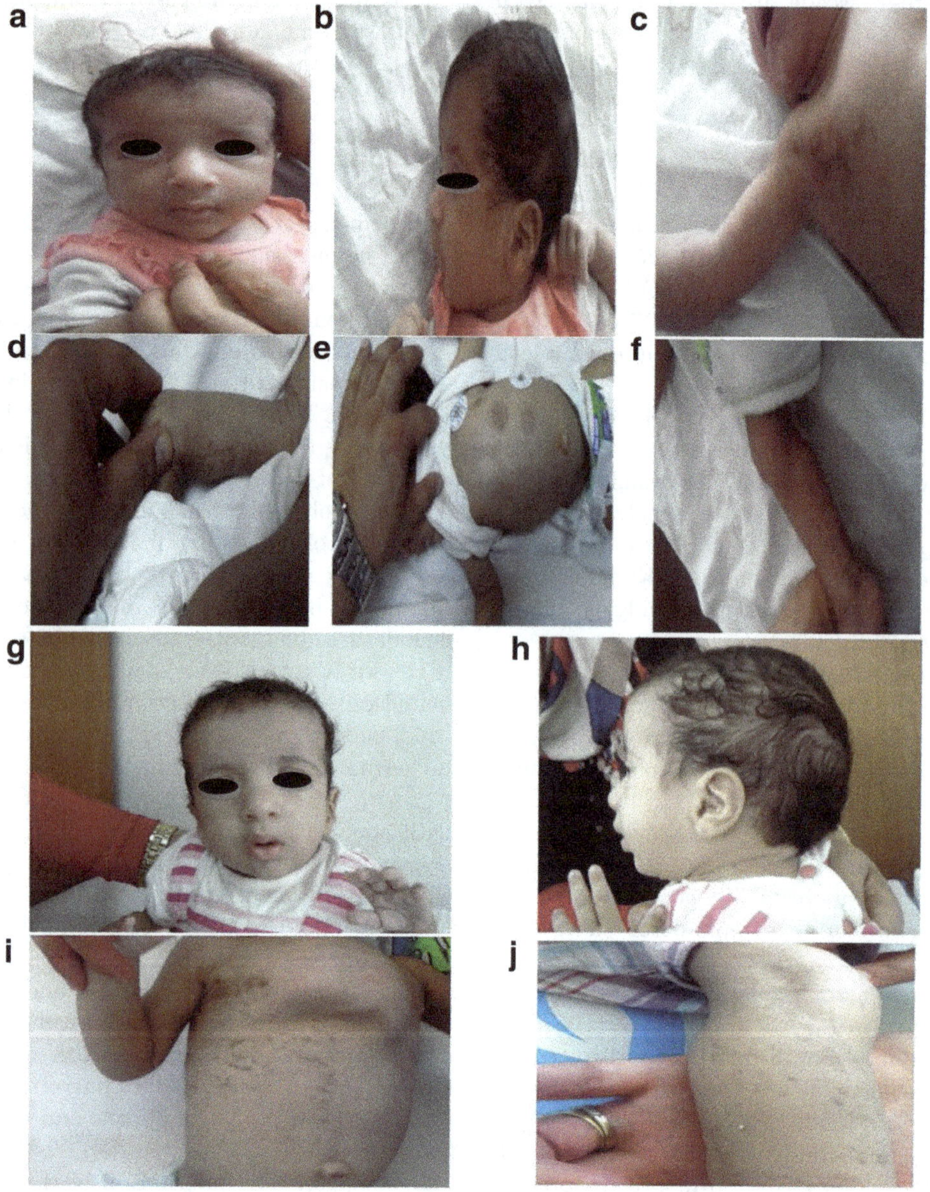

Fig. 1 Photographs of the patient showing NS and IP manifestations. **a, b** front and profile photo respectively pointing facial dysmophism at the age of 1 month with broad forehead, hypertelorism, down-slanting palpebral fissures, a high arched palate, bifid uvula and low set posteriorly rotated ears, long philtrum and epicanthal folds; **c-f** typical IP manifestations at the age of 1 month showing linear brownish pigmentation involving the trunk and the extremities; **g, h** front and profile photo of the patient at the age of 1 year highlights the evolution of NS phenotype; **i, j** evolution of the IP manifestations at the age of 1 year, pectus excatavum becomes more pronounced

visually inspected using the Integrative Genomic Viewer (IGV) before validation by Sanger Sequencing using the manufacturer's protocol for BigDye ® Terminator sequencing kits. Segregation analysis was performed in both parents by Sanger sequencing.

Genes were named following the Hugo gene nomenclature committee guidelines (https://www.genenames.org/); DNA mutations and predicted protein changes were named following the HGVS nomenclature guidelines available at http://www.hgvs.org/mutnomen/. The NS-Euronet mutation database was used to check for mutation description at https://nseuronet.com/php/.

PCR amplification method

We used an improved PCR protocol amplification which provides a robust detection of the recurrent intragenic deletion that removes exon4–10. This protocol has been previously described by Guevara et al. [28].

Results

A total of 184 variants were detected across the 29 genes analyzed. Filtering these results using in silico software predictors of a mutation's impact such as UMD predictor, Mutation-taster, PolyPhen and others, whose algorithms are integrated into the Varaft software, issued only one heterozygous variant as potentially pathogenic: a heterozygous SNV in exon 7 of the *RAF1* gene predicted to lead to a missense amino acid change (NM_002880: c.788 T > G, p. Val263Gly) (Fig. 2a). This was retained since it was correlated to the phenotypic description of the patient and was already reported [29].We confirmed this alteration in the patient by Sanger Sequencing. The analysis of transmission in the patients' parents confirmed that it occurred as de novo mutation (Fig. 2b).

Presence of a de novo exon 4–10 deletion of *IKBKG* gene was demonstrated by PCR amplification in the proband (Fig. 3a) and was confirmed in the proband's DNA using Sanger Sequencing of the 1045-bp band confirming a breakpoint in intron 3.(Fig. 3b).

Discussion and conclusion

To the best of our knowledge, this is the first reported clinical case of NS associated with IP in a non-consanguineous female patient. As previously discussed, several causal genes

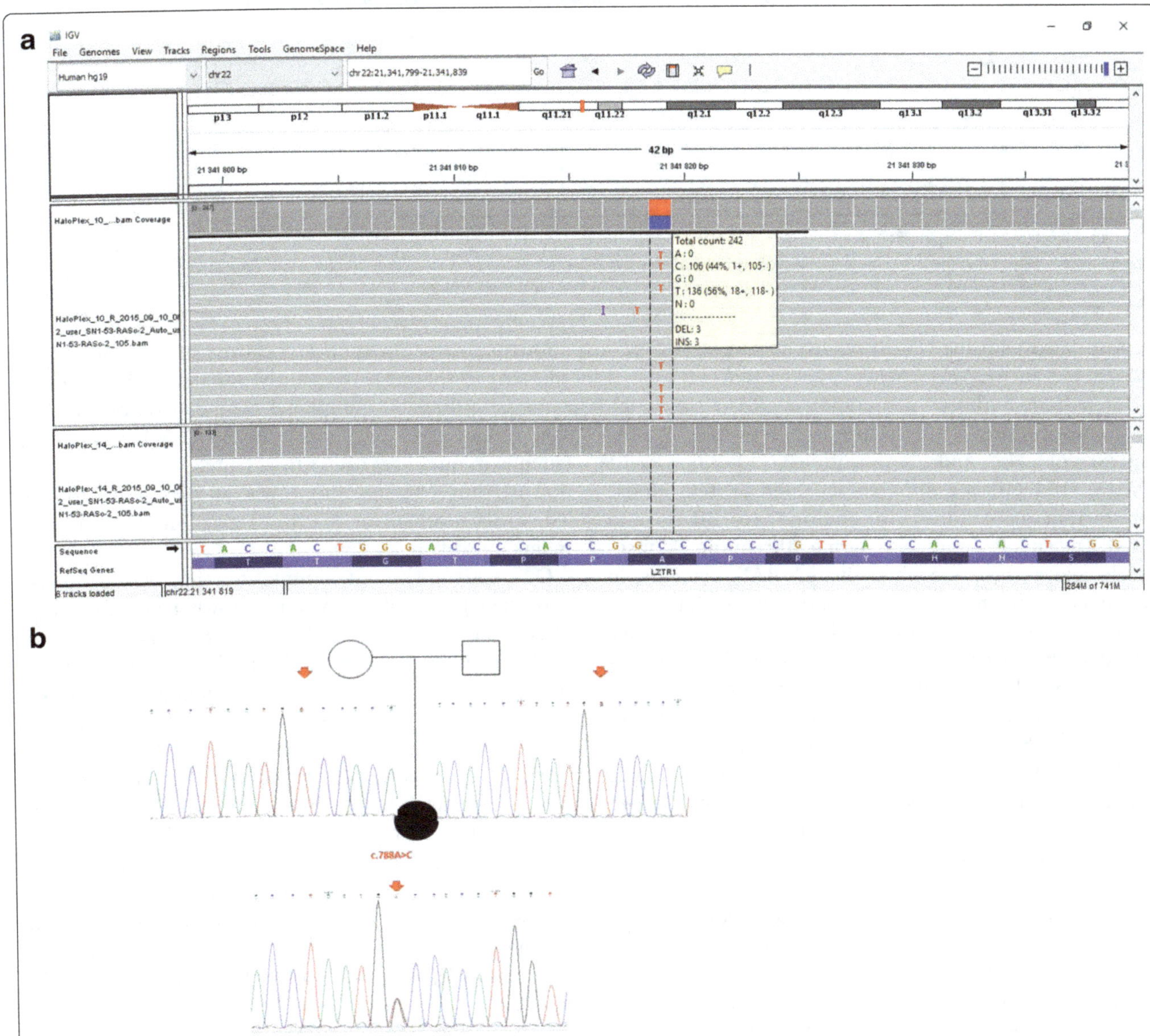

Fig. 2 Sequencing results. **a** IGV browser visualization of the targeted NGS sequencing results showing the heterozygous c.788 T > G substitution in the RAF1 gene in the patient, (reverse sequence) which is absent in another NS patient (used as a control); **b** Sanger sequencing confirming the de novo appearance of the mutation in the patient, given its absence in the parents' DNA samples

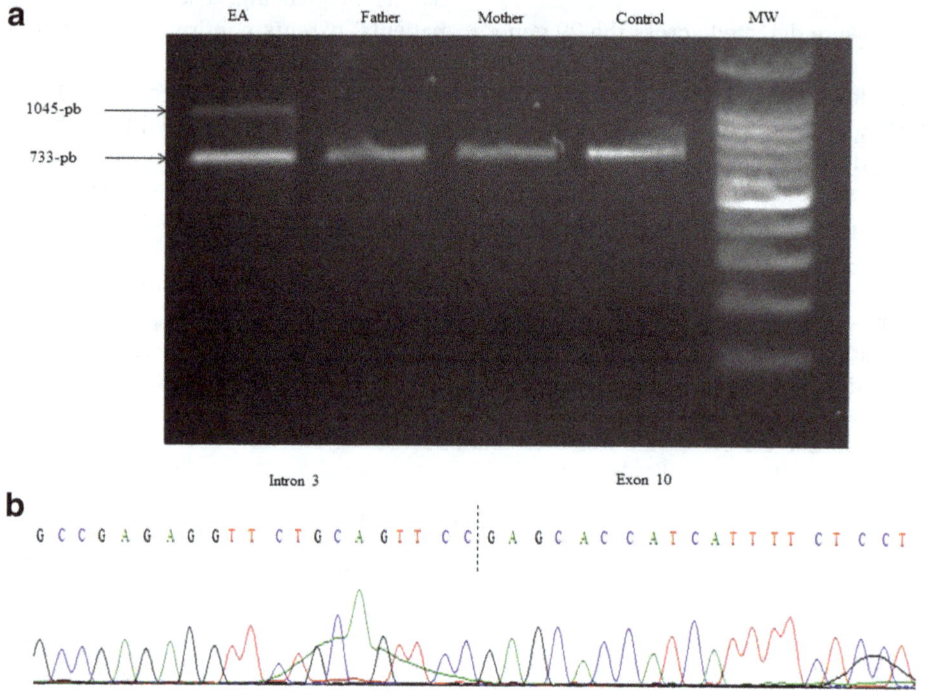

Fig. 3 Molecular confirmation of IP. **a** Polymerase Chain Reaction (PCR) amplification of peripheral blood genomic DNA confirms the presence of the intragenic deletion in the *IKBKG* gene in the proband (the 1045 bp band) but not in her parents and in the control (the 733 bp band). **b** Sanger sequencing of the 1045 bp band from the proband's amplified DNA confirms a breakpoint in intron 3

are associated with the NS phenotype, including *PTPN11, SOS1, RAF1, BRAF, NRAS, SHOC2, CBL*, and *RIT1*.

Our patient harbored a mutation in *RAF1*, in which rare substitutions were previously reported in the context of NS and RASopathies [30–32]. RAF1 (OMIM, 164760) is a mitogen activated protein kinase kinase that constitutes, in addition to BRAF and ARAF, a small family of serine threonine kinases which relays signals from activated RAS proteins to the major effectors of this pathway, ERK1/2 via MEK1/2. Compared to BRAF, RAF1 and ARAF have considerably lower MEK kinase activity, different expression profiles and also distinct regulatory mechanisms: missense mutations in these two genes are thus rarely observed in malignancies [10]. The ubiquitously expressed *RAF1* encodes a 648 amino acids protein containing three functional and conserved domains: the N-terminal CR1 (amino acids residues 61–192), *CR2* (residues 251–266),, and CR3 kinase domain (residues 333–625) [33].

About 70% of all the *RAF1* mutations identified to date are amino acid substitutions located in the *CR2* domain. The second group of mutations, identified in 15% of NS or LS-causing *RAF1* mutations, affects the kinase domain and the last 15% of *RAF1* mutations affects two adjacent residues, located at the C-terminus. None of the mutations causing NS or LS are reported in a cancer context.

Our patient's mutation is localized at position Val263, adjacent to the most frequently mutated residues, in the same CR2 domain. Functional characterizations support that mutations which affect the 14–3-3 binding motif (such is in our case) cause an enhanced kinase activity in downstream *RAS* signaling (*MEK* and *ERK*) [10, 29, 34]. The exact mechanism of *RAF1* activation in mutants remains unexplained.

Our patient showed a mutation that was previously described prenatally in a fetus showing evocative signs of Noonan syndrome (fetal hydrops and cystic hygroma-colli) together with hypoplastic left heart syndrome (HLHS), one of the most severe congenital heart defects, characterized by underdevelopment of the structures in the left-aorta complex and detectable by ultrasound at prenatal sonography between 18 and 22 weeks of gestation of the fetal heart. In Noonan syndrome patients, HLHS has only been described twice [35]. The same mutation caused in our patient one of the two most frequent congenital heart defects observed in NS: pulmonic stenosis, suggesting that other factors (genetic or environmental) are involved in the determination of the cardiac anomaly, in addition to the *RAF1* p.Val263Gly mutation.

Gain of function mutations in *RAF1* were identified for the first time in 2007 in patients with NS and negative for *PTPN11, KRAS* and *SOS1* mutations and two of six patients with LEOPARD syndrome [31, 36], with a frequency ranging between 10 and 30%. Examination of detailed clinical manifestations of these patients showed a strong association among *RAF1* mutations and congenital cardiac defects (94% of children carrying *RAF1* gene mutation), namely hypertrophic cardiomyopathy (HCM) in 70–80% of the patients, which is significant compared to the 18% HCM prevalence observed in the general NS population [10], but atrial septal defects (28%), pulmonary valve stenosis (12%), and arrhythmia are also observed [37].

Craniofacial characteristics, skeletal abnormalities and mental retardation can also be present. Skin and hair anomaly are less marked, but multiple *naevi*, café-au-lait spots and lentigines were present in one-third of NS patients with *RAF1* mutations, that suggests a predisposition to hyperpigmented cutaneous lesions [10, 34, 38–40]. In IP affected females, major linear skin hyperpigmentation can be associated with a variety of ophthalmic disorders (strabismus, retinopathy, congenital cataract...), nail and teeth dysplasia and occasionally central nervous system disease ranging from seizures to severe motor and intellectual delay [21]. Differently to NS, skin lesions of IP occur in 4 classic cutaneous stages, observed in our patient: stage 1 is characterized by erythema, vesicles, and pustules; stage 2 by papules, verrucous lesions, and hyperkeratosis; stage 3 by hyperpigmentation; and stage 4 by pallor, atrophy, and scarring [41]. Nail dystrophy is frequent but usually mild [25].

The relatively low incidence of *RAF1* gene mutations in patients with NS and the much rarer onset of cutaneous disorders within this category of patients make it difficult to establish a clear genotype/phenotype correlation and to better explain the possible underlying mechanism of such a rare association of NS phenotypes. The association between NS due to a RAF1 mutation and another disease in one patient has been rarely reported. Cerebrovascular anomalies [42], Burkitt lymphoma [43] and usually cardiomyopathies [34, 44] have been associated to NS.

Conclusion

The Co-occurence of two or several diseases has been recently reported in Tunisian population. This phenomenon has been observed mainly for autosomal recessive diseases and is due to the high rate of consanguinity [45, 46]. Nevertheless, the association we report between NS and IP is probably coincidental since no link has been established among the 2 pathophysiological pathways and high rates of consanguinity in the Tunisian patients' population are not likely to influence the appearance of IP nor NS, whose inheritance patterns are not autosomal recessive.

Abbreviations

CNV : Copy Number variation; HCM: Hypertrophic Cardiomyopathy; HLHS: Hypoplastic Left Heart Syndrome; IP : Incontinentia Pigmenti; NS: Noonan Syndrome; PCR : Polymeras Chain Reaction; RAS MAPK: Ras Mitogen Activated Protein Kinase

Acknowledgments

We thank the patient and her family for participating in this research. We would like to thank also both the personnel of the Department of intensive care and neonatal medicine, CHU Fattouma Bourguiba, Monastir, Tunisia and all members of the team of the INSERM unit UMR_S910, GMGF, Aix Marseille University, Marseille, France (Karim Harhouri, Cathy Bartoli, Guy Longepied, Françoise Merono). We also thank Pr Moncef Rassas for his helpful comments.

Funding

This study was partially funded by the University Foundation A*MIDEX by providing the Haloplex kit and the reagents needed for this study.

Authors' contributions

NG, AL SE and EK carried out experimental work and result interpretation. Clinical details and evaluation were carried out by KBA, MK and RS. NL, ADG, SO and VD supervised research work. JPD has refined the software used in this work.NL had contributed to the discussion and scientific evaluation of this work and approved all results. NG, ADG, FZC and SA refined the manuscript for publication. SO and VD have provided technical resources essential for the realization of this work. All authors read and approved the final manuscript for publication.

Competing interests

The authors declare that they have no competing interests.

Author details

[1]Research Unit 01/UR/08-14, Faculty of Medicine of Monastir, University of Monastir, Avenue Avicenne, 5019 Monastir, Tunisia. [2]Aix Marseille University, INSERM, GMGF, Marseille, France. [3]Department of Intensive Care and Neonatal Medicine, Fattouma Bourguiba University Hospital, Monastir, Tunisia. [4]Departement of Medical Genetics, Childrens' Hospital La Timone, 264 Rue Saint Pierre, Marseille, France. [5]Groupe Ramsay Générale de Santé, Hôpital Clairval, Marseille, France. [6]Institut Pasteur de Tunis, Laboratoire de Genomique Biomedicale et Oncogenetique LR11IPT05, Tunis, Tunisia.

References

1. Roberts AE, Allanson JE, Tartaglia M, Gelb BD. Noonan syndrome. Lancet. 2013;381:333–42.
2. Turner AM. Noonan syndrome. J Paediatr Child Health. 2014;50:E14–E20.
3. Romano AA, Allanson JE, Dahlgren J, Gelb BD, Hall B, Pierpont ME, et al. Noonan syndrome: clinical features, diagnosis, and management guidelines. Pediatrics. 2010;126:746–59.
4. Van der Burgt I, Berends E, Lommen E, Van Beersum S, Hamel B, Mariman E. Clinical and molecular studies in a large Dutch family with Noonan syndrome. Am J Med Genet. 1994;53:187–91.
5. Zenker M. Genetic and pathogenetic aspects of Noonan syndrome and related disorders. Horm Res. 2009;72:57–63.
6. Allanson JE, Bohring A, Dörr H-G, Dufke A, Gillessen-Kaesbach G, Horn D, et al. The face of Noonan syndrome: does phenotype predict genotype. Am J Med Genet A. 2010;152A:1960–6.
7. Bhambhani V, Muenke M. Noonan syndrome. Am Fam Physician. 2014;89: 37–43.
8. AAL J, Malaquias AC, IJP A, Mendonca BB. Noonan syndrome and related disorders: a review of clinical features and mutations in genes of the RAS/ MAPK pathway. Horm Res. 2009;71:185–93.

9. Narumi Y, Aoki Y, Niihori T, Sakurai M, Cavé H, Verloes A, et al. Clinical manifestations in patients with SOS1 mutations range from Noonan syndrome to CFC syndrome. J Hum Genet. 2008;53:834–41.
10. Tartaglia M, Zampino G, Gelb BD. Noonan syndrome: clinical aspects and molecular pathogenesis. Mol Syndromol. 2010;1:2–26.
11. Nshuti S, Hategekimana C, Uwineza A, Hitayezu J, Mucumbitsi J, Rusingiza EK, et al. Patients with Noonan Syndrome phenotype : spectrum of clinical features and congenital heart defect. Rwanda Medical Journal 2010;68:26–312010;68:26–31.
12. Tumurkhuu M, Saitoh M, Sato A, Takahashi K, Mimaki M, Takita J, et al. Comprehensive genetic analysis of overlapping syndromes of RAS/RAF/MEK/ERK pathway. Pediatr Int. 2010;52:557–62.
13. Gelb BD, Tartaglia M. Noonan syndrome and related disorders: dysregulated RAS-mitogen activated protein kinase signal transduction. Hum Mol Genet. 2006;15:R220–6.
14. Tidyman WE, Rauen KA. The RASopathies: developmental syndromes of Ras/MAPK pathway dysregulation. Curr Opin Genet Dev. 2009;19:230–6.
15. Tartaglia M, Kalidas K, Shaw A, Song X, Musat DL, van der Burgt I, et al. PTPN11 mutations in Noonan syndrome: molecular spectrum, genotype-phenotype correlation, and phenotypic heterogeneity. Am J Hum Genet. 2002;70:1555–63.
16. Tartaglia M, Martinelli S, Stella L, Bocchinfuso G, Flex E, Cordeddu V, et al. Diversity and functional consequences of germline and somatic PTPN11 mutations in human disease. Am J Hum Genet. 2006;78:279–90.
17. Aoki Y, Niihori T, Narumi Y, Kure S, Matsubara Y. The RAS/MAPK syndromes: novel roles of the RAS pathway in human genetic disorders. Hum Mutat. 2008;29:992–1006.
18. Tartaglia M, Gelb BD, Zenker M. Noonan syndrome and clinically related disorders. Best Pract Res Clin Endocrinol Metab. 2011;25:161–79.
19. Rauen KA, Huson SM, Burkitt-Wright E, Evans DG, Farschtschi S, Ferner RE, et al. Recent developments in neurofibromatoses and RASopathies: management, diagnosis and current and future therapeutic avenues. Am J Med Genet Part A. 2015;167:1–10.
20. Bardaro T, Falco G, Sparago A, Mercadante V, Molins EG, Tarantino E, et al. Two cases of misinterpretation of molecular results in incontinentia pigmenti, and a PCR-based method to discriminate NEMO/IKKγ gene deletion. Hum Mutat. 2003;21:8–11.
21. Fusco F, Paciolla M, Conte MI, Pescatore A, Esposito E, Mirabelli P, et al. Incontinentia pigmenti: report on data from 2000 to 2013. Orphanet J Rare Dis. 2014;9:93.
22. Ormerod AD, White MI, McKay E, Johnston AW. Incontinentia pigmenti in a boy with Klinefelter's syndrome. J Med Genet. 1987;24:439–41.
23. Fusco F, Bardaro T, Fimiani G, Mercadante V, Miano MG, Falco G, et al. Molecular analysis of the genetic defect in a large cohort of IP patients and identification of novel NEMO mutations interfering with NF-κB activation. Hum Mol Genet. 2004;13:1763–73.
24. Conte MI, Pescatore A, Paciolla M, Esposito E, Miano MG, Lioi MB, et al. Insight into IKBKG/NEMO locus: report of new mutations and complex genomic rearrangements leading to incontinentia pigmenti disease. Hum Mutat. 2014;35:165–77.
25. Minić S, Trpinac D, Obradović M. Incontinentia pigmenti diagnostic criteria update. Clin Genet. 2014;85:536–42.
26. Wang K, Li M, Hakonarson H, et al. Nucleic Acids Res. 2010;38(16):e164. https://doi.org/10.1093/nar/gkq603.
27. Salgado D, Desvignes JP, Rai G, Blanchard A, Miltgen M, Pinard A, et al. UMD-predictor: a high-throughput sequencing compliant system for pathogenicity prediction of any human cDNA substitution. Hum Mutat. 2016;37:439–46.
28. Guevara BEK, Hsu CK, Liu L, Feast A, Alabado KLP, Lacuesta MPM, et al. Improved molecular diagnosis of the common recurrent intragenic deletion mutation in IKBKG in a Filipino family with incontinentia pigmenti. Aust J Dermatol. 2016;57:150–3.
29. Schulz S, Fröber R, Kraus C, Schneider U. Prenatal diagnosis of hypoplastic left heart syndrome associated with Noonan syndrome and de novo RAF1 mutation. Prenat Diagn. 2012;32:1016–8.
30. Ko JM, Kim JM, Kim GH, Yoo HW. PTPN11, SOS1, KRAS, and RAF1 gene analysis, and genotype-phenotype correlation in Korean patients with Noonan syndrome. J Hum Genet. 2008;53:999–1006.
31. Razzaque MA, Nishizawa T, Komoike Y, Yagi H, Furutani M, Amo R, et al. Germline gain-of-function mutations in RAF1 cause Noonan syndrome. Nat Genet. 2007;39:1013–7.
32. Kuburović V, Vukomanović V, Carcavilla A, Ezquieta-Zubicaray B, Kuburović N. Two cases of LEOPARD syndrome - RAF1 mutations firstly described in children. Turk J Pediatr. 2011;53:687–91.
33. Wellbrock C, Karasarides M, Marais R. The RAF proteins take Centre stage. Nat Rev Mol Cell Biol. 2004;5:875–85.
34. Sana ME, Spitaleri A, Spiliotopoulos D, Pezzoli L, Preda L, Musco G, et al. Identification of a novel de novo deletion in RAF1 associated with biventricular hypertrophy in Noonan syndrome. Am J Med Genet Part A. 2014;164:2069–73.
35. Antonelli D, Antonelli J, Rosenfeld T. Noonan's syndrome associated with hypoplastic left heart. Cardiology. 1990;77:62–5.
36. Kobayashi T, Aoki Y, Niihori T, Cavé H, Verloes A, Okamoto N, et al. Molecular and clinical analysis of RAF1 in Noonan syndrome and related disorders: dephosphorylation of serine 259 as the essential mechanism for mutant activation. Hum Mutat. 2010;31:284–94.
37. Pandit B, Sarkozy A, Pennacchio LA, Carta C, Oishi K, Martinelli S, et al. Gain-of-function RAF1 mutations cause Noonan and LEOPARD syndromes with hypertrophic cardiomyopathy. Nat Genet. 2007;39:1007. https://doi.org/10.1038/ng2073.
38. Kneitel AW, Norby A, Vettraino I, Treadwell MC. A novel mutation on *RAF1* in association with fetal findings suggestive of Noonan syndrome. Fetal Pediatr Pathol. 2015;34:361–4.
39. Wu X, Simpson J, Hong JH, Kim K, Thavarajah NK, Backx PH, et al. MEK-ERK pathway modulation ameliorates disease phenotypes in a mouse model of Noonan syndrome associated with the Raf1 L613V mutation. Differences. 2011;121:1009–25.
40. Tartaglia M, Gelb BD. Disorders of dysregulated signal traffic through the RAS-MAPK pathway: phenotypic spectrum and molecular mechanisms. Ann N Y Acad Sci. 2010;1214:99–121.
41. Young I, Wilkie A. Syndrome of the month. J Med Genet. 1994;31:744.
42. Zarate YA, Lichty AW, Champion KJ, Clarkson LK, Holden KR, Matheus MG. Unique cerebrovascular anomalies in Noonan syndrome with RAF1 mutation. J Child Neurol. 2013;29:1–6.
43. Cianci P, Tono V, Sala A, Locatelli L, Carta C, Rizzari C, et al. A boy with Burkitt lymphoma associated with Noonan syndrome due to a mutation in RAF1. Am J Med Genet A. 2013;161A:1401–4.
44. Gelb BD, Roberts AE, Tartaglia M. Cardiomyopathies in Noonan syndrome and the other RASopathies. Prog Pediatr Cardiol. 2015;39:13–9.
45. Ben Abdallah LC, Lakhoua Y, Nagara M, Khiari K, Elouej S, Messaoud O, et al. A tunisian patient with two rare syndromes: triple a syndrome and congenital hypogonadotropic hypogonadism. Horm Res Paediatr. 2014;82:338–43.
46. Romdhane L, Messaoud O, Bouyacoub Y, Kerkeni E, Naouali C, Cherif Ben Abdallah L, et al. Comorbidity in the Tunisian population. Clin Genet. 2016;89:312–9.

15

Maternal depression and child severe acute malnutrition

S. Haithar[1], M. W. Kuria[2], A. Sheikh[3], M. Kumar[1,2]* and A. Vander Stoep[4]

Abstract

Background: Depression is the leading cause of disease-related disability in women and adversely affects the health and well-being of mothers and their children. Studies have shown maternal depression as a risk factor for poor infant growth. Little is known about the situation in Sub-Saharan Africa. The aim of our study was to examine the association between maternal depression and severe acute malnutrition in Kenyan children aged 6–60 months.

Methods: A matched case-control study was conducted in general paediatric wards at the Kenyatta National Hospital. The cases were children admitted with severe acute malnutrition as determined by WHO criteria. The controls were age and sex-matched children with normal weight admitted in the same wards with acute ailments. Mothers of the cases and controls were assessed for depression using the PHQ-9 questionnaire. Child anthropometric and maternal demographic data were captured. Logistic regression analyses were used to compare the odds of maternal depression in cases and controls, taking into account other factors associated with child malnutrition status.

Results: The prevalence of moderate to severe depression among mothers of malnourished children was high (64.1%) compared to mothers of normal weight children (5.1%). In multivariate analyses, the odds of maternal depression was markedly higher in cases than in controls (adjusted OR = 53.5, 95% CI = 8.5–338.3), as was the odds of having very low income (adjusted OR = 77.6 95% CI = 5.8–1033.2).

Conclusions: Kenyan mothers whose children are hospitalized with malnutrition were shown in this study to carry a significant mental health burden. We strongly recommend formation of self-help groups that offer social support, counseling, strategies to address food insecurity, and economic empowerment skills for mothers of children hospitalized for malnourishment.

Keywords: Maternal depression, Child malnutrition, Kenya, Case control study, Poverty

Background

The health and well-being of children is inextricably tied to their early social and emotional experiences. Since feeding and caring for the young is primarily the mother's responsibility, poor maternal physical or mental health can adversely affect nutrition, health, and psychological well-being of children [1]. The impact of maternal mental health on children's long-term emotional, cognitive and behavioral problems has been well studied in high income countries [2–4]. However, the impact on child physical health and development has received less attention, especially in low and middle income countries (LMIC) where poor growth due to under-nutrition is a major problem.

Globally, nearly 50.6 million children under the age of five are malnourished; 90% of these children reside in LMIC [5]. Physical growth is a key indicator of child health and nutritional status [6]. Rapid physical growth and development occur in the first two years of life when children are the most dependent on caregivers for meeting their nutritional needs [7]. Studies have shown that healthy maternal behavior and attitude have an essential role in maintaining healthy nutrition in children [5–7].

Depression is the leading cause of disease-related disability among reproductive aged women, globally [8]. The first year after a woman gives birth to an infant is a particularly high risk time for the occurrence of

* Correspondence: manni_3in@hotmail.com
[1]Department of Psychiatry, College of Health Sciences, University of Nairobi, P.O. Box 103140, Nairobi 00101, Kenya
[2]Research Department of Clinical, Health and Educational Psychology, University College London, London WC1E 7HB, UK

depression. Postpartum depression (PPD) prevalence estimates vary from 15 to 57% [9–13]. An estimated 10–15% of mothers who reside in high income countries are affected [13], with nearly double the prevalence reported in South Asia (Pakistan 28%, India 23%) [9, 11, 14–16]. PPD prevalence estimates from sub-Saharan Africa range from 6 to 30% [17].

Most research on maternal depression and child nutritional outcomes in LMIC has been conducted in S. Asia, where the majority of the world's underweight children reside [9, 10, 14, 18]. The South Asian studies suggest that poor maternal mental health, particularly maternal depression, is a risk factor for inadequate growth in young children. A case-control study conducted in South India reported a significant association between current major depression in mothers and malnutrition in children (OR = 3.2, 95% CI 1.1–9.5) [16, 19]. A cohort study conducted by Rahman et al. (2007) [20] in rural Pakistan found that perinatal depression in mothers predicted poorer growth and higher risk of diarrhea in infants [21].

In Brazil de Miranda et al. (1996) conducted a case-control study of women of San Paulo and found high levels of psychiatric morbidity among women with protein energy malnourished children, with 63% of cases having high levels of mental distress compared to 38% in controls (OR = 2.8;95% CI =1.2–6.9) [22]. In Rio de Janeiro Hassan et al. (2016) found that maternal mental health was associated with the nutritional status of infants at six months [23]. Infants of depressed mothers were reportedly two standard deviations below average height on WHO norms [12, 24].

A number of studies of child nutritional status in under-fives conducted in sub-Saharan Africa have examined related demographic, socioeconomic and cultural factors [25–29], while a small literature focuses on maternal mental health (Table 1). Adewuya et al. (2008) conducted a case-control study in Nigeria and found that at both three and six months, infants of depressed mothers had statistically significantly poorer growth than infants of non-depressed mothers, with odds ratios of 3.28 and 3.34 for length and 3.21 and 4.21 for height [30]. Depressed mothers reported that they discontinued breastfeeding earlier, and their infants had more episodes of diarrhea and other infectious illnesses [30]. Other sub-Saharan African studies have shown that maternal depression is associated with compromised parenting behavior, non-responsive care- giving practices and decrease in breast feeding, all of which contribute to childhood malnutrition [17, 21, 22]. Ashaba et al. (2015), who conducted a case-control study in Uganda, reported that 42% of mothers of malnourished children were depressed, compared to 12% of mothers of normal weight children admitted to hospital for chronic illness (OR = 2.4; 95% CI =1.18–4.79) [31]. A recent cross-sectional study conducted in Kenya with mothers attending a maternal and child clinic reported a strong association between maternal depression and both non-exclusive breastfeeding (OR = 7.1; 95% CI = 2.9–17.6) and infant underweight status (OR = 4.4; 95%CI = 1.8–11.0) [17]. To date no Kenyan studies have examined the association between severe acute malnutrition (SAM) in infants and depression in mothers. By testing the hypothesis that mothers of children hospitalized with SAM would have a significantly higher likelihood of suffering from depression than children hospitalized with other medical conditions, our research was designed to fill this gap.

Methods

Study design

We carried out a matched case-control study to examine differences in the prevalence of depression in mothers with young children hospitalized for severe acute malnutrition (SAM) and mothers with young children hospitalized for other health problems.

Sample

Sample size was determined using open Epi formula for matched case control studies. The minimum number was determined as 74 (37 cases and 37 controls). Estimates from the Husain et al. study (2000) were used to ascertain expected prevalence of maternal depression in children with SAM, and the meta-analytic study by O'Hara et al. (1996) [13] for the expected prevalence of maternal depression in normal children [9, 13].

Recruitment and consenting procedures

The study was approved by the Kenyatta National Hospital/University of Nairobi ethical review committee (approval no. KNH/ERC/A/180). Consent was administered in English or Kiswahili, depending on the mother's language preference, and written informed consent was obtained from the participants. Cases were malnourished children ages 6–60 months admitted with severe acute malnutrition at Kenyatta National Hospital pediatric wards between May and June 2014. The controls were gender and age-matched children who were normal weight and admitted to the same hospital for acute ailments. For each case found at the pediatric ward, the first author matched the control on age (up to +/−three months) and sex (except for two pairs). Sampling for the cases and controls was done sequentially in all the pediatric wards at the ratio of one to one. Malnourished children who were admitted for duration longer than 7 days or not within the age range were excluded. Mothers who could not communicate in either English or Kiswahili or were unable to give informed consent were also excluded. Consecutive convenience sampling was applied to obtain cases and controls until the desired sample size was achieved.

Table 1 Summary of Key SAM and Maternal Depression Studies in LMIC Contexts

Study	Design	Sample size & methods	Population & setting	Tools & mode of administration	Outcomes (ORs with 95% CI)
Ashaba et al. (2015) [31] Maternal depression and malnutrition in SW Uganda	Matched case control study Not blinded	$N = 166$ children (83 cases and 83 controls); Controls were age and gender-matched chronically ill children.	Rural population from low socioeconomic background. Hospital-based study.	MINI (Mini International Neuropsychiatric Interview) Clinician administered. Children aged 6–60 months.	Prevalence of depression 42% among cases versus 12% among controls OR 2.4 (95% CI = 1.18–4.79; $p = 0.015$)
Ross & Hanlon et al. (2010) [35] Perinatal mental distress & infant morbidity in Ethiopia	Cohort study	$N = 954$ mother child pairs.	Rural population of low socio-economic status. Population-based study.	SRQ 20 (Self- Reporting Questionnaire) Self-administered. Followed up from 3rd trimester through first 2 months postpartum.	Prevalence of High CMD (SRQ20 score > 6) was 9.8% in pregnancy, 2.1% post- natally: persistent high CMD was 2.5% Persistent perinatal CMD was associated with RR 2.15 (95% CI = 1.39–3.24) increased risk of infant diarrhea.
Ejaz et al. (2012) [37] Maternal psychiatric morbidity & childhood malnutrition in Pakistan	Matched case control study Not blinded	$N = 100$ (50 cases, 50 controls with significant co-morbidities were excluded. Controls were children with normal weight. Admitted with common childhood illnesses, like acute respiratory infections, diarrhea.	Urban population in Karachi of low socio-economic status. Hospital based study.	HADS (Hamilton Anxiety and Depression Scale) Clinician administered at time of hospital admission.	Cases were more likely than controls to have depressed mothers OR 0.85 (95% CI = 0.38–1.86; $p = 0.68$)
Rahman et al. (2004) [38] Maternal mental health & childhood growth in Rawalpindi, Pakistan	Case control study Interviewer blinded to case-control status of infant.	$N = 172$(82 cases, 90 controls) Controls were children from same locality whose weight for age was above the 10th percentile.	Urban and peri-urban. Mainly of low SES. Immunization clinic based.	SRQ 20 (Self- Reporting Questionnaire), Self- administered Administered to mother when she came to clinic for child's 9-mo. immunization	Strong association between maternal depression and poor weight gain. Adjusted OR 2.8 (95% CI 1.2–6.8, $p < 0.05$)
Patel et al. (2003) [14] Maternal depression & infant growth in Goa, India	Cohort study Hospitalized controls.	171 infants age > 9 months 22% with depressed mothers.	Rural population in Goa, India of low SES. Hospital based.	EPDS (Edinburgh Perinatal Depression Scale) Clinician administered at 6–8 week immunization visit.	Babies under the 5th percentile for weight were more likely to have depressed mothers Risk ratio 2.3 (95% CI = 1.1–4.7, $p = 0.01$)
Anoop et al. (2004) [19] Maternal depression as risk factor for malnutrition in children 6–12 months in Kaniyambadi Block, Nadu	Case control study Interviewer blind to child nutritional status.	72 cases and 72 controls, matched. Cases were children 50–80% of expected weight. Controls matched for age, sex, and locality were > 80% of expected weight.	Rural and peri-urban of low SES Community based.	SCID (Structured Clinical Interview for DSM-IV) Clinician administered.	Mothers with malnourished babies were more likely to have post- natal depression OR 7.4 (95% CI = 1.6–3.85; $p = 0.01$)

Study procedures

Once consent was given by the mothers, the anthropometric measures of the children were taken using the normogram to ascertain weight and height. Usually the cases had files which categorized these children as SAM. Research data were collected on site in the hospital ward. Two medical students who were trained by first author assisted in the collection of anthropometric data. The mother's socio-demographic data was captured in the study questionnaire, and the mother was invited for depression assessment. According to study protocol, all mothers whose PHQ-9 scores indicated that they were experiencing severe depression or suicidality were referred to the KNH mental health unit for treatment.

Data collection instruments

Socio-demographic information

We collected information about family income and size, maternal age, education, occupation including spouses', maternal empowerment and control over finances, HIV status, exposure to chronic illnesses, and family and social support.

Measurement of child's weight and height to confirm case and control status

Once recruited, the children were undressed, and their weights were measured using a digital compression scale and recorded to one decimal point (in kilograms). The height of each child was measured (in centimetres) from crown to heel with the child in prone position using a tape measure. Weight for height scores was generated from WHO normograms, and these were used to confirm the case definition. Children were classified according to WHO criteria (severe wasting (< 70% weight for length or < − 3 Z score) and/or oedema [12]. The cases stood out clearly; therefore there were no changes in classification after anthropometric measurements were taken, and none of the mothers were excluded from the study.

Measurement of maternal depression

Maternal depression was assessed using the PHQ-9 which was developed in the U.S. [32]. The PHQ-9 is a self-administered depression scale with nine items that asks about past two weeks with response options ranging from "not at all" to "nearly every day." The items reflect the nine criteria on which the diagnosis of DSM-V major depressive disorder is based [32]. In this study we used the PHQ-9 to grade depressive symptom severity as none (score of 0–4), mild (5–9), moderate (10–14), or moderately severe/severe (11–27), as recommended by the scale developers [32]. The validity and usefulness of the PHQ-9 in East Africa has been discussed by Gelaye et al. 2014 [33]. The PHQ-9 has been widely used in Kenya, and there is a translated version available in Kiswahili language. Monahan et al. 2009 [34] validated the tool in a Kenyan sample.

The PHQ-9 was administered orally by the lead author or one of her medical school assistants when the mother was unable to complete it (mainly due to poor literacy level) or by herself with the choice of filling the Kiswahili or English version. A high percentage of participants preferred it to be administered orally due to their low literacy level. Quality assurance criteria were instated in training the study assistants in collecting maternal depression information including instructing them to stay close to the tonal/semantic reference of the questionnaire.

Data analytic approach

The data were entered, cleaned, and analyzed with SPSS version 17. Continuous and categorical variables were analyzed using descriptive statistics. Logistic regression analyses estimated the ratio of the odds of moderate to severe depression (PHQ-9 score ≥ 10) among the cases compared to controls. Adjusted odds ratios were calculated to take into account other risk factors of malnutrition. In analysis of variables with missing data, participants with missing values were excluded.

Results

We recruited seventy-eight mother-child dyads (39 cases and 39 controls) during the study period. The mean ages of the cases and controls were similar (20.4 months (SD = 12.2) vs 20.3 months (SD = 20.3)), while the mean height (72.8 (SD = 10.4) vs 78.8 (SD = 10.5) and weights (7.2 (SD = 2.2 and 10.1 (SD = 2.8)) of the cases were significantly lower than that of the controls with t (76) = − 2.5, $p < 0.005$ (height) and t (76) = − 5.2, $p < 0.001$(weight). We recruited 19 girls and 19 boys as cases and 22 boys and 17 girls as controls.

The participating mothers ranged from 16 to 46 years of age, with a mean age of 27.7 (SD = 6.4). With regard to their marital status, 81.2% of the mothers were married; half had had some secondary schooling; and 45.1% were employed. Of the children, 35.1% were firstborn. For those with siblings, the number ranged from 1 to 5. As shown in Table 2, mothers of children hospitalized with malnutrition had significantly lower levels of family income ($X^2 = 14.1$, df = 2, $p = .001$) than mothers of children hospitalized with other conditions. Among those who were married, mothers with children with SAM were more likely to have spouses who were unemployed. There were no statistically significant differences in mothers of cases and controls with respect to age, marital status, educational attainment, employment status, chronic health conditions, or number of children under age 5 years. Similar proportions of mothers of malnourished children (43.6%) and control children (38.5%) had breastfed their infants for 12 months or more. The

Table 2 Baseline Social and Demographic Characteristics of the Mother-child Dyads

Variable	Mothers of Hospitalized Severely Malnourished Children (Cases)	Mothers of Hospitalized Normal Weight Children (Controls)	Difference Statistic	Significance
Mean age (SD)	28.4 (7.6)	27.0 (5.0)	$t\ (75) = 1.032$	0.32
Mean number of children under age 5 yrs (SD)	1.2 (0.38)	1.3 (0.57)	t (75) = .741	0.46
Marital status N (%)				
Single/divorced/ widowed	9 (23.7)	5 (12.8)	$X^2\ (1) = 2.110$	0.28
Married	29 (76.3)	34 (87.2)		
Unknown	1	0		
Mother's education level				
None	0	1 (2.6)	$X^2\ (3) = 3.24$	0.35
Primary	22 (56.4)	15 (38.5)		
Secondary	13 (33.3)	18 (46.2)		
Post-secondary	4 (10.3)	5 (12.8)		
Spouse's education level*				
Primary	10 (34.5)	11 (32.4)	$X^2\ (3) = 1.97$	0.37
Secondary	16 (55.2)	15 (44.1)		
Post-secondary	3 (10.3)	8 (23.5)		
Chronic illnesses (i.e. hypertension, diabetes)				
Yes	5 (12.8)	5 (12.8)	$X^2\ (1) = 0.00$	1.00
No	34 (87.2)	34 (87.2)		
Self-reported HIV status				
Positive	7 (17.9)	2 (5.1)	$X^2\ (2) = 3.35$	0.20
Negative	31 (79.5)	35 (89.7)		
Unknown	1 (2.6)	2 (5.1)		
Duration of breastfeeding				
≤12 months	22 (56.4)	24 (61.5)	$X^2\ (1) = 0.21$	0.64
> 12 months	17 (43.6)	15 (38.5)		
Mother's occupation				
Unemployed	28 (73.7)	24 (61.5)	$X^2\ (1) = 1.29$	0.25
Employed	10 (26.3)	15 (38.5)		
Spouse's occupation*				
Unemployed	15 (51.7)	8 (23.5)	$X^2\ (1) = 5.37$	*0.02*
Employed	14 (48.3)	26 (76.5)		
Family income per annum				
< 36,000	14 (36.8)	1 (2.8)	$X^2(2)\ 14.15$	0.001
36,000–150,000	16 (42.1)	18 (52.8)		
> 150,000	8 (21.1)	16 (44.4)		
Social support from others				
Yes	28 (71.8)	33 (84.6)	$X^2(1) = 1.88$	0.17
No	11 (28.2)	6 (15.6)		
Mother's level of control over family finances				
Total control	16 (53.3)	14 (45.2)	$X^2(1) = 0.41$	0.52
Partial control	14 (46.7)	17 (54.8)		
None	9 (23.1)	8 (20.5)		

• No data for mothers who are not married ($N = 14$) or marital status is unknown ($N = 1$)

self-reported prevalence of HIV was 17.9% among mothers of the cases and 5.1% among mothers of the controls. The majority of the mothers of cases (71.8%) and controls (84.6%) reported that they were receiving social support from family members or friends. Over three quarters of mothers in both groups reported having some control over family finances.

The prevalence of mild, moderate, or moderately severe depression was 64.1% ($N = 25$) among mothers of severely malnourished children. This statistically significantly higher than the 5.1% ($N = 2$) prevalence of depression identified in mothers of normal weight children, OR = 33.0; 95% CI 6.9–158.2, $p < 0.001$ (Fig. 1). Among the 25 case mothers who were depressed, 13 had mild depression, 9 had moderate depression and 3 had moderately severe depression. In the control group one mother had mild depression, and the other had moderately severe depression (Fig. 1).

Results of multivariate logistic models showed child nutrition to be significantly associated with maternal depression (AOR = 53.5; 95% CI: 8.5–338.3) and low family income (AOR = 77.6; 95% CI: 5.8–1033.2). Besides family income, none of the covariates were statistically significantly associated with child malnutrition in multivariate analyses (see Tables 2 and 3).

Table 3 Logistic Regression Model: Depression Status of Mothers with Children Hospitalized with Severe Acute Malnutrition or Other Health Conditions

Model	Variable	OR (95% CI)	*p* value
1	Depression Status		
	Depressed	33.0 (6.9–158.2)	< 0.001
	Not depressed	1.0	
2	Depression Status		
	Depressed	53.5 (8.5–338.3)	< 0.001
	Not depressed	1.0	
	Family income per annum		
	< 36,000	77.6 (5.8–1033.2)	0.001
	36,000-150,000	3.3 (0.6–18.0)	0.162
	> 150,000	1.0	

Discussion

Our study demonstrated that infant malnutrition is significantly associated with both maternal depression and family income. Several studies in low income countries such as India, Pakistan, Ethiopia and Uganda have shown similar findings [19, 21, 31, 35]. In a meta-analysis of seventeen studies from eleven different countries, Sukran et al. reported an OR of 2.2 in the association between maternal depression and underweight and an OR of 2.0 in the association between maternal depression and stunting [36]. Our study findings stand out in both the high prevalence of depression in mothers of hospitalized malnourished children and in the discrepancy between the prevalence of depression in these mothers compared to mothers of children hospitalized with other illnesses.

The hospital-based case control study conducted in Pakistan by Ejaz et al. reported high psychiatric morbidity of 50% in the cases, but with nearly as high a prevalence of depression (46%) in controls who were mothers of hospitalized normal weight children [37]. This high mental health morbidity in both cases and controls reflected the generally high prevalence of mental health problems amongst women in Pakistan [38]. Although the prevalence of depression in cases in the current study (64.1%) is higher than estimates of 15–63% reported among mothers in other LMICs, what is more striking in our study is the low prevalence of depression (5.1%) in the controls [14, 16, 21, 30, 31, 39]. A prior Kenyan study conducted by Madeghe et al. (2016) with women with infants attending well-child visits reported a PPD prevalence (EPDS score of 10 or higher) of 13% [17].

Several features of our study sample and methods may have contributed to differences between our findings and those of previous studies of hospitalized children.

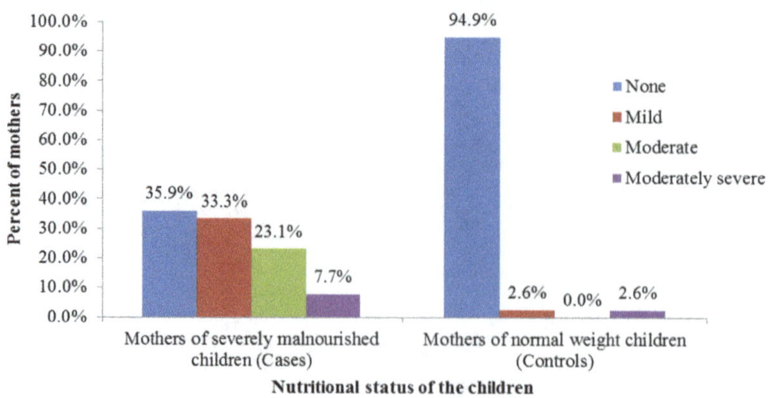

Fig. 1 Severity of depression among mothers of cases and controls

Our study sample was restricted to mothers whose children had been hospitalized for seven days or less, whereas the children in Ashaba et al. (2015) were not restricted to those with brief length of hospitalization and, subsequently, their control mothers may have been suffering psychological effects of their children's long hospital stays (as high as 2–3 months) [31]. We only include those children admitted fewer than seven days previously in order to mitigate this potential contributor to maternal distress. The higher prevalence of depression in mothers of our cases may be due to differences in study populations, with the current sample being predominantly urban slum dwellers of low socio economic status, while the Ashaba et al. sample was mainly rural. Table 1 highlights that a variety of tools, including the MINI, EPDS, HADS etc., were used in different studies. We administered the PHQ-9 because it has been validated in Kenya.

Our study had several limitations. Although the study was adequately powered to evaluate the primary study question, the small sample size contributed to the very wide confidence intervals around estimated odds ratios for maternal depression and family income. We were not able to draw conclusions about the contribution to child malnutrition status of factors such as mother's HIV status and father's unemployment status that may have distinguished cases from controls in a larger study. Researchers were aware of the case-control status of the mother at the time they administered the depression questionnaire. A high proportion of participating mothers requested that the questionnaire be administered orally. While the medical students were carefully trained to administer the PHQ-9 in a systematic way to both case and control mothers, there may have been errors in understanding the intent of the questions or in the data collectors' sensitivity, based on the health status of the child or if the mother was perceived as highly distressed. Additionally, because the case-control study was organized around the outcome of the child's hospitalization, it is difficult to establish temporal sequence between maternal depression and the child's nutritional status. We were not able to determine which mothers in this study suffered from depression before or during pregnancy. In addition we did not gather information about which children were born preterm or were underweight at the time of their birth. Knowledge of the date of onset and temporal ordering of depression in the mother and malnourishment in the infant would help to determine the optimal timing for targeting intervention strategies.

Having a child who is severely malnourished and who is undergoing hospitalization requires high reserves of parental energy. From what we know about how depression affects functioning, a mother with moderate depression will have difficulty in carrying out ordinary work and social activities. Maternal depression may contribute to undernutrition in children by compromising parenting behavior. Depression can adversely affect the mother's ability to perform caregiving activities such as breast feeding, stimulation, hygiene and overall care [27]. This interferes with formation of a secure early attachment and bonding behaviors with the baby [19, 21] which, in turn affect a child's physical and emotional well-being. Conversely, having a child who is severely malnourished is highly distressing. In the current study the malnourished children had been ill intermittently with general deterioration of health that could trigger sustained psychological distress in the mothers. Additionally, the fact that the infant was physically extremely fragile, and this was visually apparent to the mother as she waited for the infant to recover, could heighten feelings of hopelessness and helplessness in the mother. Children in the hospital wards where the study was conducted have high mortality rates with consequences for the mothers' level of stress and low mood. In contrast, the controls may have been ill for a shorter window of time, so the mothers may not have been subjected to sustained distress.

Our study illustrates the juxtaposition of two health conditions that have serious adverse effects on large segments of populations in low income countries. In this case-control study, we draw attention to tremendous challenges parents face in caring for malnourished children and the burgeoning challenges children face when their caregivers are debilitated with depression. While our study is inconclusive regarding the temporal sequence in the causal association between mother's depression and child's nutritional status, the empirical evidence regarding the etiology of depression would support the argument that there is considerable reciprocity, with maternal depression affecting feeding and other child-rearing practices, and the stress of caring for a malnourished child affecting the mental health status of the caregiver [31, 40, 41]. Hospitalization is an added burden on caregiving resources. By matching cases and controls on the condition of hospitalization and by taking family income into account in multivariate analyses, our study was able to control for these sources of parental stress.

Our study findings suggest that mothers of malnourished children are a very vulnerable group for whom emotional health support and economic empowerment programs are warranted. Mothers of malnourished infants are discharged from hospital to carry out feeding protocols that require time, effort, new skills, and financial resources. It may be difficult for mothers with depression and low income to comply with recommendations. Our findings strongly suggest that the need for clinicians who care for families with malnourished infants should learn to recognize and treat maternal mental health conditions that can impede attainment of desired nutritional goals. In addition, the association between malnourishment and very low income calls for measures to ensure that families have adequate economic resources so that mothers and infants do not suffer the health consequences of having insufficient food.

Promising findings have emerged from a trial of the WHO endorsed Thinking Healthy Program conducted in rural Pakistan, where mothers with depression who received cognitive behavioral therapy experienced significant reduction in depression. Additionally their infants had fewer episodes of diarrhea in the first year, compared to women whose depression was not treated [21, 42]. The Thinking Healthy Program targets maternal depression and infant health promotion and has been endorsed by WHO [43] for use in LMIC. The intervention can be offered by lay health workers and could be implemented in Kenya to provide greater support to vulnerable women.

Conclusions

The prevalence of depression in Kenyan mothers of children under five years of age who were hospitalized for malnutrition was found to be significant. We found maternal depression in these women significantly and markedly higher than in mothers of children hospitalized for other conditions. We strongly recommend formation of hospital-based support and self-help groups for mothers of children hospitalized with severe acute malnutrition. The implementation of WHO endorsed Thinking Healthy Program at community and health care levels to strengthen mothers' ability to shoulder and share the heavy burden of rearing children who are at risk of life-threatening malnutrition may be considered. In this model, lay health workers including health facility staff can be trained in basic psychosocial support to bolster maternal mental health.

Abbreviations

DSM: Diagnostic and statistical manual of mental disorders; EPDS: Edinburgh postnatal depression inventory; HADS: Hamilton anxiety and depression scale; LMIC: Lower and middle-income countries; MINI: Mini international neuropsychiatric interview; PHQ-9: Patient health questionnaire 9; PPD: Post partum depression; SAM: Severe acute malnutrition; WHO: World Health Organization

Acknowledgements

Kenneth Mutai assisted with statistical analyses and Winnie Sharon Kiche for help with referencing. The authors wish to acknowledge our participants, both children and their mothers.

Funding

The design, field work, and writing for the study were supported through a Medical Education Partnership Initiative (MEPI) Award from the U.S. National Institute of Mental Health/Fogarty International Center, R25 MH099132.

Authors' contributions

The work was carried out by SH as part of the Masters degree in Psychiatry at the department of Psychiatry University of Nairobi. SH with support from AS collected data and wrote the findings, MK and MK were her University mentors and helped in conceptualization, writing up and conducting statistical analysis. AVS was her third mentor who assisted during planning of the research concept, reviewed the writing and data analysis and helped shape the manuscript for submission. All authors read and approved the final manuscript.

Competing interests

The authors declare that they have no competing interests.

Author details

[1]Department of Psychiatry, College of Health Sciences, University of Nairobi, P.O. Box 103140, Nairobi 00101, Kenya. [2]Research Department of Clinical, Health and Educational Psychology, University College London, London WC1E 7HB, UK. [3]Department of Clinical Medicine and Therapeutics, College of Health Sciences, University of Nairobi, P.O. Box 19676, Nairobi 00202, Kenya. [4]Psychiatry & Behavioral Sciences and Epidemiology, 6200 NE 74th Street, Suite 210, Seattle, WA 88115-1538, USA.

References

1. Cummings EM, Kouros CD. Maternal depression and its relation to Children's development and adjustment. In: Tremblay RE, Boivin M, RDeV P, editors. Encycl early child dev; 2007. p. 1–10.
2. Haas JD, Murdoch S, Rivera J, Martorell R. Early nutrition and later physical work capacity. Nutr Rev. 2009;54:S41–8. https://doi.org/10.1111/j.1753-4887.1996.tb03869.x.
3. Victora CG, Adair L, Fall C, Hallal PC, Martorell R, Richter L, et al. Maternal and child undernutrition: consequences for adult health and human capital. Lancet (London, England). 2008;371:340–57. https://doi.org/10.1016/S0140-6736(07)61692-4.
4. Pollitt E, Gorman KS, Engle PL, Rivera JA, Martorell R. Nutrition in early life and the fulfillment of intellectual potential. J Nutr. 1995;125(4 Suppl):1111S–8S. http://www.ncbi.nlm.nih.gov/pubmed/7536831. Accessed 15 July 2017.
5. Faruque ASG, Ahmed AMS, Ahmed T, Islam MM, Hossain MI, Roy SK, et al. Nutrition: basis for healthy children and mothers in Bangladesh. J Health Popul Nutr. 2008;26:325–39. http://www.ncbi.nlm.nih.gov/pubmed/18831228. Accessed 15 July 2017.
6. Black RE, Allen LH, Bhutta ZA, Caulfield LE, de Onis M, Ezzati M, et al. Maternal and child undernutrition: global and regional exposures and health consequences. Lancet. 2008;371:243–60. https://doi.org/10.1016/S0140-6736(07)61690-0.
7. Semba RD, Victora CG. Low birth weight and neonatal mortality. In: Nutrition and health in developing countries. Totowa, NJ: Humana Press; 2008. p. 63–86. https://doi.org/10.1007/978-1-59745-464-3_3.
8. Kessler RC. Epidemiology of women and depression. J Affect Disord. 2003;74:5–13. http://www.ncbi.nlm.nih.gov/pubmed/12646294. Accessed 15 July 2017.
9. Husain N, Creed F, Tomenson B. Depression and social stress in Pakistan. Psychol Med. 2000;30:395–402. http://www.ncbi.nlm.nih.gov/pubmed/10824659. Accessed 15 July 2017.
10. Gelaye B, Rondon MB, Araya R, Williams MA. Epidemiology of maternal depression, risk factors, and child outcomes in low-income and middle-income countries. Lancet Psychiatry. 2016;3:973–82. https://doi.org/10.1016/S2215-0366(16)30284-X.
11. Mirza I, Jenkins R. Risk factors, prevalence, and treatment of anxiety and depressive disorders in Pakistan: systematic review. BMJ. 2004;328:794–7. http://www.bmj.com/content/328/7443/794. Accessed 15 July 2017.
12. WHO child growth standards and the identification of severe acute malnutrition in infants and children. http://apps.who.int/iris/bitstream/10665/44129/1/9789241598163_eng.pdf?ua=1. Accessed 15 July 2017.
13. O'hara MW, Swain AM. Rates and risk of postpartum depression—a meta-analysis. Int Rev Psychiatry. 1996;8:37–54. https://doi.org/10.3109/09540269609037816.
14. Patel V, DeSouza N, Rodrigues M. Postnatal depression and infant growth and development in low income countries; a cohort study from Goa, India. Arch Dis Child. 2003;88(1):34–7.
15. Afzal S, Khalid R. Social Support and Postnatal Depression in Pakistani Context. Pakistan J Soc Clin Psychol. 2014;12(1):34–8. www.gcu.edu.pk/Fulltextjour/PJSCS/2014/5.sidra Afzal.pdf

16. Rahman A, Iqbal Z, Harrington R. Life events, social support and depression in childbirth: perspectives from a rural community in the developing world. Psychol Med. 2003;33:1161–7. http://www.ncbi.nlm.nih.gov/pubmed/14580070. Accessed 15 July 2017.
17. Madeghe BA, Kimani VN, Vander Stoep A, Nicodimos S, Kumar M. Postpartum depression and infant feeding practices in a low income urban settlement in Nairobi-Kenya. BMC Res Notes. 2016;9:506. https://doi.org/10.1186/s13104-016-2307-9.
18. The State of the world's children 1998. 1998;16–9. https://www.unicef.org/sowc/archive/ENGLISH/The%20State%20of%20the%20World%27s%20Children%201998.pdf .
19. Anoop S, Saravanan B, Joseph A, Cherian A, Jacob KS. Maternal depression and low maternal intelligence as risk factors for malnutrition in children: a community based case-control study from South India. Arch Dis Child. 2004;89:325–9. http://www.ncbi.nlm.nih.gov/pubmed/15033840. Accessed 15 Jul 2017
20. Rahman A, Creed F. Outcome of prenatal depression and risk factors associated with persistence in the first postnatal year: prospective study from Rawalpindi, Pakistan. J Affect Disord. 2007;100:115–21. https://doi.org/10.1016/j.jad.2006.10.004.
21. Rahman A, Iqbal Z, Bunn J, Lovel H, Harrington R. Impact of maternal depression on infant nutritional status and illness. Arch Gen Psychiatry. 2004;61:946–52. https://doi.org/10.1001/archpsyc.61.9.946.
22. de Miranda CT, Turecki G, de Jesus Mari J, Andreoli SB, Marcolim MA, Goihman S, et al. Mental health of the mothers of malnourished children. Int J Epidemiol. 1996;25:128–33. http://www.ncbi.nlm.nih.gov/pubmed/8666480. Accessed 15 July 2017.
23. Hassan BK, Werneck GL, Hasselmann MH. Maternal mental health and nutritional status of six-month-old infants. Rev Saude Publica. 2016;50:7. https://doi.org/10.1590/S1518-8787.2016050006237.
24. Patel V, Rahman A, Jacob KS, Hughes M. Effect of maternal mental health on infant growth in low income countries: new evidence from South Asia. BMJ. 2004;328:820–3. https://doi.org/10.1136/bmj.328.7443.820.
25. Reed BA, Habicht JP, Niameogo C. The effects of maternal education on child nutritional status depend on socio-environmental conditions. Int J Epidemiol. 1996;25:585–92. http://www.ncbi.nlm.nih.gov/pubmed/8671560. Accessed 15 July 2017.
26. Madise NJ, Matthews Z, Margetts B. Heterogeneity of child nutritional status between households: a comparison of six sub-saharan African countries. Popul Stud (NY). 53:331–43. https://doi.org/10.2307/2584703.
27. Gwatkin DR, Rutstein S, Johnson K, Suliman E, Wagstaff A, Amouzou A. Socio-economic differences in health, nutrition, and population within developing countries: an overview. https://siteresources.worldbank.org/INTPAH/Resources/IndicatorsOverview.pdf. Accessed 15 July 2017.
28. Owor M, Tumwine JK, Kikafunda JK. Socio-economic risk factors for severe protein energy malnutrition among children in Mulago hospital, Kampala. East Afr Med J. 2000;77:471–5. http://www.ncbi.nlm.nih.gov/pubmed/12862136. Accessed 15 July 2017.
29. Pongou R, Ezzati M, Salomon JA. Household and Community Socioeconomic and Environmental Determinants of Child Nutritional Status in Cameroon. 2006. https://doi.org/10.1186/1471-2458-6-98.
30. Adewuya AO, Ola BO, Aloba OO, Mapayi BM, Okeniyi JAO. Impact of postnatal depression on infants' growth in Nigeria. J Affect Disord. 2008;108:191–3. https://doi.org/10.1016/j.jad.2007.09.013.
31. Ashaba S, Rukundo GZ, Beinempaka F, Ntaro M, LeBlanc JC. Maternal depression and malnutrition in children in Southwest Uganda: a case control study. BMC Public Health. 2015;15:1303. https://doi.org/10.1186/s12889-015-2644-y.
32. Kroenke K, Spitzer RL, Williams JB. The PHQ-9: validity of a brief depression severity measure. J Gen Intern Med. 2001;16:606–13. http://www.ncbi.nlm.nih.gov/pubmed/11556941. Accessed 15 July 2017
33. Gelaye B, Williams MA, Lemma S, Deyessa N, Bahretibeb Y, Shibre T, et al. Validity of the patient health questionnaire-9 for depression screening and diagnosis in East Africa. Psychiatry Res. 2013;210:653–61. https://doi.org/10.1016/j.psychres.2013.07.015.
34. Monahan PO, Shacham E, Reece M, Kroenke K, Ong'or WO, Omollo O, et al. Validity/reliability of PHQ-9 and PHQ-2 depression scales among adults living with HIV/AIDS in western Kenya. J Gen Intern Med. 2009;24:189–97. https://doi.org/10.1007/s11606-008-0846-z
35. Ross J, Hanlon C, Medhin G, Alem A, Tesfaye F, Worku B, et al. Perinatal mental distress and infant morbidity in Ethiopia: a cohort study. Arch Dis Child - Fetal Neonatal Ed. 2010;96:F59–64. https://doi.org/10.1136/adc.2010.183327 .
36. Sukran P, Kennedy C, Hurley K, Black MWHOJ. Maternal depression and early childhood growth in developing countries: systematic review and meta-analysis. Bull World Health Organ. 2011;89:545–620. https://doi.org/10.2471/BLT.11.088187.
37. Ejaz M, Sarwat A, Aisha T. Maternal psychiatric morbidity and childhood malnutrition. Pak J Med Sci. 2012;28:874–8. http://pjms.com.pk/index.php/pjms/article/viewFile/2747/942. Accessed 15 July 2017.
38. Rahman A, Lovel H, Bunn J, Iqbal Z, Harrington R. Mothers' mental health and infant growth: a case-control study from Rawalpindi, Pakistan. Child Care Health Dev. 2004;30:21–7. https://doi.org/10.1111/j.1365-2214.2004.00382.x.
39. Makoka D. The Impact of Maternal Education on Child Nutrition : Evidence from Malawi,Tanzania and Zimbabwe. DHS Work Pap. 2013;84:1–32. www.dhsprogram.com/pubs/pdf/WP84/WP84.pdf
40. Martins C, Gaffan EA. Effects of early maternal depression on patterns of infant-mother attachment: a meta-analytic investigation. J Child Psychol Psychiatry. 2000;41:737–46. http://www.ncbi.nlm.nih.gov/pubmed/11039686. Accessed 15 July 2017.
41. Murray L, Cooper P. Effects of postnatal depression on infant development. Arch Dis Child. 1997;77:99–101. https://doi.org/10.1136/ADC.77.2.99.
42. Rahman A, Patel V, Maselko J, Kirkwood B. The neglected "m" in MCH programmes - why mental health of mothers is important for child nutrition. Trop Med Int Heal. 2008;13:579–83. https://doi.org/10.1111/j.1365-3156.2008.02036.x.
43. Thinking healthy: A manual for psychosocial management of perinatal depression WHO generic field-trial version 1.0, 2015 Series on Low-Intensity Psychological Interventions – 1. http://apps.who.int/iris/bitstream/10665/152936/1/WHO_MSD_MER_15.1_eng.pdf?ua=1&ua=1. Accessed 15 July 2017.

16

Sexual and physical abuse and its determinants among street children in Addis Ababa, Ethiopia 2016

Ayana Chimdessa[1*] and Amsale Cheire[2]

Abstract

Background: The life and health of street children is becoming a global concern. Street children are vulnerable to a variety of problems including physical, psychological and sexual exploitations as well as social isolation. Therefore, it was the purpose of this study to point out the experience of sexual and physical exploitation and its determinant factors among street children in Addis Ababa, the capital city of Ethiopia.

Methodology: A phenomenological qualitative method was conducted from March to June 2016 in Addis Ababa, Ethiopia. Data were collected from street children by focus group discussion (FGD) and in-depth interview. Open code was used to analyze data. The transcribed note was translated. Following this coding was done. Based on a coding book, major themes and main categories were developed and analyzed.

Result: The study has explored the life experience of street children in the city. Deaths of parents/unhealthy relationship of extended families forced them be on a street. Thus, flee to street to search for work was the main reason for joining to a street. Street children are vulnerable to sexual and physical exploitations on a daily basis. For street children, street is the world characterized by misery deprivation, physical, verbal and sexual abuse and become daily victims of violence. There is no safe place for the children of on-street. Most street children are involved in all types of sex; heterosexual, bisexual, homosexual and group sex are common among themselves and out siders. They are involved highly in transactional sex for survival. Drug use, stress and depression are common experiences. Thus, they were socially isolated. The main challenges of living on a street are lack of basic needs, social isolation, lack of safety and security and being out of school are the common problems these vulnerable groups are facing.

Conclusions: Street children are at high risk of sexual and physical exploitation. Interventions targeting integration and reunion with families, reduction of physical and sexual exploitation, access to education, mental health promotion and reduction of drug use behavior should be taken in to considerations.

Keywords: Street children, Sexual and physical abuse, Drug use, Addis Ababa, Ethiopia

Background

The life and health of street children is becoming a global concern. Street children are vulnerable to a variety of problems including physical, psychological, sexual and social isolation. Children who spend time on the street are at risk of increased aggression, hopelessness, drug use, and informal sex work [1].

Though street children are hard to count, a recent global estimate showed that nearly 150 million street children are living in the urban and semi-urban areas [2, 3]. The number of street children is increasing worldwide for various reasons [3]. Factors related to family disruption and lack of basic needs has been strongly associated with these marginalized groups of people [2, 3]. HIV/AIDS is the most significant global factor to increase the number of orphans, particularly in sub-Saharan Africa. Studies indicated that there were 17.3 million orphans due to HIV/AIDS globally. Out of these, the majority of orphan and vulnerable children (OVC) are found in sub-Saharan Africa

* Correspondence: ayanayoom@gmail.com
[1]School of Nursing and Midwifery, College of Health Sciences, Wollega University, P.O Box: 395, Nekemte, Ethiopia

and Southern and Southeastern Asia [4]. Children who lost their parents are at increased risk of physical, psychological, social, health, and economic problems. Lack of parental protection, guidance and support may predispose children to street life and made them highly vulnerable group [5–7].

In Ethiopia, over 4 million children are estimated to live under difficult circumstances of poverty and health problems. It is estimated that 600,000 children are taking part in street life. As many as 500,000 children are at high risk of becoming involved in street life in Ethiopia [2].

Studies conducted in different part of sub-Saharan countries showed that street children are one of the high risk groups to acquiring sexually transmitted infections including HIV/AIDS. They are prone to sexual abuse, rape, prostitution, sexual bartering and exchange, casual sex and early exposure to both heterosexual and homosexual behaviors [1, 5, 8].

Thus, exploring the magnitude of sexual and physical exploitation among street children is a pivotal to address the needs of street adolescent and mitigating the negative outcomes of the growing street children population worldwide. Therefore, it was the aim of this study to assess the experience of sexual and physical exploitations among street children in Addis Ababa, Ethiopia.

Methods

Study design and period

The study was conducted in Addis Ababa, the capital city of Ethiopia using phenomenological qualitative study design. All on and off street children age 10–18 years old were involved in the study. The phenomenological inquiry consisted of in-depth interview and focus group discussion (FGD) for both on and off street children. The study was conducted from March to June 2016.

Sample and sampling techniques

Snowball and purposive sampling strategies were employed in recruiting participants into the study. Both FGD and in-depth interview were conducted up to the level of information saturation. Both on and off street children were participated in FGD and in-depth interview. Totally six FGDs each consisting of 4–10 members ($n = 41$) and in-depth interviews ($n = 20$) were conducted.

Data collection procedure

Semi- structured FGD and in-depth interview guides (Additional file 1) were used to explore the life experience of study subjects. Both FGD and in-depth interview lasted for an average of 60–70 min. Study subjects were separated into two based on their sex in order to get more insight of physical and sexual experience as well as factors affecting it. All FGDs and in-depth interviews were conducted in a private place for the purpose of concentration and privacy of participants. Permission to use a tape recorder was obtained from the participants prior to actual data collection. Six trained BSc nurses and two supervisors who have experience in qualitative data collection have taken part in data collection.

In this study, children off-street were those who were working or begging on street but, either living with their parents/relatives or visiting their parents/relatives regularly. Children on the street were those who live and work on a street without any kind of supervision from parents or relatives. They were both economically and socially dependent on a street life.

Data processing and analysis

Data inquiry was analyzed using content analysis software. The transcribed note was translated. Following this coding was done. Based on a code book, major themes and main categories were developed following the research objectives and questions of the study. Researchers identified the major themes and main categories of the research. After the themes and categories are identified intuiting the data was done. Analysis of data includes coding, categorizing and making sense of the essential meanings of the phenomenon. Researchers came to understand and describe the phenomenon. Results were written by reorganizing, summarizing and quoting when needed.

Ethical clearance was received from Addis Ababa University. A formal letter was written to all concerned authorities and permission was secured at all levels. Since the study subjects were younger than 18 years, written assent was taken from study subjects and written consent was taken from guardians or nongovernmental organizations (NGO) who were responsible to look after them. To compensate the study participants' time, the researchers provided them 15 birr (USD 0.5) per person. Participation in the study was voluntary and information that was collected from the study subjects assured confidentiality.

Results

Demographic characteristics of study participants

In this study, snowball sampling strategy was employed in recruiting the study participants. Data collectors interviewed available on and off-street children throughout the data collection period which resulted in different numbers of male and female study participants. Thus, a total of 40 on-street and 21 off-street children aged 10–18 years were participated in the study. Of which, 46 were male and 15 were female street children. Among these ($n = 61$), 20 street children (on-street $n = 12$) and (off-street $n = 8$) were participated in the in-depth interview. Whereas, a total of 41 street children from both categories (on-street $n = 28$) and (off-street $n = 13$) were involved in the six FGDs.

During data collection period, data collectors had registered participants who were in and out of school on their field notes. Based on the field note memo the number of children in and out of school were well noted. Of the total study participants ($n = 37$) had never been to school, ($n = 9$) were dropped their schooling and ($n = 15$) were in school during data collection period. The finding showed that there was a huge gap of schooling between on and off-street children. The result shows that the number of off-street children who were in school was higher than on-street children. Out of 40 on-street children about ($n = 31$) of respondents had never been to school. Whereas, out of 21 off-street children ($n = 6$) of them had never been to school during data collection period. About ($n = 9$) of on-street children reported that they were dropped their primary education. Whereas, ($n = 15$) off-street children were in primary education during data collection. Out of 40 on-street study participants about ($n = 12$) of them were informally married to one another in order to cope with the stressful street life. However, all off-street children were reported never married (Table 1).

Determinants of being on street, life on street and challenges of being a street child

The findings of in-depth interview and FGD on the factors that exposed children to street life, their life experiences and challenges they were facing by being on street is shown in Table 2.

Theme 1 determinants of being street children

Participants pointed that there are different factors to practice street life. Out of these, respondents have given stress to factors like death of the family, extended family relation destruction and poverty. After the death of their parents, they were being on street or flee to extended family to search for daily basic needs. From their experience participants revealed that most of the time they flee to extended family. If the relation with their extended family become unhealthy, they would be forced to join a street life. The other factor forced them to join a street life was poverty. Respondents indicated that when their family face challenges of poverty, unable to educate and cloth their children, the children flee from home and search for jobs in the near towns. Later fled to more industrialized and urbanized cities.

Category 1.1: Death of parents and other relatives

The deaths of parents were one of the main reasons forcing them to street life. Discussants said that most of them joined street life after the death of one or both of their parents. They revealed that *"if you don't have parents you will not have any one to fulfill the daily basic needs. You don't have anyone to take care of you, to support you, to protect you and to love you"* (FGD 1, 3).

Interviewees pointed that death of their mothers was more severe and have affected their life significantly. The interviewees pointed their reason of being on street was; *"following my mother's death my father married another woman. This step mother was not friendly, she was unloving, she insults and beats me every day and she was not giving me enough food. Because of this I run away. I joined a street life"* (Interview 5, 7, 19).

The FGD discussants and other interviewees also shared the same experiences. They said loss of parents was the main reason for a considerable number of children to be on street. *"If your parents die, you will lose everything: parental love, means of survival, shelter and*

Table 1 Demographic characteristics of street children in Addis Ababa, Ethiopia 2016

Research tools used	Category of study participants	Number of participants	Sex		Educational level			Marital status	
			Male	Female	Never been to school	Grade 1–6	Grade 7–8	Single	Informally married
FGD									
FGD 1	On street children	7	7	–	6	1	–	4	3
FGD 2		9	9	–	7	2	–	7	2
FGD 3		8	8	–	7	1	–	5	3
FGD 4		4	–	4	3	1	–	3	1
	Total	28	24	4	23	5	–	19	9
FGD 5	Off street children	5	–	5	1	2	2	5	–
FGD 6		8	8	–	2	5	1	8	–
	Total	13	8	5	3	7	3	13	–
In-depth interview	On street children	12	9	3	8	3	1	9	3
	Off street children	8	5	3	3	3	2	8	–
	Total	20	14	6	11	6	3	17	3

A total of 41 discussants participated in FGD: on-street ($n = 28$) and off-street ($n = 13$)
A Total of 20 children participated in in-depth interview: On-street ($n = 12$) and off-street ($n = 8$)

Table 2 Major thematic areas and main categories of in-depth interviews and FGDs of street children in Addis Ababa, Ethiopia 2016

Theme	Categories
Theme 1: Determinants of being street children	1.1. Death of parents and other relatives 1.2. Searching for work
Theme 2: Context of living on a street	2.1. Sexual practice: Early initiation of sex, coercive sex, transactional sex, heterosexual, bisexual and homosexual sex, nonuse of condom, multiple partners 2.2. Drug use behavior and mental illness 2.3. Involving in income generating activity 2.4. Low knowledge of STIs and HIV
Theme 3: Challenges of living on a street	3.1. Lack of basic needs, social isolation and lack of safety and security 3.2. Being out of school

security. You and you alone, you have to struggle to survive by using all means you know, like surviving through scavenging garbage and sharing experience from friends how to survive street life"(FGD 5 and interview 10, 14).

Category 1.2: Searching for jobs

Focus group discussants reported that most street children drifted to Addis Ababa and other big cities to search for a job. Some of the street children migrated to Addis Ababa hoping that they could get a better job to change their life unfortunately, the situation was quite different. What they experienced was not what they dreamed and expected. Participating in manual work was common practice. *"Doing this manual work with empty stomach and beyond your age was sometimes difficult to bear. Then you will be involved in any other activities that helps you to get your daily basic needs"* (FGD 1, 6).

Theme 2: Context of living on street

Participants reported that context of living on street was hard to survive. Sexual activity among street children was common practice to survive this harsh life. On daily basis, these situations exposed to risky sexual behaviors and positioned them under various health problems.

Category 2.1: Sexual practices among street children

Street children were highly involved in risky sexual behaviors in order to survive. These situations exposed them to sexually transmitted infections (STIs) and HIV/AIDS.

This study shows that street children articulated experiencing sexual exploitation that could predisposed them to various health problems. For the street children, environment does not provide protection against such vulnerability. The study also revealed that new arrivals on streets especially girls are used as sex objects by older boys and watchmen of shops at night. Mostly, such sexual relationships were for protection to the newcomers. In the case of those newcomers that refused such sexual advances, they were beaten up and chased away from that particular area of the street. From the six groups of FGD two groups reported that they have a girl friend or wife; which is an informal arrangement made by the homeless street children. However, being under informal agreement, their wives used to go for sex work with strangers to get money and comes back to her informal husband **(FGD 4 and 2)**.

Transactional sex All discussants pointed that street children participate in risky sexual behaviors on daily basis for their survival. They reported that if they do not involve in survival sex, living on street will be unbearable. They indicated that no one is there to provide them with basic needs like food, cloths rather than dying from hunger. ***"We sell flesh to survive on street"*** **(FGD 1 and 2).**

Condom use Participants reported that inconsistent and nonuse of condom were common practices among street children during sexual intercourse. Interviewees said that condom usage depends on their partner's interest. Most partners particularly, strangers prefer to have sex without condom. Respondents said that ***"we were unable to negotiate to use condom with strangers instead of doing what they want and get money for our survival. We obey to our partners' interest/decisions to survive on street"*** **(Interviewees 1, 4 and FGD 3).**

Types of sex The study revealed that sexual intercourse among street children and outsiders were common. The discussants articulated that ***"most of us are involved in all types of sexual intercourses: heterosexual, bisexual, homosexual and group sex were common practice among us and outsiders"*** **(FGD 2 and 4).** There is no safe place for children of on-street. Study participants indicated that no safer places to spend the night, both boys and girls sleep in the same quarter. The focus group participants pointed that all types of sexual relation does exist on a street ***"Sexual relationship among street children and with outsiders is widespread. Thus, multiple partnership is a common practice"*** **(FGD 2, 3, 6).**

Coercive sex Forced sex was common within a street group and from outsider communities. Interviewees pointed that the most difficult challenge they were facing was older street children forces the younger ones to have either vaginal or anal sex. ***"We street children have no one to stand for us. As far as you are in the loop, you cannot escape except, accepting whether***

***forced homosexual or heterosexual and even physical and sexual misuse. You don't have any one to protect you. For whom would you cry?*"** (**interviewee 5, 8, 19**).

Two groups indicated that ***"we try to defend ourselves from unwanted sex with strangers by sleeping in a group. If we get a job and paid money, we may spend the night at the bed room called DC (low price and poorly cleaned hotel around Merkato) which we have been paying 15 birr (USD 0.5) per night. Since it was difficult to get money to spend the night at DC we sleep in a group to protect ourselves from strangers over the night. Our dogs are also with us every night. If somebody came to hurt us at night our dogs alerts us"*** (**FGD 1 and 4**). The study also revealed that female street children who spend a night over street face another challenge called **'gelbo'**. "Gelbo" means in their language female street children being a victim of forced sex while sleep on a street during night time (**FGD 4, 6**).

Category 2.2: Drug use behaviors and mental illnesses

Living on a street had direct relation to being exposed to drugs. Participants pointed that ***"life on street is misery. You feel hopelessness, your current and future life is dark. We cry out for help but from where? There is no one by our side. At times we feel lonely, suffer from lack of sleep, anxiety, isolation and face mood depressions. To subsist all these; we use variety of substances: like glue, hashish, cannabis, khat and local alcoholic drinks such as arekie and tej" (FGD 1, 4, 5, 6).*** Discussants indicated that the use of substances helps them to temporarily relieve themselves from the hurdles they were facing on a street. They said ***"Even dogs and cats have their shelter but, we …we have to hide ourselves from our selves by taking different substances. We use variety of substances to temporarily mask our problems and relive from the pain of it. By taking these substances, we enjoy the temporary pleasure of it and forget the disgustful life we are facing on a street"*** (**FGD 2, 3, 5 and 6) and interviewees (12, 13, 17 and 19)**.

Category 2.3: Engagement in income generating activities (IGA) on a street

Street children get basic needs through different ways. The study participants pointed that they were generating income through begging, participation in informal sex work, survival sex and manual work. These all activities were the main income generating methods to subsist.

Begging Begging on a street was one of the strategies to survive. Discussants pointed that ***"Although we don't like it, we beg to get our daily bread. This is our day to day activity. If we have a family or anybody who care for us, rather than begging by this age; we prefer to go to school"*** (**FGD 2, 6 and interviewee 7, 11**).

Transactional sex/survival sex All study participants extensively discussed that transactional sex was the major income generating activity in easy approach. Interviewees pointed that ***"We sell our flesh just to survive"*** (**Interviewees 8, 13, 20**).

An interviewee stated that ***"you don't have option rather than living this ugly life; I had anal sex with strangers in exchange of food and other goods. If my parents were alive this would not happen to me. But I have to live this way and face the ugly life for subsistence".*** Some discussants and interviewees shared the same experiences (**Interviewees 3, 7, 15**).

Out of the six groups, two groups reported ***"The other most intricacy we street children facing is; rich people who have cars come and talk with us, give us cloth, food, money or other goods and takes us to their home. After you reach home, they force you to have sex with them"*** (**FGD 1, 3**).

There were countless street children who were forced to have either anal or vaginal sex with strangers. One focus group participants cited one example: ***"one day one of our friend was taken by a rich person who had been driving his own car to his home. After our friend reached home, the man forced him to have anal sex. Although I cited this example, it is a common experience of numerous street children"*** (**FGD 1**).

Three of the interviewees also expressed their deep sorrow with their eyes filled of tears: ***"You don't have right on yourself; you simply permit those who have money and power to play on your flesh. You allow them to do whatever they want because they have money. You need to survive. This is what happens to me in most instances".*** Other interviewees shared similar sorrow in their life (**Interviewee 2, 3, 18**).

Manual work Street children use different mechanisms to survive on a street and at the same time their life style endanger their health. The other issues that exposed street children to health problems was participating in heavy manual work in order to survive on a street. They participate in heavy manual work in exchange of breads or cloths in daily basis.

In this study, participants cited that ***"we participate in sifts through garbage in order to collect recyclable materials such as plastics, paper and metal, cleaning cars, petty vending, selling small items, shining shoes, digging, carrying heavy loads which compromise our health and schooling. We usually rise before sunrise and carry our heavy load by bag over our shoulder and change it with basic needs like bread, money and cloths"*** (**FGD 3, 5**). All study participants, both on and off-street children share the same experience of manual work.

Category 3.4: Knowledge of STIs and HIV/AIDS

Misconception about STIs and HIV transmission and prevention was widespread among street children. Study participants said that they heard about STIs and HIV/AIDs. However, discussants had misconceptions about transmission and prevention of HIV. Most of them responded that HIV can be transmitted by lice, sputum expectoration, and drinking water with unclean or used cup. Most of participants cited that ***"walking on bare foot is one of the way to transmit HIV"*** **(FGD 2, 5).**

Theme 3: Challenges of living on a street

Respondents were glowing up that they were facing different challenges while they were living on a street.

Category 3.1: Lack of basic needs, safety, security and social isolation

The challenge of living on a street was described by discussants as: ***"Street is our home, it is our social abode. We live in the streets and eat on streets. Street life means hunger, deprivation of basic necessities, being homeless, sleeping on the ground, passing the day on the sun and suffering from the cold at night". "We face begging, physical and sexual exploitation on the daily basis. Living on a street means lack of belongingness, being neglected, lack of protection, discrimination, social exclusion, drug addiction, and participation in prostitution"*** **(FGD 1, 2 and interviewees 1, 7).**

All categories agreed that the most challenges of living on street were ***"hunger, cold and rain. In addition to this, police men consider us a pickpocket person and abuse us physically every day"*** **(FGD 4, 5, 6).** Streets children were victimized on a daily basis. Focus group discussants pointed that police men consider them as criminals/ pickpocket person and strike them without any reason and had been taking their things (jalbo). As participants indicated sometimes police men had been taking them to jail without any legal background. ***"Street children are not criminals rather than people who live with their own problems on a street. I am facing different challenges by being on street: hunger, cold, sleep on a street while flood flows under the place where I sleep on a street"*** **(FGD 5, and Interviewees 12, 17, 20).**

Female participant revealed that the other most challenge of living on a street was ***"suffering of rain during rainy season; there is no any roof to sleep under and no enough cloth to wear. Imagine, the hunger you face during rainy time! Sleeping on a street with the agony of hunger since you do not get enough food is another hurt we are facing on a street"*** **(Interviewees 16, 18).**

Category 3.2: Being out of school

On-street children have not got any opportunity to attend their educational endeavor. To attend the school basic needs are obligatory. Thus, they devoted their time in searching of basic needs rather than attending school.

Most of children on-street never attempt to join school due to lack of school requirements, food and other basic needs. They had nobody to support them for their schooling. Those who attempt school, forced to drop their school due to lack of money for school requirements such as school fees, uniform and shoes. Incapability to concentrate to attend school due to hunger. Thus, regular absenteeism from the school results in the loss of interest to continue their education was another tricky situation that these young vulnerable groups were facing.

Participants' highlighted that ***"Living on a street means being out of school. We are created simply to watch other children who have parents, home and going to school. Even if we want to go to school, we can't. We don't have the pre requisite for learning. It is difficult to be enrolled, to get teaching materials, to be accepted by other students in the school. We blame our hard luck"*** **(FGD 1, 3).**

Off-street children reported that ***"We have opportunity to be in school when we compare ourselves with our colleagues. However, absenteeism from school is the challenge we are facing. To survive you should search for daily manual work" (FGD 5, 6).***

Discussion

This study provided the opportunity to look at the life experience of street children related to determinant of being on street, context of living on a street and challenges of living on a street of this young vulnerable group in Ethiopia, Addis Ababa city.

The findings of this study revealed that death of parents (single or double orphan) or conflict with extended relatives were determinant factors to be street child. Thus the death/conflict with extended family resulted in poverty. As the consequence, they were forced to participate in transactional sex and risky sexual behaviors. Lack of basic needs was perceived to lead to engage in survival sex. It is strategy to meet such need. This finding is similar with the study conducted in Malawi and Kenya [3, 9].

This phenomenological inquiry revealed that socio-economic factor puts street children at elevated risk of sexual behaviors. To resist the economic problem, street children initiate early sexual engagement. Thus, multiple sexual partners is perhaps in their life. This is consistent with the study conducted in Liberia and Uganda [10, 11].

The result shows prominent report on context of living on a street. The context is full of risky sexual behaviors, early sexual initiation, multiple sexual partners and physical exploitation were common practices. The finding of this study is similar with the study conducted in sub-Saharan countries [9, 12, 13]. The finding revealed that street children have been found to be at higher likelihood of being sexually active, initiate sex at an earlier age, have unprotected sex and multiple partners. In this study participants reported that street children are involved in high risk sexual behaviors every day for survival. The studies conducted in southern Africa, Uganda and HIV report on global have documented higher rates of STIs and HIV/AIDS among street children [9, 14–16].

This study revealed that street children are facing sexual abuse, rape, prostitution, sexual bartering from day to day which is the same trend with the study conducted in sub-Saharan African countries [12, 14].

This finding shows that street children are high risk group for STIs and HIV. Both male and female street children spent their night at same domicile. Being out of school and insecurity life on a street are the challenges they are facing in their day to day life. Thus, it makes sexual relationships wide spread among themselves and with outsiders. This is similar with the study conducted in Malawi and other sub-Saharan countries [3, 12, 16].

This report shows that street children are using different substances to be out of depression and mood fluctuation. Inline to this finding, the study conducted in south Africa shows (30.3%) of street children had reported clinical depression [14].

There was poor knowledge of STIs and HIV/AIDS among street children. Similarly, different studies shows that respondents' knowledge about STIs and HIV/AIDS is very low [10, 15].

Conclusion

The study has explored the life experience of street children. In different aspects street children are vulnerable to sexual and physical exploitations on the daily basis. The study verified that street children are the most vulnerable group of young people that their life style put them under the circuit of risky sexual behaviors, sexual abuse and physical exploitations.

Rapes, anal sex, unprotected sex and survival sex are common factors that increase healthy problem of them. On-street children has no safe sleeping place over the night. Thus, street environments do not offer protection to them from sexual and physical abuse. Lack of safe night shelter places street children on high risk of sexual and physical exploitations and added an advantage of prostitutes for strangers. This study showed that children off-street is less likely to be sexually exploited compared to children on-street as they share night shelter with their families or extended families.

Recommendations

Physical and sexual exploitation reduction programmes targeting both on-street and off-street children should be taken in to considerations through multi-cultural and community involvement perspectives. Creating income generating activities should be considered for these young vulnerable groups. Creating social protection systems under the collaboration of governments and non-government organizations should be considered. Forming temporary residency and try to re-unite with their families has sufficient advantage in their healthy. Not only for their health, has indisputable credibility to avoid social isolation. Additionally efforts should be targeted to increase street children schooling and opportunity for safe shelter (separate quarter for male and female street children) over the night. (Government organizations and NGOs like Hope Enterprise should work on it).

The researchers recommend mega researches on both on and off-street children that can identify their STIs and HIV/AIDS statuses by using large sample size. Large sample size that allow mixed qualitative and quantitative researches recommended to understand the life experience of street children in different cities of Ethiopia.

Limitation of the study

This study used only phenomenological qualitative research design that used small number of study participants up to the level of information saturation from a single city.

Abbreviations

BSc: Bachelor of Science; FGD: Focus Group Discussion; IGA: Income Generating Activities; NGO: Non-Government Organization; OVC: Orphan and Vulnerable Children; STIs: Sexually Transmitted Infections

Acknowledgements

The author would like to heart fully thank the study participants who dedicated to participate in the study and contribute their valuable responses.

Authors' contributions

Both authors, FAC and CA involved from the inception of idea to the design and analysis of the study and preparation of manuscript. Both authors read and approved the final manuscript.

Ethics approval and consent to participate

Ethical clearance and permission was obtained from Addis Ababa University Institutional Research Review Board.

Since the study subjects were younger than 18 years, written assent was taken from study subjects and written consent was taken from guardians or nongovernmental organizations (NGO) who were responsible to look after them. To compensate the study participants' time, the researchers provided them 15 birr (USD 0.5) per person. Participation in the study was voluntary and information that was collected from the study subjects assured confidentiality.

Competing interests
The authors declare that they have no competing interests.

Author details
[1]School of Nursing and Midwifery, College of Health Sciences, Wollega University, P.O Box: 395, Nekemte, Ethiopia. [2]College of Health Science, Addis Ababa University, Addis Ababa, Ethiopia.

References

1. Laura K. Murray, Namrita S. Singh: A qualitative study of Georgian youth who are on the street or institutionalized. Int J Pediatr. 2010;2012:11. Article ID 921604.
2. Demelash H, Addisie A. Assessment of sexual and reproductive health status of street children in Addis Ababa. J Sex Transm Dis. 2013;2013:524076.
3. Street children's vulnerability to HIV and Sex Transm Infect in Malawian cities.
4. Boston University Center for Glob Health, Nigeria August 2009. (Effect of Economic Assets on Sexual Risk- Taking Intentions Among Orphaned Adolescents in Uganda).
5. Amuyunzu-Nyamongo M, Biddlecom AE, Ouedraogo C, Woog V. Qualitative Evidence on Adolescents' Views of Sexual and Reproductive Health in Sub-Saharan Africa Occasional Report. New York: The Alan Guttmacher Institute; 2005. p. 16.
6. Ljungqvist B. Millennium dream campaign, UNICEF Representative in Ethiopia 2007.
7. Assche VMaSB-V: Orphans and Vulnerable Children in High HIV-Prevalence Countries in Sub-Saharan Africa 2008.
8. Juma M, LKB JA, Askew I, Van den Born B. Understanding orphan and non-orphan adolescents' sexual risks in the context of poverty: a qualitative study in Nyanza Province, Kenya. BMC Int Health Hum Rights. 2013;13:32.
9. Puffer ES, Drabkin AS, Stashko AL, Broverman SA, Ogwang-Odhiambo RA, Sikkema KJ. Orphan status, HIV risk behavior, and mental health among adolescents in rural Kenya. J Pediatr Psychol. 2012;37(8):868–78.
10. Atwine B, Cantor-Graae E, Bajunirwe F. Psychological distress among AIDS orphans in rural Uganda. Soc Sci Med. 2005;61:555–64.
11. Kathryn Whetten, Jan Ostermann, Rachel A, et al. Comparison of the Wellbeing of Orphans and Abandoned Children Ages 6–12 in Institutional and Community-Based Care Settings in 5 Less Wealthy Nations. PLoS One. 2009;4(12):e8169. https://doi.org/10.1371/journal.pone.0008169.
12. Ssewamala FM, Han CK, Neilands TB, Ismayilova L, Sperber E. Effect of Economic Assets on Sexual Risk-Taking Intentions Among Orphaned Adolescents in Uganda. Am J Public Health. 2010;100(3):483–8.
13. Atwood KA, Kennedy SB, Shamblen S, Taylor CH, Quaqua M, Bee EM, Gobeh ME, Woods DV, Dennis B. Reducing sexual risk taking behaviors among adolescents who engage in transactional sex in post-conflict Liberia. Vulnerable Child Youth Stud 2012; 1(7):55-65.
14. Case A, Paxson C, Ableidinger J. Orphans in Africa: parental death, poverty, and school enrollment. Demography. 2004;41(3):483–508.
15. UNAIDS report on the global AIDS epidemic 2013.
16. Whetten K, Ostermann J, Rachel Whetten, Karen O'Donnell, Nathan Thielman:. More than the loss of a parent: potentially traumatic events among orphaned and abandoned children. J Trauma Stress 2011;24(2):174-182.

17

Prevalence of pain reports in pediatric primary care and association with demographics, body mass index, and exam findings

Randall W. Grout[1,3*], Rachel Thompson-Fleming[1,4], Aaron E. Carroll[2,3] and Stephen M. Downs[1,3]

Abstract

Background: Pediatric pain is associated to patient weight and demographics in specialized settings, but pain prevalence and its associated patient attributes in general pediatric outpatient care are unknown. Our objective was to determine the rate of positive pain screenings in pediatric primary care and evaluate the relationship between reported pain and obesity, demographics, and exam findings during routine pediatric encounters.

Methods: Cross-sectional observational study of 26,180 patients ages 2 to 19 seen in five urban pediatric primary care clinics between 2009 and 2016. Data were collected from systematic screening using a computerized clinical decision support system. Multivariable logistic regressions were used to analyze the association between pain reporting and obesity (body mass index), age, sex, race, season, insurance status, clinic site, prior pain reporting, pain reporting method, and exam findings.

Results: Pain was reported by the patient or caregiver in 14.9% of visits. In adjusted models, pain reporting was associated with obesity (Odds Ratio (OR) 1.23, 95% Confidence Intervals (CI) 1.11–1.35) and severe obesity (OR 1.32, CI 1.17–1.49); adolescents (OR 1.47, CI 1.33–1.61); and females (OR 1.21, CI 1.12–1.29). Pain reported at the preceding visit increased odds of pain reporting 2.67 times (CI 2.42–2.95). Abnormal abdominal, extremity, ear, nose, throat, and lymph node exams were associated with pain reporting. Pain reporting increased in minority races within clinics that predominantly saw a concordant race.

Conclusions: Pain is common in general pediatric encounters, and occurs more frequently in obese children and those who previously reported pain. Pain reporting may be influenced by seasonal variation and clinic factors. Future pediatric pain screening may be guided by associated risk factors to improve identification and targeted healthcare interventions.

Keywords: Pain, Obesity, Ambulatory care, Clinical decision support

Background

Despite over 16 years of Joint Commission standards to assess and address patient pain, data are sparse regarding the prevalence, demographics, and body metrics associated with pain in general pediatrics. Prior studies have assessed pain in general practice or family practice, but only a fraction of those patients were children. [1, 2] Epidemiological studies in adults describe significant differences in pain prevalence among racial, socioeconomic, sex, and age categories, [3–5] however, comparable studies in pediatrics are sparse. Current scientific knowledge of outpatient pediatric pain is limited to non-routine/emergency [6] or subspecialty/disease-specific [7, 8] settings (e.g., emergency room, obesity clinic, pain clinic), or when pain is the primary complaint/diagnosis. [2, 9] Additionally, epidemiologic studies have focused on chronic pain, [10] especially through surveys at

* Correspondence: rgrout@iu.edu
[1]Children's Health Services Research, Department of Pediatrics, Indiana University School of Medicine, 410 W. 10th Street, HS 2000, Indianapolis, IN 46202, USA
[3]Regenstrief Institute, Inc, 1101 W. 10th Street, Indianapolis, IN 46202, USA

the school, [11] national, [12] or international [13] levels. Among these, general pain estimates ranged between 5% (report of chronic pain at the time of the survey) and 88% (at least one pain episode within the 3 previous months). Site-specific specific pain (e.g., headache, abdominal pain, musculoskeletal pain) rates varied nearly as much, but were also subject to many differences in assessment windows. [10] Few studies assessed the prevalence of pain assessed at the instant of data collection, but these were in school settings. None measured the prevalence of general pain at routine clinical encounters—the largest portion of pediatric healthcare. Even less is known of how clinicians respond to pain reports among children and physical exam findings from visits where pain is reported.

In a 2011 report, the Institute of Medicine requested better data on pain incidence, prevalence, and characteristics, specifically among vulnerable subpopulations, including children, people with low income, and racial and ethnic minorities. [14] This study responds, in part, to this call. Our objective was to determine prevalence of reported pain during a general pediatric encounter, and

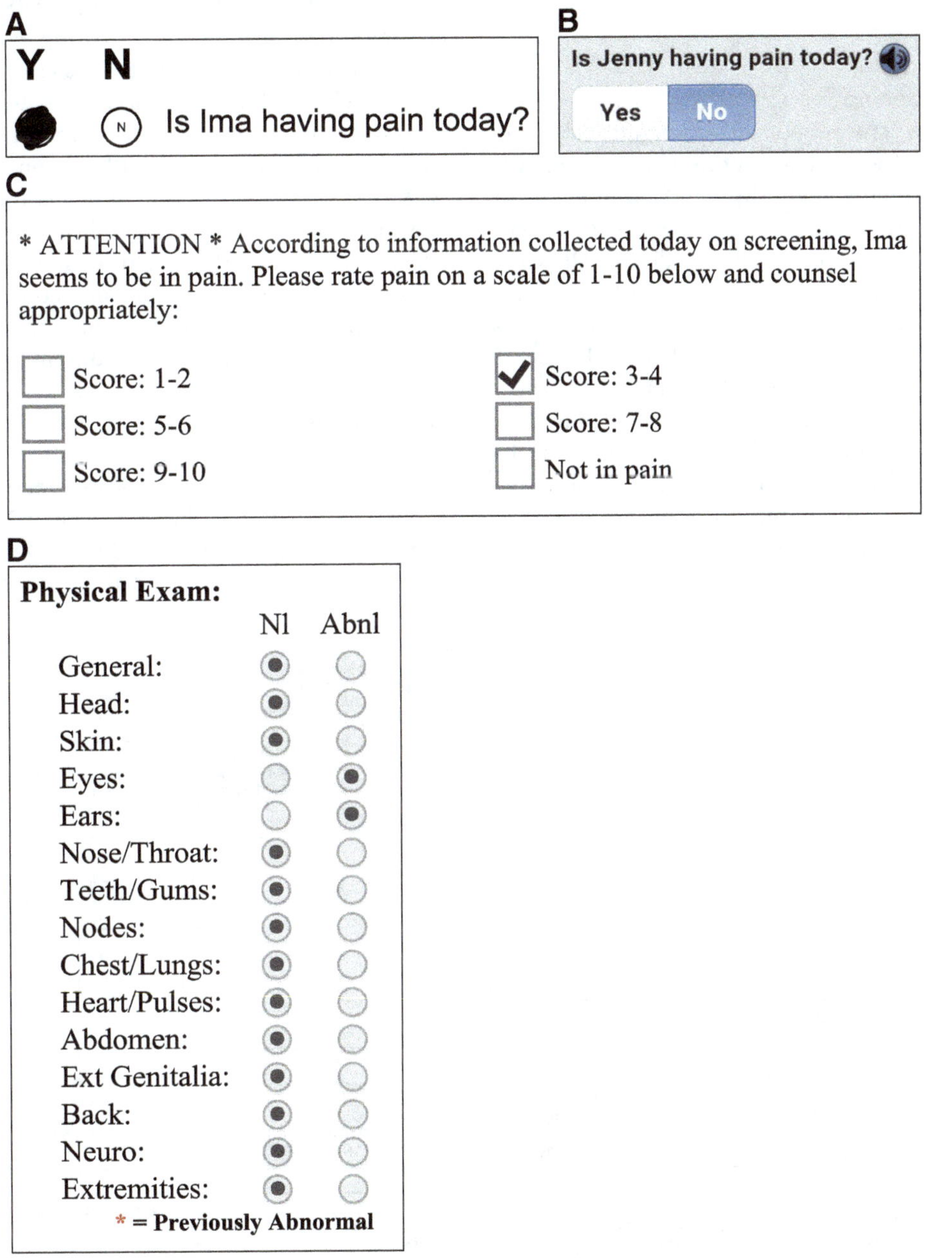

Fig. 1 Parts **a-d**: User interfaces for CHICA forms. **a** Paper PSF question to assess pain in child. **b** Tablet PSF question to assess pain in child. **c** Positive PSF pain response alert to provider on PWS. **d** Exam documentation template on PWS

its relationship with body mass index (BMI) percentile, demographics, socioeconomic status, and season, using records from a clinical decision support system used in pediatric primary care clinics. As secondary outcomes, we investigated physician documentation of pain, and normal versus abnormal physical exam findings associated with reports of pain. Given the existing findings in adults and, to a lesser degree, children, we hypothesized differences in pain exist in pediatric patients based on obesity, sex, age, socioeconomic status, and race, and that pain is associated with an abnormal physical exam and previous pain reports.

Methods

Study design and setting

We conducted a cross-sectional observational study using data gathered as part of routine clinical care with the Child Health Improvement through Computer Automation system (CHICA), a clinical decision support system used by five urban, outpatient pediatric clinics in Indianapolis, IN. CHICA was launched in 2004, and has been in continuous use since. CHICA houses data for over 50,000 patients and nearly 350,000 clinical encounters. All clinics are staffed by pediatricians (the majority) or advanced practitioners, referred to as "providers" or "clinicians" herein. These providers receive initial training on CHICA, and have ongoing onsite technical support available. Data and usage patterns are reviewed weekly by the informatics team, and targeted outreach is conducted as needed.

CHICA collects data about patients via two primary means. One is a Pre-Screener Form (PSF), available in English or Spanish, completed by parents or patients in the waiting room. The PSF includes 20 yes/no questions concerning the child's health and risk factors (e.g., household violence, maternal depression). The questions on the PSF are derived algorithmically [15] based on the child's age, responses on previous screeners, information from previous clinic visits, and data in the child's medical record. While initially printed on paper forms, the PSF is now administered on an electronic tablet. [16]

The Provider Worksheet (PWS) is the second source of data in CHICA. The PWS contains up to six reminder prompts for treating clinicians that are also algorithmically-generated based on the responses on the child's PSF(s), data in the electronic medical record, and age-appropriate care guidelines. Each of the six reminders on the PWS contains checkboxes, with which the providers indicate their responses to the prompt. If the patient indicated pain on the PSF screening, the PWS would prompt the provider to document the level of pain and counsel appropriately (Fig. 1c). In addition to decision support, the PWS offers a method to quickly document normal or abnormal exams across 15 body systems, according to each clinician's assessment (Fig. 1d).

Patients in the clinics using CHICA are diverse, with significant proportions of African American and Hispanic children. CHICA distributes nearly 1000 PSF forms and generates between 2000 and 3000 patient-specific prompts for the various providers on the PWS each month. The

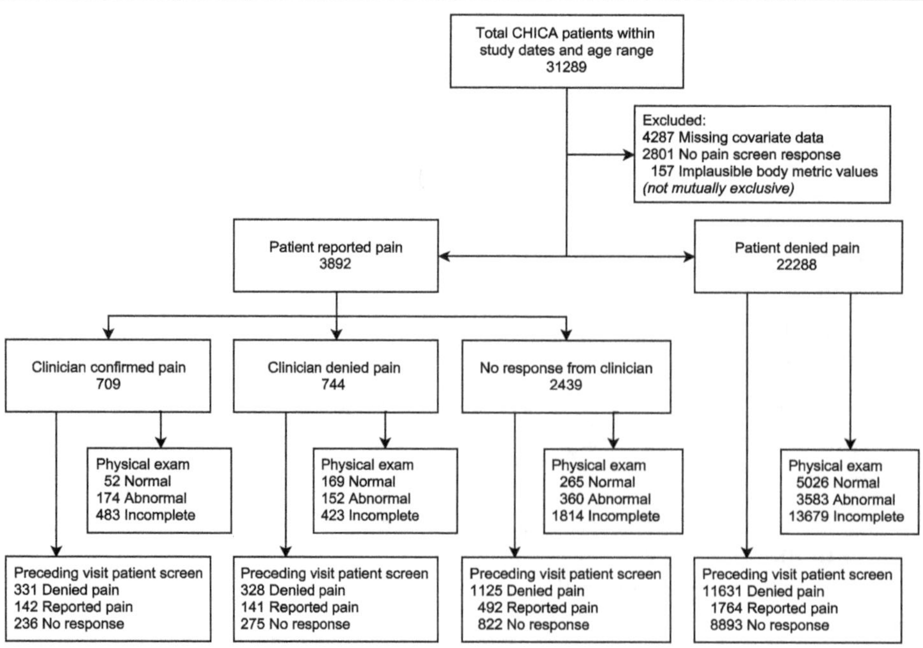

Fig. 2 Patient flow and counts through study

overall patient-response rates on the PSF are greater than 85%. CHICA has been used to study a variety of phenomena, such as improved developmental screening [17], infant television viewing and maternal depression [18], and mental health outcomes of children exposed to violence or depression [19].

Procedure

In this study, we relied on a specific PSF prompt assessing pain that was asked as a routine part of all patient encounters. For patients less than 12 years old, the question was directed to the parent/guardian, reading, "Is [child's name] having pain today?" (Fig. 1a and b). For patients 12 years and older, with the intention that the child would complete the PSF himself or herself, the question reads, "Are you in pain today?" If the patient reported pain, the physician received the alert in Fig. 1c, with a numeric pain scale reporting option. We recorded the physician responses to the alert and physical exam documented on the PWS at these encounters. We also collected each patient's pain report from the preceding visit, if available.

We extracted sociodemographic data from CHICA, including race/ethnicity, sex, age, and the payer source at the index encounter. We determined the PSF delivery method—paper versus electronic tablet—based on the date of the visit and the date each clinic transitioned to tablets. Additionally, we classified each visit date by season, using the calendar months as break points (e.g., December through February as winter). We coded age groups based on National Institute of Child Health and Human Development recommendations: 2 to less than 6 years; 6 to less than 12 years; and 12 to less than 20 years of age. We coded race/ethnicity as Black, White, Hispanic, or Other/Unknown. We coded payer source as commercial/private, public (Medicaid/Medicare), and other (self-pay or no insurance).

CHICA records each child's clinic-measured height and weight. We calculated BMI as weight in kilograms divided by height in meters squared. We determined BMI percentile using Centers for Disease Control and Prevention (CDC) 2000 growth chart parameters. To eliminate biologically implausible values, we discarded data from patient encounters with height, weight, or BMI percentile modified z-score values beyond pre-determined limits by age, following a technique recommended and validated by the CDC. [20]

BMI category was stratified into underweight (less than 5th percentile), normal BMI (5th to less than 85th percentile), overweight (85th to less than 95th percentile), obese (95th to less than 120% of the 95 percentile), and severely obese (120% of the 95th percentile or greater) classes, again following recommendations for stratifying extreme BMI values. [21]

Data collection

Data were gathered from all patient encounters between July 2009 and February 2016. Eligibility criteria for this study were age between 2 and 19 years, inclusive, and having a PSF pain question response, height, and weight at the same visit. Patient encounters were excluded if

Table 1 Demographic and patient variables

	Pain reported at index visit		Overall
	No	Yes	
No. with data	22,288	3892	26,180
BMI Class, No. (%)			
Normal BMI	12,793 (57.4)	2037 (52.3)	14,830 (56.6)
Underweight	888 (4.0)	148 (3.8)	1036 (4.0)
Overweight	3636 (16.3)	653 (16.8)	4289 (16.4)
Obese	3233 (14.5)	659 (16.9)	3892 (14.9)
Severely Obese	1738 (7.8)	395 (10.1)	2133 (8.1)
Age, No. (%)			
2–5 years old	7311 (32.8)	1006 (25.8)	8317 (31.8)
6–11 years old	8845 (39.7)	1672 (43.0)	10,517 (40.2)
12–19 years old	6132 (27.5)	1214 (31.2)	7346 (28.1)
Sex = Female, No. (%)	10,808 (48.5)	2064 (53.0)	12,872 (49.2)
Race/ethnicity, No. (%)			
Black	11,711 (52.5)	1878 (48.3)	13,589 (51.9)
Hispanic	6202 (27.8)	1125 (28.9)	7327 (28.0)
White	2145 (9.6)	427 (11.0)	2572 (9.8)
Other/Unknown	2230 (10.0)	462 (11.9)	2692 (10.3)
Insurance type, No. (%)			
Public	19,903 (89.3)	3461 (88.9)	23,364 (89.2)
Commercial	1355 (6.1)	237 (6.1)	1592 (6.1)
Other	1030 (4.6)	194 (5.0)	1224 (4.7)
Clinic site, No. (%)			
Clinic 1	6126 (27.5)	923 (23.7)	7049 (26.9)
Clinic 2	2335 (10.5)	373 (9.6)	2708 (10.3)
Clinic 3	5077 (22.8)	954 (24.5)	6031 (23.0)
Clinic 4	3868 (17.4)	698 (17.9)	4566 (17.4)
Clinic 5	4882 (21.9)	944 (24.3)	5826 (22.3)
Used tablet interface, No. (%)	14,116 (63.3)	2915 (74.9)	17,031 (65.1)
Season, No. (%)			
Autumn	6644 (29.8)	1158 (29.8)	7802 (29.8)
Winter	5299 (23.8)	1131 (29.1)	6430 (24.6)
Spring	3788 (17.0)	736 (18.9)	4524 (17.3)
Summer	6557 (29.4)	867 (22.3)	7424 (28.4)
Pain indicated in preceding visit, No. (%)			
No	11,631 (52.2)	1784 (45.8)	13,415 (51.2)
Yes	1764 (7.9)	775 (19.9)	2539 (9.7)
Unknown (no response)	8893 (39.9)	1333 (34.2)	10,226 (39.1)

any covariate data were missing; no data were imputed. For patients with multiple visits in the CHICA system, we used the last clinical encounter that met eligibility criteria (index encounter).

The study protocol was approved by the Indiana University Institutional Review Board, and included a waiver of informed consent because no interventions were being implemented, impracticability, and minimal risk.

Statistical analysis

We tested for association between potential variables using Pearson's chi-squared, with Cramer's V to measure effect size. Unadjusted (univariable) logistic regression was used to identify variables associated with patient-reported pain, with a threshold of $P < 0.10$ to be retained in an adjusted model. Despite not meeting this cutoff, we retained payer source in the adjusted model as a means-tested proxy for income, and in turn, socioeconomic status (SES). [22] We used multivariable logistic regression models to identify factors associated with positive pain reports. Variables included were BMI category, age category, sex, race, payer source, clinic site, PSF delivery method, season, and pain reported on the PSF at the preceding visit. The most common levels of each variable was chosen as the reference level for the models, except for age, where we chose the youngest group as a chronologic baseline. Due to the association between clinic site and race, we also included an interaction term between clinic and race. We chose to use an interaction fixed effect instead of a random effect for clinic due to the limited number of clinics and to describe the clinic-race mechanisms more deeply. Two models were prepared: the first included all patients at their most recent qualifying visit, and the second was a subset limited to patients for which there was a preceding visit with a response to the pain question. Separately, we created a multivariable logistic regression model to determine the odds ratio of reporting pain based on abnormal exam variables. All multivariable regressions were two-sided tests with alpha = 0.05. We used R 3.3.1 [23] to conduct the analyses.

Results

Over the study period, 31,289 patients within the appropriate age range were seen; 26,180 met eligibility criteria and their most recent encounter was selected for analysis (see Fig. 2 for patient flow in study).

Table 1 describes patient demographic data. Approximately half of the patients were male (50.8%), and Black patients were the largest race/ethnicity group (51.9%). There were fewer adolescent patients (28.1%) than other age groups. Most visits were covered by public payers (89.2%). Clinics 2 and 3 had more Black patients (87.1 and 82.9%, respectively). Clinic 4 had approximately twice as many Hispanic (45.2%) as Black patients (22.7%). See Table 2 for proportions of clinic populations by race.

The majority of patients had normal BMI percentile (56.6%). The distribution of BMI percentile was skewed left (indicating relatively more frequent obesity); 4% were underweight and 23% obese or severely obese. Approximately 15% of patients reported pain at the index encounter. More than half (15,954 or 60.9%) of all patients had completed pain screening at the preceding visit, and 15.9% of that subset reported pain. There were on average 293 days (SD 269 days) between the index and preceding visits.

All potential variables showed weak or small associations with one another, except for race versus clinic (Cramer's V = .291, medium correlation). Table 3 presents regression model data. All the variables except payer source were significantly associated with reporting pain in unadjusted models. In the adjusted model, obese and severely obese children had 1.22 and 1.31 times higher odds of reported pain than normal weight children, respectively. Adolescent and middle-childhood patients were each more likely to report pain than younger patients (OR 1.47 and 1.34, respectively). There were higher odds of pain reporting (1) among females, (2) during winter and spring seasons, and (3) when using a tablet interface to record responses. Pain reported at the preceding visit was strongly associated (OR 2.67, CI 2.42–2.95) with pain reports at the index visit.

There were significant interactions on pain reporting between clinic and race. At the reference site, Black patients had lower odds of reporting pain than other races. Compared to the reference clinic, Black patients at a

Table 2 Clinic and race/ethnicity distribution

Variable	Overall (*n* = 26,180)	Clinic 1 (*n* = 7049)	Clinic 2 (*n* = 2708)	Clinic 3 (*n* = 6031)	Clinic 4 (*n* = 4566)	Clinic 5 (*n* = 5826)
Race/ethnicity, No. (%)						
Black	13,589 (51.9)	2526 (35.8)	2359 (87.1)	5000 (82.9)	1037 (22.7)	2667 (45.8)
Hispanic	7327 (28.0)	2764 (39.2)	157 (5.8)	372 (6.2)	2066 (45.2)	1968 (33.8)
White	2572 (9.8)	1034 (14.7)	124 (4.6)	413 (6.8)	435 (9.5)	566 (9.7)
Other	2692 (10.3)	725 (10.3)	68 (2.5)	246 (4.1)	1028 (22.5)	625 (10.7)

Table 3 Unadjusted and adjusted models predicting a pain report

	Unadjusted Models		Adjusted Model 1[a] (n = 26,180)		Adjusted Model 2[b] (*n* = 15,954)	
	OR	90% CI	OR	95% CI	OR	95% CI
BMI Class						
Normal Weight (Ref)						
Underweight	1.05	(0.9–1.21)	1.14	(0.95–1.37)	1.26	(1–1.58)**
Overweight	1.13	(1.04–1.22)*	1.09	(0.99–1.2)	1.12	(0.99–1.27)
Obese	1.28	(1.18–1.39)*	1.23	(1.11–1.35)**	1.2	(1.06–1.36)**
Severely obese	1.43	(1.29–1.58)*	1.32	(1.17–1.49)**	1.26	(1.08–1.48)**
Age						
2–5 years old (Ref)						
6–11 years old	1.37	(1.28–1.47)*	1.33	(1.22–1.45)**	1.13	(1.02–1.26)**
12–19 years old	1.44	(1.33–1.55)*	1.47	(1.33–1.61)**	1.25	(1.11–1.41)**
Sex						
Male (Ref)						
Female	1.2	(1.13–1.27)*	1.21	(1.12–1.29)**	1.2	(1.1–1.3)**
Race/ethnicity						
Black (Ref)						
Hispanic	1.13	(1.06–1.21)*	1.19	(1–1.41)**	1.28	(1.02–1.6)**
White	1.24	(1.13–1.37)*	1.52	(1.23–1.88)**	1.58	(1.18–2.11)**
Other	1.29	(1.18–1.42)*	1.3	(1.02–1.65)**	1.25	(0.89–1.75)
Insurance type						
Public (Ref)						
Commercial	1.01	(0.89–1.13)	1.02	(0.88–1.18)	1.04	(0.86–1.25)
Other	1.08	(0.95–1.23)	1.1	(0.94–1.29)	1.02	(0.81–1.28)
Clinic site						
Clinic 1 (Ref)						
Clinic 2	1.06	(0.95–1.18)	1.13	(0.95–1.35)	1.12	(0.88–1.42)
Clinic 3	1.25	(1.15–1.35)*	1.29	(1.11–1.51)**	1.36	(1.11–1.68)**
Clinic 4	1.2	(1.1–1.31)*	0.75	(0.59–0.96)**	0.98	(0.69–1.39)
Clinic 5	1.28	(1.18–1.39)*	1.01	(0.85–1.21)	1.18	(0.94–1.49)
Pre-screener form (PSF) medium						
Paper (Ref)						
Tablet	1.73	(1.62–1.84)*	1.77	(1.62–1.93)**	1.73	(1.53–1.96)**
Season						
Autumn (Ref)						
Winter	1.22	(1.14–1.32)*	1.21	(1.1–1.32)**	1.2	(1.08–1.35)**
Spring	1.11	(1.02–1.21)*	1.15	(1.04–1.27)**	1.18	(1.04–1.35)**
Summer	0.76	(0.7–0.82)*	0.76	(0.69–0.83)**	0.72	(0.64–0.82)**
Pain reported at preceding visit						
No (Ref)						
Yes	2.86	(2.64–3.11)*			2.67	(2.42–2.95)**
Clinic:Race interaction terms						
Clinic 2:Hispanic			0.71	(0.41–1.17)	0.66	(0.3–1.31)
Clinic 2:White			0.93	(0.54–1.53)	0.86	(0.41–1.7)
Clinic 2:Other			0.55	(0.22–1.19)	0.33	(0.05–1.16)

Table 3 Unadjusted and adjusted models predicting a pain report *(Continued)*

	Unadjusted Models		Adjusted Model 1[a] (n = 26,180)		Adjusted Model 2[b] (*n* = 15,954)	
	OR	90% CI	OR	95% CI	OR	95% CI
Clinic 3:Hispanic			0.89	(0.63–1.23)	1.01	(0.66–1.51)
Clinic 3:White			0.78	(0.55–1.09)	0.86	(0.55–1.35)
Clinic 3:Other			0.71	(0.45–1.08)	0.92	(0.51–1.62)
Clinic 4:Hispanic			1.44	(1.08–1.93)**	1.21	(0.81–1.83)
Clinic 4:White			0.87	(0.58–1.29)	0.74	(0.42–1.31)
Clinic 4:Other			1.38	(0.97–1.96)	1.31	(0.8–2.18)
Clinic 5:Hispanic			0.91	(0.72–1.15)	0.83	(0.62–1.12)
Clinic 5:White			0.93	(0.68–1.28)	0.84	(0.57–1.25)
Clinic 5:Other			0.89	(0.64–1.25)	0.85	(0.55–1.32)

[a]Model 1: Adjusted for BMI class, age, sex, race/ethnicity, insurance type, pre-screener form medium, season, with race:clinic interaction terms
[b]Model 2: In addition to Model 1 covariates, includes pain report at prior visit. Limited to patients for whom a pain screen exists at the preceding visit
*$P < 0.1$, **$P < 0.05$

large clinic that saw primarily (> 80%) Black patients had 29% (CI 1.11–1.51) higher odds of reporting pain. In contrast, Black patients at Clinic 4, a Spanish-English fully bilingual clinic, had lower odds of reporting pain (OR 0.75, CI 0.59–0.96) than at the reference clinic. Within that bilingual clinic, Hispanic patients were 1.72 times (CI 1.36–2.18) more likely to report pain than Black patients.

To confirm this finding, we built a secondary model (not reported in detail here) where the race-clinic interaction was replaced by a variable indicating race-clinic concordance, which was positive when the patient's race and the predominant race of the clinic were the same. There was a significant 27% increase odds of pain reporting in race-concordant clinics. However, when re-creating Adjusted Model 2 from Table 3 (which includes pain reported at the preceding visit), the effect was not significant.

Clinicians documented a scaled pain assessment for 1453 (37%) of the 3892 patients who reported pain, but listed 744 (51%) of those as 0/10 pain (Table 4).

A physical exam for at least one body system was documented through the CHICA PWS on 9781 (37%) of eligible encounters, and a full physical exam (all 15 systems) was documented in 3149 (12%). Table 5 reports descriptive data on abnormal exams for that subset of subjects with a full exam documented.

Table 4 Clinician pain assessment responses for patients reporting pain

Clinician pain assessment (scale 0–10)	No. (%)
0	744 (19.1)
1–2	321 (8.2)
3–4	187 (4.8)
5–6	114 (2.9)
7–8	52 (1.3)
9–10	35 (0.9)
No response documented	2439 (62.7)

In a multiple logistic regression model including only patients with full exams documented, an abnormal exam of the abdomen, ears, extremities, lymph nodes, or nose/throat was associated with higher odds of pain reporting (Table 6). In contrast, heart/pulses and teeth/gum abnormal findings were independently associated with lower odds of pain reporting.

Discussion

We examine the prevalence of undifferentiated pain in general pediatric outpatient care. We found about 15% of patients reported pain in our setting, which falls within prior limited clinical and non-clinical estimates among similar age groups or time frames. Previous studies in general or family practice across several countries used pain as the visit reason to estimate prevalence between 5.1 and 36%. [24–26] Within school-based surveys of varying age ranges, point prevalences have been reported between 4.8 and 27.1%. [27–29]

The obesity rates in our study sample were similar to nationally reported statistics. Obesity is linked to several pain outcomes, notably musculoskeletal complaints, headache, and chronic pain. [7, 8] A previous convenience sample showed a positive relationship between BMI and general pain report in an obesity clinic. [30] We show that obesity and severe obesity were associated with higher pain report prevalence in a pediatric population visiting a general outpatient clinic. However, underweight and overweight children did not report more pain. The correlation between obesity and pain may reflect a cycle of decreased exercise due to pain, and pain due to increased BMI from lack of exercise. [31] Unfortunately, many parents do not perceive this association in their own children. [32] Perhaps providers can use

Table 5 Abnormal exams documented in CHICA

	Pain reported at index visit[a]		Overall[a]
	No	Yes	
No. with complete exam documented in CHICA	2838	311	3149
Abnormal Exam component, No. (%)			
Abdomen	87 (3.1)	22 (7.1)	109 (3.5)
Back	43 (1.5)	10 (3.2)	53 (1.7)
Chest/Lungs	73 (2.6)	16 (5.1)	89 (2.8)
Ears/Hearing	98 (3.5)	28 (9.0)	126 (4.0)
External Genitalia	107 (3.8)	18 (5.8)	125 (4.0)
Extremities	87 (3.1)	30 (9.6)	117 (3.7)
Eyes/Vision	97 (3.4)	16 (5.1)	113 (3.6)
General	153 (5.4)	25 (8.0)	178 (5.7)
Head	68 (2.4)	15 (4.8)	83 (2.6)
Heart/Pulses	61 (2.1)	7 (2.3)	68 (2.2)
Neurologic	49 (1.7)	13 (4.2)	62 (2.0)
Nodes	56 (2.0)	20 (6.4)	76 (2.4)
Nose/Throat	190 (6.7)	61 (19.6)	251 (8.0)
Skin	492 (17.3)	73 (23.5)	565 (17.9)
Teeth/Gums	119 (4.2)	12 (3.9)	131 (4.2)

[a]Columns do not sum to total because exam components are not mutually exclusive

this knowledge to incentivize weight reduction to try to reduce pain. However, other psychosocial determinants of health may independently lead to pain and obesity, complicating this relationship.

Our findings are consistent with prior research on characteristics related to pain in children. Females reported pain more often than males, [2, 10] perhaps for psychosociocultural reasons, as the difference is noted across experimental pain response studies, [33] survey instruments, [12] and several pain subtypes. [10, 13] Older children generally report more location specific pain (except for abdominal pain). [10] The lower same-day pain reporting here among younger children may represent a true decrease in pain reports or sensation, a difference between acute and chronic pain among childhood ages, or even a known phenomenon of surrogates (e.g., parents or caregivers) underestimating pain. [34] Insurance at the time of visit was not associated with any change in pain reporting. Past studies demonstrate mixed findings of associations between SES and chronic pain. [10, 35, 36] However, the vast majority of our study population was on public insurance, limiting our power to assess this association. Additionally, the prevalence here includes both chronic and acute pain, and that combination may mask the prior associations with an isolated chronic pain. Increased pain reporting in winter months may reflect known seasonality of common complaints like abdominal pain, headache and respiratory complaints. [37]

Table 6 Multivariable Logistic Regression Model Predicting a Pain Report from Abnormal Exam Components

Abnormal Exam Component	Adjusted OR[a]	95% CI
Abdomen	1.83	(0.99–3.22)*
Back	0.56	(0.18–1.54)
Chest/Lungs	1.30	(0.63–2.47)
Ears/Hearing	2.32	(1.39–3.73)*
External Genitalia	0.93	(0.47–1.7)
Extremities	3.44	(2.03–5.66)*
Eyes/Vision	0.88	(0.45–1.6)
General	1.22	(0.72–1.96)
Head	1.05	(0.5–2.03)
Heart/Pulses	0.22	(0.06–0.69)*
Neurologic	1.50	(0.58–3.46)
Nodes	2.34	(1.21–4.35)*
Nose/Throat	3.15	(2.21–4.44)*
Skin	1.32	(0.98–1.77)
Teeth/Gums	0.31	(0.13–0.64)*

[a]Adjusted model included all terms in this table
$^*P < 0.05$

In a subset analysis, the strongest predictor of pain reporting was pain reported at the preceding visit. Chronic pain is a notable burden in pediatrics, and it is possible the consecutive pain reports reflect ongoing symptoms. However, it may also be a characteristic of certain patients who are more likely to voice concerns of various common pains.

The largest racial minority in our population reported more pain when in a clinic that predominantly saw patients of that same race. We suspect the social context of patient-clinic racial and cultural concordance may offer a comfort with which to disclose more medical symptoms. Hsieh et al. [38] found increased affective and nonverbal pain expressions when there was both cultural milieu (including language) and race concordance between participants and experimenters – a context similar to the clinics in this population. While it is possible that the race of the treating provider may play a role in pain reporting, we feel this factor is minimized in our data, since the pain question was assessed in the waiting room before interaction with the provider. Further clinical research is needed in facility-level interactions on pain reporting, especially within a new era of computerized clinical decision support systems.

An electronic PSF medium was notably associated with increased pain reports, even when controlling for question response rates. We expected the patient-reported outcomes to be generally equivalent between paper and electronic reporting interfaces. [39] We are uncertain why our experience differs, and it is possible that caregivers and adolescents are more inclined to report pain when the responses go directly to the server instead of on paper, which is handed to clinic personnel. We recommend this topic for future research efforts.

Only 37% of providers rated their patients' pain after an alert reporting a patient's positive response. Although the provider response rate to positive pain screens appears low, it is reasonable within the context of historical [40], local [41], and other voluntary clinical reminder system precedent. [42–46] About half (51.2%) of the completed provider assessments confirmed the patient's pain report, and these were generally rated at low pain levels. It is possible that clinicians were more inclined to respond to the prompt in order to negate what they observed was an erroneous report, which would lead to an artificially depressed rate of providers confirming a patient's pain report. This perceived error may come from a difference between what the patients are trying to report on the screening question and what providers want to know from the alert. Or, it may simply reflect the disparity between patient, caregiver, and clinician pain assessments. Previous research on concordance of pain assessments by clinicians and patients indicate that providers significantly underestimate pain intensity in both adults and children. [47–49] Pain assessment is just the first step in a pain treatment pathway; one study showed clinicians administered pain relief to fewer than half the patients they determined to be in severe pain. [47] Clinical decision support systems aid in pain screening, but further work is needed enhance provider attention and response. Beyond alerting the clinician, decision support and provider training should focus on pain recognition disparities, and actionable and appropriate treatment recommendations.

Exam findings positively correlated with increased pain may come from common painful conditions within pediatrics, such as acute otitis media, gastroenteritis, extremity injuries, and pharyngitis. The negative correlations may result from routinely documenting an abnormal finding that is not usually painful, like heart murmur or dentition with multiple fillings. It is important to note that our sample of patients with full physical exams is a minority, since clinicians may have documented their exams elsewhere, and it is not routine practice to perform a full physical exam when evaluating a targeted chief complaint. Since our screening question assessed general, undifferentiated pain, it is possible many of the reports were for localized concerns.

The Joint Commission accreditation standard in 2001 described a "patient right" to have pain assessed and addressed. Over the past 16 years, many studies and editorials have discussed the difficulties and outcomes of the universal pain assessment intervention. Authors of these studies/editorials often find little or no effect on pain control attributable to systematic pain assessment, and there is controversy over the timing of an "opioid crisis" and the Joint Commission mandate to assess and address pain. [50] Whether systematic pain assessment improved outcomes for the patients in our study is uncertain, but pain was associated with a subset of physical findings, suggesting that there is diagnostic information in the pain measure.

Our study is not without limitations. First, CHICA PSF questions have binary (yes/no) responses, and clinicians are not required to follow-up with a standardized pain assessment. Since pain reports were generally rated by parents or providers, it is possible our findings underestimate the true pain prevalence in this population. It is possible that clinicians were documenting pain or physical exams independently in their notes, which would not be captured with our clinical decision support system. Our observational, cross-sectional study design is unable to identify causal relationships; for example, physical exam findings may be from other abnormalities that are not painful. We do not have data to differentiate well visits versus sick visits, or acute versus chronic pain, which is likely to affect pain reporting, and we emphasize our results are from routine, systematic screening. At the time of this study, the medical record data did not differentiate between race and ethnicity, and so the effect of these two distinct constructs is blurred. Finally, our data come from five urban pediatric primary care clinics serving predominantly low-income and minority families living in a single metropolitan area, so readers should exercise caution in generalizing these results.

Conclusions

Using a large diverse sample, we establish the first data on prevalence of pain and associated characteristics in general pediatric primary care. We show that previously reported trends in pain epidemiology in fact extend to the ambulatory practice environment. More than one in seven patients reported pain at these encounters. Our data suggest that females, White children, children 5 years of age or older, and obese or severely obese children had higher odds of reporting pain at the time of a clinical encounter. In addition, Black and Hispanic patients reported more pain in clinics with concordant majority races. Pain reports were also positively associated with electronic reporting interfaces, certain seasons, and specific exam findings. Our study answers an Institute of Medicine request for better data on childhood pain, especially within a minority and low socioeconomic status population, and provides a springboard for research into such a common symptom in primary care. Future studies should apply methods [51] that improve pain assessment workflows and efficiency in general pediatric practice, and assess clinical outcomes associated with pain assessment in children.

Abbreviations

ADHD: Attention deficit hyperactivity disorder; BMI: Body mass index; CHICA: Child Health improvement through computer automation; PSF: Pre-screener form; PWS: Provider worksheet

Acknowledgements

We thank Htaw Htoo and Tammy Dugan for their assistance with data extraction for this study. We also thank users of the CHICA system at Eskenazi Health and members of Child Health Informatics Research and Development Laboratory (CHIRDL).

Funding

This study was not grant supported, although the CHICA system receives support from the Department of Health and Human Services [grant numbers R01DK092717, R01HS017939, R01HS018453, R01HS020640]. The funding bodies had no role in the design, conducting, or reporting of this study.

Authors' contributions

RG, RTF, AC, and SD designed the study, interpreted results, and reviewed and revised the manuscript. RG and SD coordinated data extraction and conducted the analyses. RG prepared the manuscript, and all authors approved the final manuscript.

Authors' information

AC and SM are co-creators of the CHICA clinical decision support system, which was developed at Indiana University, a non-profit state university.

Competing interests

In 2016, SD co-founded a company to disseminate the CHICA technology. AC is a co-inventor of CHICA. There is no patent, and at this time, there is no licensing agreement. The other authors declare that they have no competing interests to disclose.

Author details

[1]Children's Health Services Research, Department of Pediatrics, Indiana University School of Medicine, 410 W. 10th Street, HS 2000, Indianapolis, IN 46202, USA. [2]Pediatric and Adolescent Comparative Effectiveness Research, Department of Pediatrics, Indiana University School of Medicine, 410 W. 10th Street, HS 2000A, Indianapolis, IN 46202, USA. [3]Regenstrief Institute, Inc, 1101 W. 10th Street, Indianapolis, IN 46202, USA. [4]Present address: Children's Hospital of Wisconsin, 8915 W Connell Ct, Milwaukee, WI 53326, USA.

References

1. Hasselström J, Liu-Palmgren J, Rasjö-Wrååk G. Prevalence of pain in general practice. Eur J Pain. 2002;6:375–85.
2. Knapp DA, Koch H. The management of new pain in office-based ambulatory care: National Ambulatory Medical Care Survey, 1980 and 1981. Adv Data. 1984;97:1–9. https://www.ncbi.nlm.nih.gov/pubmed/10266817.
3. Nahin RL. Estimates of pain prevalence and severity in adults: United States, 2012. J Pain Off J Am Pain Soc. 2015;16:769–80.
4. Riskowski JL. Associations of socioeconomic position and pain prevalence in the United States: findings from the National Health and nutrition examination survey. Pain Med. 2014;15:1508–21.
5. Campbell CM, Edwards RR. Ethnic differences in pain and pain management. Pain Manag. 2012;2:219–30.
6. Drendel AL, Brousseau DC, Gorelick MH. Pain assessment for pediatric patients in the emergency department. Pediatrics. 2006;117:1511–8.
7. Wilson AC, Samuelson B, Palermo TM. Obesity in children and adolescents with chronic pain: associations with pain and activity limitations. Clin J Pain. 2010;26:705–11.
8. Smith SM, Sumar B, Dixon KA. Musculoskeletal pain in overweight and obese children. Int J Obes. 2014;38:11–5.
9. Caudill-Slosberg MA, Schwartz LM, Woloshin S. Office visits and analgesic prescriptions for musculoskeletal pain in US: 1980 vs. 2000. Pain. 2004;109:514–9.
10. King S, Chambers CT, Huguet A, MacNevin RC, McGrath PJ, Parker L, et al. The epidemiology of chronic pain in children and adolescents revisited: a systematic review. Pain. 2011;152:2729–38.
11. Roth-Isigkeit A, Thyen U, Stöven H, Schwarzenberger J, Schmucker P. Pain among children and adolescents: restrictions in daily living and triggering factors. Pediatrics. 2005;115:e152–62.
12. Perquin CW, Hazebroek-Kampschreur AAJM, Hunfeld JAM, Bohnen AM, van Suijlekom-Smit LWA, Passchier J, et al. Pain in children and adolescents: a common experience. Pain. 2000;87:51–8.
13. Swain MS, Henschke N, Kamper SJ, Gobina I, Ottová-Jordan V, Maher CG. An international survey of pain in adolescents. BMC Public Health. 2014;14:447.
14. Institute of Medicine (US) Committee on Advancing Pain Research, Care, and Education. Relieving Pain in America: A Blueprint for Transforming Prevention, Care, Education, and Research. Washington (DC): National Academies Press (US); 2011. http://www.ncbi.nlm.nih.gov/books/NBK91497/. Accessed 16 Apr 2016.
15. Anand V, Carroll AE, Biondich PG, Dugan TM, Downs SM. Pediatric decision support using adapted Arden syntax. Artif Intell Med. 2015. https://doi.org/10.1016/j.artmed.2015.09.006.
16. Anand V, McKee S, Dugan TM, Downs SM. Leveraging electronic tablets for general pediatric care: a pilot study. Appl Clin Inform. 2015;6:1–15.
17. Carroll AE, Bauer NS, Dugan TM, Anand V, Saha C, Downs SM. Use of a computerized decision aid for developmental surveillance and screening: a randomized clinical trial. JAMA Pediatr. 2014;168:815–21.
18. Anand V, Downs SM, Bauer NS, Carroll AE. Prevalence of infant television viewing and maternal depression symptoms. J Dev Behav Pediatr JDBP. 2014;35:216–24.
19. Bauer NS, Gilbert AL, Carroll AE, Downs SM. Associations of early exposure to intimate partner violence and parental depression with subsequent mental health outcomes. JAMA Pediatr. 2013;167:341–7.

20. Freedman DS, Lawman HG, Pan L, Skinner AC, Allison DB, McGuire LC, et al. The prevalence and validity of high, biologically implausible values of weight, height, and BMI among 8.8 million children. Obes Silver Spring Md. 2016;24:1132–9.
21. Flegal KM, Wei R, Ogden CL, Freedman DS, Johnson CL, Curtin LR. Characterizing extreme values of body mass index-for-age by using the 2000 Centers for Disease Control and Prevention growth charts. Am J Clin Nutr. 2009;90:1314–20.
22. Cheng TL, Goodman E, Committee on Pediatric Research. Race, ethnicity, and socioeconomic status in research on child health. Pediatrics. 2015;135: e225–37.
23. R Core Team. R: a language and environment for statistical computing. Vienna: R Foundation for Statistical Computing; 2018. https://www.R-project.org/
24. Zailinawati AH, Teng CL, Kamil MA, Achike FI, Koh CN. Pain morbidity in primary care - preliminary observations from two different primary care settings. Med J Malaysia. 2006;61:162–7.
25. Mäntyselkä P, Kumpusalo E, Ahonen R, Kumpusalo A, Kauhanen J, Viinamäki H, et al. Pain as a reason to visit the doctor: a study in Finnish primary health care. Pain. 2001;89:175–80.
26. Frølund F, Pain in General Practice FC. Pain as a cause of patient-doctor contact. Scand J Prim Health Care. 1986;4:97–100.
27. van Dijk A, McGrath PA, Pickett W, VanDenKerkhof EG. Pain prevalence in nine- to 13-year-old school children. Pain Res Manag J Can Pain Soc 2006; 11:234–240.
28. Huguet A, Miró J. The severity of chronic pediatric pain: an epidemiological study. J Pain. 2008;9:226–36.
29. Barajas C, Bosch F, Baños J-E. A pilot survey of pain prevalence in schoolchildren. Pain Clin. 2001;13:95–102.
30. Hainsworth KR, Miller LA, Stolzman SC, Fidlin BM, Davies WH, Weisman SJ, et al. Pain as a comorbidity of pediatric obesity. Infant Child Adolesc Nutr. 2012;4:315–20.
31. Rabbitts JA, Holley AL, Karlson CW, Palermo TM. Bidirectional associations between pain and physical activity in adolescents. Clin J Pain. 2014;30:251–8.
32. Hainsworth KR, Jastrowski Mano KE, Stoner AM, Anderson Khan K, Ladwig RJ, Davies WH, et al. "What does weight have to do with it?" parent perceptions of weight and pain in a pediatric chronic pain population. Child Aust. 2016;3. https://doi.org/10.3390/children3040029.
33. Boerner KE, Birnie KA, Caes L, Schinkel M, Chambers CT. Sex differences in experimental pain among healthy children: a systematic review and meta-analysis. Pain. 2014;155:983–93.
34. Chambers CT, Reid GJ, Craig KD, PJ MG, Finley GA. Agreement between child and parent reports of pain. Clin J Pain. 1998;14:336–42.
35. Perquin CW, Hazebroek-Kampschreur AA, Hunfeld JA, van Suijlekom-Smit LW, Passchier J, van der Wouden JC. Chronic pain among children and adolescents: physician consultation and medication use. Clin J Pain. 2000;16: 229–35.
36. Korterink JJ, Diederen K, Benninga MA, Tabbers MM. Epidemiology of pediatric functional abdominal pain disorders: a meta-analysis. PLoS One. 2015;10. https://doi.org/10.1371/journal.pone.0126982.
37. Schrijver TV, Brand PLP, Bekhof J. Seasonal variation of diseases in children: a 6-year prospective cohort study in a general hospital. Eur J Pediatr. 2016; 175:457–64.
38. Hsieh AY, Tripp DA, Ji L-J. The influence of ethnic concordance and discordance on verbal reports and nonverbal behaviours of pain. Pain. 2011; 152:2016–22.
39. Muehlhausen W, Doll H, Quadri N, Fordham B, O'Donohoe P, Dogar N, et al. Equivalence of electronic and paper administration of patient-reported outcome measures: a systematic review and meta-analysis of studies conducted between 2007 and 2013. Health Qual Life Outcomes. 2015; 13:167.
40. McDonald CJ. Protocol-based computer reminders, the quality of care and the non-perfectability of man. N Engl J Med. 1976;295:1351–5.
41. Bauer NS, Carroll AE, Saha C, Downs SM. Experience with decision support system and comfort with topic predict clinicians' responses to alerts and reminders. J Am Med Inform Assoc. 2016;23:e125–30.
42. Zheng K, Padman R, Johnson MP, Diamond HS. Understanding technology adoption in clinical care: clinician adoption behavior of a point-of-care reminder system. Int J Med Inf. 2005;74:535 43.
43. Meigs JB, Cagliero E, Dubey A, Murphy-Sheehy P, Gildesgame C, Chueh H, et al. A controlled trial of web-based diabetes disease management: the MGH diabetes primary care improvement project. Diabetes Care. 2003;26:750–7.
44. van Wyk JT, van Wijk MAM, Sturkenboom MCJM, Mosseveld M, Moorman PW, van der Lei J. Electronic alerts versus on-demand decision support to improve dyslipidemia treatment: a cluster randomized controlled trial. Circulation. 2008;117:371–8.
45. Green LA, Nease D, Klinkman MS. Clinical reminders designed and implemented using cognitive and organizational science principles decrease reminder fatigue. J Am Board Fam Med. 2015;28:351–9.
46. Litzelman DK, Dittus RS, Miller ME, Tierney WM. Requiring physicians to respond to computerized reminders improves their compliance with preventive care protocols. J Gen Intern Med. 1993;8:311–7.
47. Brudvik C, Moutte S-D, Baste V, Morken T. A comparison of pain assessment by physicians, parents and children in an outpatient setting. Emerg Med J. 2017;34:138–44.
48. Singer AJ, Gulla J, Thode HC Jr. Parents and practitioners are poor judges of young children's pain severity. Acad Emerg Med. 2002;9:609–12.
49. Mäntyselkä P, Kumpusalo E, Ahonen R, Takala J. Patients' versus general practitioners' assessments of pain intensity in primary care patients with non-cancer pain. Br J Gen Pr. 2001;51:995–7.
50. Baker DW. Joint Commission Statement on Pain Management. http://www.jointcommission.org/joint_commission_statement_on_pain_management/. Accessed 19 Dec 2017.
51. Simons LE, Smith A, Ibagon C, Coakley R, Logan DE, Schechter N, et al. Pediatric pain screening tool: rapid identification of risk in youth with pain complaints. Pain. 2015;156:1511–8.

Seroprevalence of diphtheria and pertussis immunoglobulin G among children with pneumonia in Ji'nan, China

Qinghong Meng[1†], Lijun Li[1†], Wei Shi[1], Qing Wang[1], Mingjie Ding[2], Yanqin Liu[2], Xiang Ma[2*] and Kaihu Yao[1*]

Abstract

Background: Vaccination is still one of the most important methods to control and prevent childhood infections including diphtheria and pertussis. This study evaluated the level of diphtheria (DT) and pertussis (PT)-related antibodies among children with pneumonia in Ji'nan, China.

Methods: A total of 484 sera of children from 1 day to 13 years of age were collected from 2014 to 2015 in Ji'nan. Children with recent history of pertussis were excluded from this study. Anti-DT and PT IgG concentrations were measured by ELISA (Euroimmun, Lübeck, Germany).

Results: Of the 484 subjects tested, the overall positivity rate of anti-DT IgG (≥0.1 IU/ml) was 48.97%, and the highest positivity rate of anti-DT IgG (68.55%) and proportion with long term protection (23.27%) were observed in children aged 6 m- < 3 y. For anti-PT IgG, 334 subjects (69.01%) had anti-PT IgG levels below the lower limit of detection (5 IU/ml). Even with detectable anti-PT antibodies, the majority (115/150, 76.67%) of them had antibody levels of 5- < 40 IU/ml. The highest proportion of subjects with detectable anti-PT IgG (≥5 IU/ml) was observed in children aged < 6 m (44.36%), then the proportion continually decreased to 15.0% at 3 y- < 6 y ($\chi^2 = 24.05$, $p < 0.0001$). The highest positivity rate (≥40 IU/ml) was only 8.27% in children aged < 6 m. Subjects with an anti-PT IgG ≥100 IU/ml were observed in all the groups and there were no significant differences in the proportions of subjects with a level ≥ 100 IU/ml among these age groups ($\chi^2 = 2.572$, $p = 0.4624$). A total of 5 subjects had anti-PT IgG ≥100 IU/ml (≥1 years post pertussis vaccination) which was considered to be indicative of a recent pertussis infection.

Conclusions: We demonstrated low antibody levels and protection against pertussis in our study population. The anti-PT IgG maintained a low level throughout all age groups, and even no immune responses were observed after the basic immunization and booster. Our study supported the need to reevaluate the immune response of DTP vaccine which was used in Shandong province after 2010.

Keywords: Pertussis, Pertussis toxin, IgG, Children

* Correspondence: maxiang0176@163.com; yaokaihu@bch.com.cn
†Qinghong Meng and Lijun Li contributed equally to this work.
[2]Respiratory department, Qilu Children's Hospital, Shandong University, Ji'nan 250022, China
[1]Beijing Key Laboratory of Pediatric Respiratory Infection Diseases, Key Laboratory of Major Diseases in Children, Ministry of Education, National Clinical Research Center for Respiratory Diseases, National Key Discipline of Pediatrics (Capital Medical University), Beijing Pediatric Research Institute, Beijing Children's Hospital, Capital Medical University, National Center for Children's Health, Beijing 100045, China

Background

Diphtheria and pertussis, caused by *Corynebacterium diphtheria* and *Bordetella pertussis*, are highly infectious and vaccine-preventable respiratory diseases [1, 2]. Diphtheria and pertussis vaccination significantly reduced the incidence of these diseases. However, pertussis has re-emerged in some developed countries that maintain high vaccine coverage [3]. For an example, there was a 50-y high of 48,277 cases of pertussis in the United States in 2012 [4]. In 2012, according to the Pan American Health Organization/World Health Organization (PAHO/WHO) estimation, there were 50 million cases of pertussis which led to 300,000 deaths worldwide [5]. Therefore, pertussis remains one of the leading causes of vaccine-preventable deaths in the world today.

In China, a combined diphtheria-tetanus-whole cell pertussis (DTwP) vaccine was introduced in 1978. From 2007, a combined diphtheria-tetanus-acellular pertussis (DTaP) vaccine was introduced in the Expanded Program on Immunization (EPI) of China, and both DTwP and DTaP were used since then. Only DTaP was administered after 2010 [6, 7]. The first immunization of DTP is administrated in the third month after birth, which is followed by another two dosages in the fourth and fifth month for the basic immunization. The children will be inoculated again for the booster immunization at 18–24 months. After that, the individuals will not get inoculation against pertussis any more in China. DTP vaccination is mandatory, and it is freely available by the public health system. According to official Chinese estimates, the immunization coverage has been over 99% since 2011. No case of diphtheria has been reported in China since 2007 [8]. However, the number of pertussis cases has increased in recent years according to reports from the Center for Disease Control and Prevention (CDC) in China, from 6658 cases in 2015 and 5584 in 2016 to 10,390 in 2017 [9]. In fact, pertussis was most likely underestimated [10], due to the lack of diagnostic testing in most community hospitals in China. In a recent prospective study conducted from 2012 through 2013 in Xi'an, China, more than half of the 313 children who had been coughing for more than 2 weeks were proven to be positive for *B. pertussis* which was determined by nasopharyngeal swab culture and PCR [11]. Therefore, pertussis is still a notifiable disease in children in China.

Vaccination is still one of the most important methods to control and prevent pertussis. Pertussis toxin (PT) is the most specific and protective antigen for pertussis. Both DTwP and DTaP vaccines contain PT. Therefore, anti-PT IgG is a good indicator for surveillance of the effectiveness of DTP vaccines in vaccinated populations. In this present study we evaluated the immune status against pertussis in different age groups of children. The present study included the data of diphtheria and pertussis in children. By comparing the 2 components in the same vaccine - diphtheria and pertussis, it will help us better understand the change of immunity level against them in children.

Methods

Serum sample

The sample size of this study was evaluated based on a recent report. A recent seroepidemiological study conducted in Beijing reported that about 15–70% of subjects between the ages of 1–14 years had detectable anti-PT IgG levels [12]. Assuming conservatively a detectable rate of 20% and a significance level of 5%, a minimum number of 94 samples are needed to reach a statistical power of 80%. According to the feasibility and situation of clinical practice, the sample size was expanded to > 400.

From August 2014 to March 2015, 484 children with pneumonia hospitalized in the respiratory department of Qilu Children's Hospital, Shandong University were included in this study. Those cases diagnosed with pertussis, suspected pertussis and immune system related diseases were not enrolled. In addition, those who had history of coughing ≥2 weeks during the previous year were also excluded in this study. For all children, basic data about age, gender, date of sampling, medical histories and DTP vaccination history were collected from their parents. All serum samples were frozen at – 20 °C until analysis.

Serological testing

Anti-DT IgG was detected using the commercially available ELISA kits (Euroimmun, Lübeck, Germany). The antibody results were expressed in international units per milli-liter (IU/ml) and referred to the "International Standard for Diphtheria Antiserum", NIBSC code: 00/496. According to the manufacturer's instructions, the results were divided to six groups: < 0.01 IU/ml (undetectable/no protection), 0.01- < 0.1 IU/ml (no protection), 0.1–1.0 IU/ml (short term protection/basic protection), > 1.0–1.5 IU/ml (long term protection/booster after 5 years), > 1.5–2.0 IU/ml (long term protection/booster after 7 years) and > 2.0 IU/ml (long term protection/booster after 10 years).

Anti-PT IgG was also detected using the commercially available ELISA kits (Euroimmun, Lübeck, Germany). The antibody results were expressed in international units per milli-liter (IU/ml) and referred to the "First International Standard for Pertussis Antiserum", NIBSC code: 06/140, World Health Organization (WHO). The lower limit of detection was 5 IU/ml. The anti-PT IgG levels ≥40 IU/ml was categorized as positive, according to the manufacturer's protocol. Anti-PT IgG ≥100 IU/ml

(≥1 years post pertussis vaccination) was considered to be indicative of a recent pertussis infection.

Quality control

After the samples were tested, we randomly chose 5% of the samples for re-testing. Then, we calculated the coefficient of variation (CV) of the results for these re-tested samples. The results were only considered valid if the CV value of each sample was < 15%, otherwise the test was repeated. Each serological test run was carried out with positives and negative serological controls.

Data analysis

The study population was divided into four age groups: < 6 m, 6 m- < 3 y, 3 y- < 6 y and ≥ 6 y. For statistical analysis, antibody concentrations below the lower limit for quantitation were assigned as half the lower limit of quantitation (0.005 IU/ml for DT, and 2.5 IU/ml for PT). The value of anti-DT level ≥ 2.0 IU/ml and anti-PT level ≥ 200 IU/ml was counted as 2.0 IU/ml and 200 IU/ml, respectively. Data were analyzed using the GraphPad Prism software (version 5; GraphPad Software, La Jolla, CA, USA) and SPSS (version 19.0). χ^2 test was used to compare positivity rate, rate of subjects with long term protection and proportions of subjects with undetectable anti-PT IgG among different age groups. The difference in antibody concentration among different age groups was tested by the Wilcoxon/Krusakal Wallis test. p values ≤0.05 were considered statistically significant.

Results

Characteristics of study population

A total of 484 subjects were enrolled in the study with the age range of 1 day to 13 y (median: 1.8 y). The ratio of male to female was 2.13:1 (324:160). Among subjects > 3 m, the rate of at least one dose of DTP vaccination was 74.4% (360/406). Among the subjects > 6 m, more than 84.3% (296/351) had a confirmed history of DTP vaccination with at least 3 doses. There were 20, 8 and 1 unvaccinated subjects identified in age groups of < 6 m, 6 m- < 3 y and 3 y- < 6 y, respectively. A total of 17 subjects were unknown for the history of vaccination against diphtheria or pertussis.

Seroprevalence of anti-DT IgG

The overall positivity rate of anti-DT IgG (≥0.1 IU/ml) was 48.97% with a mean concentration of 0.38 ± 0.53 IU/ml (median: 0.10 IU/ml). There was no significant difference in positivity rates and IgG level between males and females (Table 1). Of the 484 subjects tested, a total of 247 (51.03%) subjects lacked protection, 166 (34.30%) subjects had basic protection, and 71 (14.70%) of them showed long term protection (> 1.0 IU/ml). Fig. 1a shows more details about the distribution of anti-DT IgG in subjects from different age groups. Compared with children without full vaccinations (< 6 m), the positivity rates of anti-DT IgG in the 6 m- < 3 y group (68.55% vs 34.59%, $\chi^2 = 34.162$, $p < 0.0001$) increased significantly, while the rate of subjects with long-term protection in the 6 m- < 3 y group also increased (23.27% vs 3.76%, $\chi^2 = 22.639$, $p < 0.0001$). Then, the positivity rate and proportion with long term protection at 3 y- < 6 y decreased to 40.0% ($\chi^2 = 20.558$, $p < 0.0001$) and 12.0% ($\chi^2 = 5.346$, $P = 0.0208$), respectively. After tetanus and reduced diphtheria combined vaccine (Td) booster at 6 y, the proportion of high- level anti-DT IgG (> 2.0 IU/ml) increased significantly (5.43% vs 0%, $\chi^2 = 7.503$, $p = 0.0062$). Similar to the patterns of change in the positivity rate of anti-DT IgG, the concentration of anti-DT IgG observed in the 6 m- < 3 y ($p < 0.0001$) group increased significantly (Table 1).

Seroprevalence of anti-PT IgG

The anti-PT IgG level in 334 subjects (69.01%) was below the lower limit of detection (5 IU/ml). Even with detectable anti-PT IgG, the majority (115/150, 76.67%) of them had antibody levels of 5- < 40 IU/ml. The mean concentration of anti-PT IgG was 11.85 ± 29.51 IU/ml (median: 2.5 IU/ml) (Table 1). The highest proportion of subjects with anti-PT IgG > 5 IU/ml (44.36%) was observed in children aged < 6 m. Although there was DTP vaccination in the 3rd, 4th and 5th months and booster immunization at 18–24 months, there were no significant differences in the positivity rate among these age groups ($\chi^2 = 1.074$, $p = 0.7834$). The highest positivity rate was only 8.27%, observed in children in the < 6 m group. Meanwhile, the proportion of subjects with anti-PT IgG > 5 IU/ml decreased to 15.0% at < 6 y ($\chi^2 = 24.047$, $p < 0.0001$). Although there was no DTP booster at 6 y, the proportion of subjects with anti-PT IgG > 5 IU/ml increased (21.74% vs 15.0%, $\chi^2 = 1.461$, $p = 0.2268$). There was significant difference ($p < 0.0001$) in concentration of anti-PT IgG among different age groups (Table 1). Compared with children in 6 m- < 3 y group, the concentration of anti-PT IgG observed in the 3 y- < 6 y ($p < 0.0001$) group decreased significantly ($p = 0.0015$). Subjects with an anti-PT IgG ≥100 IU/ml were observed in all the groups, and there were no significant differences in the proportions of subjects with a level ≥ 100 IU/ml among these age groups ($\chi^2 = 2.572$, $p = 0.4624$). A total of 5 subjects (3 in the 3 y- < 6 y group and 2 in the ≥6 y group) had an anti-PT IgG ≥100 IU/ml (≥1 years post pertussis vaccination), which was considered to be indicative of a recent pertussis infection (Fig. 1b).

Table 1 Demographic and status of anti-DT and anti-PT IgG in the sera of subjects among different age groups

	N	Anti-DT Positive rate (≥0.1 IU/ml) (95% CI, %)	Anti-DT Concentration and 95% CI (IU/ml)	Anti-PT Positive rate (≥40 IU/ml) (95% CI, %)	Anti-PT Concentration and 95% CI (IU/ml)
Gender					
Male	324	48.15 (42.76–53.58)	0.37 (0.32–0.43)	8.03 (5.53–11.50)	13.44 (9.20–17.67)
Female	160	50.00 (42.34–57.66)	0.40 (0.31–0.49)	5.63 (2.99–10.34)	11.43 (6.32–16.54)
p		0.7014	0.4594	0.3376	0.7663
Age					
< 6 m	133	34.59 (27.04–43.0)	0.19 (0.14–0.24)	8.27 (4.68–14.20)	11.76 (7.88–15.65)
6 m- < 3y	159	68.55 (60.97–75.26)	0.56 (0.47–0.66)	7.55 (4.37–12.73)	12.59 (7.72–17.46)
3y- < 6y	100	40.00 (30.94–49.80)	0.62 (0.45–0.79)	5.00 (2.15–11.18)	10.34 (4.02–16.66)
≥6y	92	45.65 (35.88–55.80)	0.44 (0.31–0.57)	7.61 (3.73–14.88)	12.32 (5.47–19.17)
p		< 0.0001	< 0.0001	0.7776	< 0.0001
Total	484	48.97 (44.54–53.41)	0.38 (0.33–0.43)	7.23 (5.25–9.89)	11.85 (9.21–14.48)

Discussion

As shown in this study, the increase of anti-DT IgG was consistent with the current immunization schedule in China. However, this population was generally lacking protective immunity to pertussis. The low immunity to *B. pertussis* was associated with an increased risk of pertussis outbreak in Ji'nan. The different patterns of antibody level observed for DT and PT in one combined vaccine indicate the less-than-ideal immune response of anti-pertussis induced by the current DTP vaccine.

In China, the last diphtheria case was recorded in 2006 [8], which means natural boosting by circulating *Corynebacterium diphtheria* occurred less often [13]. Hence, anti-DT IgG levels are almost completely acquired from DTP vaccination. For safety reasons, a tenfold higher value (0.1 IU/ml) than the internationally specified minimum title for prophylaxis was recommended [13–15]. According to the standard, the overall positivity rate of anti-DT IgG in our study was 48.97%. If the lower cut off value (0.01 IU/ml) was adopted [16], the positivity rate of DT-IgG increased to 88.82%. After the implementation of basic immunization at the 3rd, 4th and 5th months of age, there was an increase of the positivity rate and proportions of long term protection observed in the 6 m- < 3 y group. No significant increase in the positivity rate was observed after the 2nd booster immunization at 6 y, however, the proportion with high concentrations (> 2 IU/ml) showed an increase in this age group. Therefore, the results of anti-DT IgG in the study showed that a certain amount of antibody response was generated after Td vaccination.

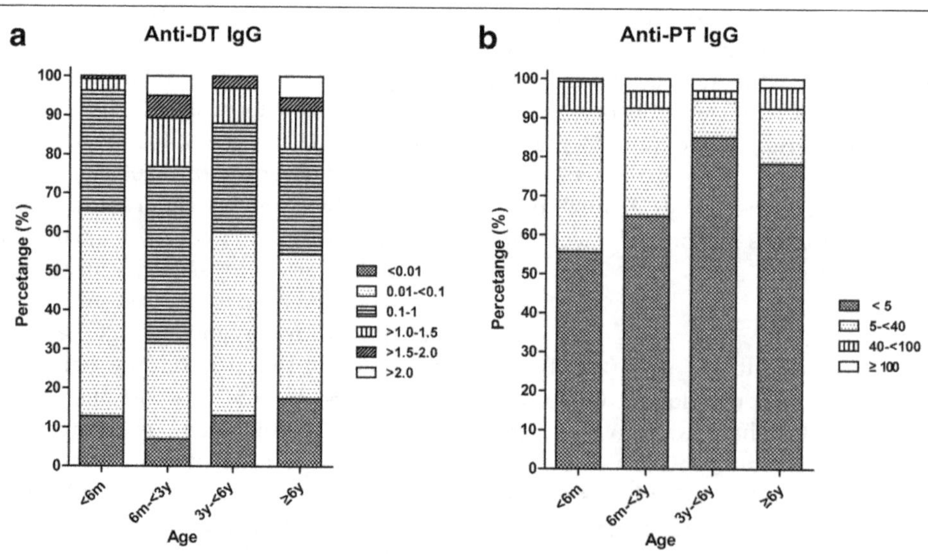

Fig. 1 The distribution of anti-DT (**a**) and anti-PT (**b**) IgG level in the sera of subjects among different age groups

Much to our surprise, the pattern of anti-pertussis immunity was quite different from diphtheria. The anti-PT IgG maintained a low-level throughout all age groups, and even no immune responses were observed after the basic immunization and booster. According to the current Immunization Program Schedule in China, children had received four doses of DTP vaccines at 2 years of age [17]. The coverage rate of three primary doses of DTwP was more than 90% since 1990, thus, theoretically, subjects 6 m- < 3 y of age should have higher anti-PT IgG than any other age groups. However, about 65.0% of children in this age group showed anti-PT IgG beyond the lower limit of detection (5 IU/ml), and only 3.14% of them had anti-PT IgG levels ≥100 IU/ml after DTP vaccination in 1 year. This pattern of anti-pertussis immunity was similar with that in another previous study carried out in Beijing [12]. As shown in that study in Beijing, even after four doses of DTP vaccination at 2 y, the proportion of subjects with undetectable anti-PT IgG increased gradually in the 3y, 4y, 5y and 6y groups. The highest proportion of subjects with undetectable anti-PT IgG (84.62%) was observed in children aged 7 y. The results of the study indicated that vaccination has limited contribution to the immunity level of pertussis in the population. Another interpretation for no immune responses after the basic immunization and the booster was that the duration of anti-PT IgG after vaccination was very limited [18, 19]. However, more than half of vaccinated children (53.1%) between 6 m–8 m of age had anti-PT IgG levels below the lower limit of detection (5 IU/ml) in our study.

During the preparation of this manuscript, the China Food and Drug Administration reported that the potency indexes of two batches (201605014–01 and 201607050-2) of DTP vaccines produced by two companies did not reach the requirements of antibody titer, on November 3, 2017. The serum samples in our study were collected in 2014–2015, therefore, these two batches had not been used for the children in our study. The highest rate of subjects with undetectable anti-PT IgG indicated less-than-ideal immune response of DTP vaccination in this study. Therefore, the phenomenon about insufficient potency of DTP vaccines may be common. The children < 4 y in this study were born after 2010, and they got DTaP vaccination. The DTwP or DTaP were used in children > 4 y in this study. The low detectable rate of anti-PT IgG among different age groups also indicated insufficient potency of both DTwP and DTaP vaccinations. As the only organization which approved vaccine products used in China, the China Food and Drug Administration should strengthen the supervision and testing of vaccines.

An Estonia study demonstrated that nearly half of subjects < 18 y had undetectable anti-PT IgG levels [20], which were also evaluated with Euroimmun ELISA kits. The author stated that the relatively high proportion of subjects with undetectable anti-PT IgG levels and the relatively low rate of officially reported pertussis cases suggested that low antibody levels did not necessarily indicate an absence of protection. There was also growing evidence that $CD4^+$ T cell-mediated cellular immunity was necessary for clearance of *B. pertussis* infection [21]. However, different from the Estonia study, no humoral immune response was observed after the basic immunization and booster. Although anti-PT IgG was not a complete indicator for immunity, the high proportion of children with undetectable anti-PT IgG indicated the less-than-ideal immunogenicity of DTP vaccine.

In our study, 5 subjects (> 3 y) had anti-PT IgG ≥100 IU/ml (≥1 years post pertussis vaccination), indicative of a recent pertussis course. Another 7 subjects had anti-PT IgG 40- < 100 IU/ml (≥1 years post pertussis vaccination), indicative of a possible pertussis course. These cases suggest that this population may be vulnerable. The cases that had diagnosed pertussis and suspected pertussis had been excluded in this study. However, there were cases of recent pertussis infection. Several seroepidemiological studies conducted in different provinces of China also indicated that the incidence of pertussis was most likely underestimated [22, 23]. There are several possible reasons for the pertussis resurgence [24]: (1) increased recognition and reporting of pertussis; (2) diagnostic techniques (such as culture, PCR assay and serologic tests) are available at lots of hospitals; (3) a decrease in vaccine efficacy; (4) antigenic variation of *B. pertussis*. The increase of pertussis cases could be linked to the adverse events of vaccine with insufficient potency, which could become evidence to challenge or deny the effectiveness of vaccination, and bring a persistent inhibition of the public's enthusiasm for vaccination. Despite the high vulnerability to pertussis, there was no large outbreak of pertussis in China in recent years. To a certain degree, the control strategy against pertussis is still effective at present. Therefore researchers and clinical workers should rationally assess the impact of vaccine titer deficiency on pertussis epidemiology, and improve the public confidence in vaccination. However, there is another possibility. It is usual for people who feel ill to get antibiotics (such as a macrolide) without a prescription in China, which may have efficacy against various bacteria, including *B. pertussis*. This may also explain the serendipitous observation of relatively few pertussis cases among patients who are not well protected by the vaccine.

There were certain limitations in this study. Firstly, one limitation is the restriction of the selected population, since all subjects were pneumonia patients and collected in only one hospital. Multi-center studies in community populations should be performed in other provinces, especially as two batches (201605014–01 and 201607050-2) of DTP vaccines were used. Secondly, there was no definitive cut-off value for single-serum serology in China. Various cut-offs values were used in different studies and countries, such as 30 IU/ml [22], 50 IU/ml [25], 62.5 IU/ml [26], 100 IU/ml [14, 27] and 125 IU/ml [28–30]. According to the manufacturer's instructions, anti-PT IgG ≥100 IU/ml (≥1 years post pertussis vaccination) was considered to be indicative of a recent pertussis infection. Levels of anti-PT IgG in children were very low in our study. The cut-off value of ≥100 IU/ml might be thus relatively harsh. Thirdly, the history of vaccination was recalled by the parents, which probably resulted in recall bias. The distribution of diphtheria antibody level by age groups also indicated the real proportion of subjects with vaccination could be probably much lower than the estimate of this study.

Conclusion

We demonstrated low antibody levels and protection against pertussis in our study population. From the epidemiological point of view, this means that these children may be susceptible to pertussis. Our study supported the need to reevaluate the immune response of DTP vaccine which was used in Ji'nan since 2010.

Abbreviations

CV: Coefficient of variation; DT: Diphtheria; DTaP: Diphtheria-tetanus-acellular pertussis; DTwP: Diphtheria-tetanus-whole cell pertussis; EPI: Expanded program on immunization; IU/ml: International units per milli-liter; PAHO/WHO: Pan American health organization/world health organization; PT: Pertussis

Acknowledgments

We thank Dr. Yaguang Peng for providing help on power calculation and statistical analysis in this study.

Funding

This work was supported by the National Natural Science Foundation of China (81701565), Ji'nan Medical and Health Science Technology Innovation Plan (201805015) and Basic-Clinical Scientific Research Cooperation Fund of Capital Medical University (17JL55).

Authors' contributions

XM and KHY designed the study, QHM and LJL conducted the experiments and wrote the manuscript, WS and QW oversaw data analysis planning and execution, reviewed and revised the manuscript, MJD and YQL designed the data collection instruments and coordinated sample collection. All authors read and approved the final manuscript.

Competing interests

The authors declare that they have no competing interests.

References

1. May ML, McDougall RJ, Robson JM. Corynebacterium diphtheriae and the returned tropical traveler. J Travel Med. 2014;21(1):39e44.
2. Syed MA, Bana NF. Pertussis. A reemerging and an underreported infectious disease. Saudi Med J. 2014;35(10):1181–7.
3. Domenech de Celles M, Magpantay FM, King AA, Rohani P. The pertussis enigma: reconciling epidemiology, immunology and evolution. Proc Biol Sci. 2016;283(1822):20152309.
4. Warfel JM, Zimmerman LI, Merkel TJ. Acellular pertussis vaccines protect against disease but fail to prevent infection and transmission in a nonhuman primate model. Proc Natl Acad Sci U S A. 2014;111(2):787–92.
5. Chen Z, Zhang J, Cao L, Zhang N, Zhu J, Ping G, et al. Seroprevalence of pertussis among adults in China where whole cell vaccines have been used for 50 years. J Inf Secur. 2016;73(1):38–44.
6. Wang L, Lei D, Zhang S. Acellular pertussis vaccines in China. Vaccine. 2012;30(50):7174–8.
7. Chen Z, He Q. Immune persistence after pertussis vaccination. Hum Vaccin Immunother. 2017;13(4):744–56.
8. World Health Organisation. Immunization, Vaccines and Biologicals: Data, statistics and graphics. http://www.who.int/immunization/monitoring_surveillance/data/en/. Accessed 19 Nov 2018.
9. National Health Commission of the People's Republic of China. http://www.nhfpc.gov.cn/jkj/s3578/201802/de926bdb046749abb7b0a8e23d929104.shtml. Accessed 19 Nov 2018.
10. He H, Yao P, Zhou Y, Deng X, Pan JI. Pertussis infection neglected in China? Evidence from a Seroepidemiology survey in Zhejiang, an Eastern Province of China. PLoS One. 2016;11(5):e0155965.
11. Wang Z, Cui Z, Li Y, Hou T, Liu X, Xi Y, et al. High prevalence of erythromycin-resistant *Bordetella pertussis* in Xi'an, China. Clin Microbiol Infect. 2014;20(11):O825–30.
12. Li X, Chen M, Zhang T, Li J, Zeng Y, Lu L. Seroepidemiology of diphtheria and pertussis in Beijing, China: a cross-sectional study. Hum Vaccin Immunother. 2015;11(10):2434–9.
13. Zasada AA, Rastawicki W, Rokosz N, Jagielski M. Seroprevalence of diphtheria toxoid IgG antibodies in children, adolescents and adults in Poland. BMC Infect Dis. 2013;13:551.
14. Tanriover MD, Soyler C, Ascioglu S, Cankurtaran M, Unal S. Low seroprevalence of diphtheria, tetanus and pertussis in ambulatory adult patients: the need for lifelong vaccination. Eur J Intern Med. 2014;25(6):528–32.
15. Zhang Q, Han F, Nie Q, Ren H, Zhang B, Liu Q, et al. Seroprevalence of antibodies to pertussis and diphtheria among healthy adults in China. J Inf Secur. 2011;63(6):441–6.
16. Yao N, Zeng Q, Wang Q. Seroepidemiology of diphtheria and pertussis in Chongqing, China: serology-based evidence of *Bordetella pertussis* infection. Public Health. 2018;156:60–6.
17. Xu Y, Wang L, Xu J, Wang X, Wei C, Luo P, et al. Seroprevalence of pertussis in China: need to improve vaccination strategies. Hum Vaccin Immunother. 2014;10(1):192–8.
18. Pertussis vaccines. WHO position paper. Wkly Epidemiol Rec. 2010;85(40):385–400.
19. Zhang Y, Huang H, Gao Z, Liu Y, Liu P, Ding Y, et al. A sera-epidemiological study on pertussis immunity levels among community populations and an analysis of the underlying factors in Tianjin China. Vaccine. 2015;33(51):7183–7.
20. Jogi P, Oona M, Toompere K, Leedo S, Epstein J, Lutsar I. Seroprevalence of IgG antibodies to pertussis toxin in children and adolescents in Estonia. Vaccine. 2014;32(41):5311–5.
21. Brummelman J, Wilk MM, Han WG, van Els CA, Mills KH. Roads to the development of improved pertussis vaccines paved by immunology. Pathog Dis. 2015;73(8):ftv067.
22. Zhang Q, Zheng H, Liu M, Han K, Shu J, Wu C, et al. The seroepidemiology of immunoglobulin G antibodies against pertussis toxin in China: a cross sectional study. BMC Infect Dis. 2012;12:138.
23. Wu Y, Zhu B, Gao Y, Shi Z, Wang J, Wang H, et al. Clustered cases of *Bordetella pertussis* infection cause high levels of IgG antibodies against pertussis toxin in adolescents in Gaobeidian city. China Epidemiol Infect. 2014;142(4):738–43.
24. Cherry JD. Pertussis: challenges today and for the future. PLoS Pathog. 2013;9(3):e1003418.

25. Guiso N, Berbers G, Fry NK, He Q, Riffelmann M, Wirsing von Konig CH, et al. What to do and what not to do in serological diagnosis of pertussis: recommendations from EU reference laboratories. Eur J Clin Microbiol Infect Dis. 2011;30(3):307–12.
26. Koh MT, Liu CS, Chiu CH, Boonsawat W, Watanaveeradej V, Abdullah N, et al. Under-recognized pertussis in adults from Asian countries: a cross-sectional seroprevalence study in Malaysia, Taiwan and Thailand. Epidemiol Infect. 2016;144(6):1192–200.
27. Plans P, Alvarez E, de Ory F, Campins M, Paya T, Balfagon P, et al. Prevalence of antibody to Bordetella pertussis in neonates and prevalence of recent pertussis infection in pregnant women in Catalonia (Spain) in 2003 and 2013. Pediatr Infect Dis J. 2014;33(11):1114–8.
28. Campbell P, McIntyre P, Quinn H, Hueston L, Gilbert GL, McVernon J. Increased population prevalence of low pertussis toxin antibody levels in young children preceding a record pertussis epidemic in Australia. PLoS One. 2012;7(4):e35874.
29. Launay O, Toneatti C, Bernede C, Njamkepo E, Petitprez K, Leblond A, et al. Antibodies to tetanus, diphtheria and pertussis among healthy adults vaccinated according to the French vaccination recommendations. Hum Vaccin. 2009;5(5):341–6.
30. Teepe J, Broekhuizen BD, Ieven M, Loens K, Huygen K, Kretzschmar M, et al. Prevalence, diagnosis, and disease course of pertussis in adults with acute cough: a prospective, observational study in primary care. Br J Gen Pract. 2015;65(639):e662–7.

19

Extracorporeal membrane oxygenation with prone position ventilation successfully rescues infantile pertussis

Jingyi Shi[1], Chunxia Wang[1,2], Yun Cui[1] and Yucai Zhang[1,2*]

Abstract

Background: *Bordetella pertussis* can cause fatal illness with severe acute respiratory distress syndrome (ARDS) and pulmonary hypertension (PHT).

Case presentation: A 6-month-old non-vaccinated boy with *B. pertussis* infection who developed ARDS was treated by extracorporeal membrane oxygenation (ECMO). During his ECMO support stage, sudden occurred decreasing of ECMO flow implied increasing intrathoracic pressure. The airway spasm followed caused sudden drop of ventilator tidal volume as well as poor lung compliance. Prone position ventilation and bundle care were conducted as lung protection ventilator strategy. After 297-h of ECMO support, the patient was weaned off ECMO, and extubated one week later.

Conclusions: In this patient with severe ARDS caused by *Bordetella pertussis*, ECMO was performed for cardiopulmonary support and rescued the infant with severe pertussis. During ECMO support period, prone position ventilation and care bundle nursing strategy contributed to the relief of continuous airway spasm.

Keywords: Pertussis, ECMO, Prone position ventilation, Airway spasm, Infant

Background

Pertussis, caused by *Bordetella pertussis* infection, is the fifth leading cause of vaccine preventable deaths in children under 5 years of age and remains a public health concern worldwide [1]. For the infant with pertussis, the prognosis is worse if the child develops pneumonia, worsening respiratory failure, PHT and requires mechanical ventilation [2]. For the critical care management of the infant with pertussis, strategies include conventional ventilation, high-frequency oscillatory ventilation, plasmapheresis, inhaled nitric oxygen, leukodepletion, and more recently, extracorporeal membrane oxygenation (ECMO) [2, 3]. Prior reports from the Extracorporeal Life Support Organization (ELSO) Registry demonstrated survival rates of 30% for pertussis patients receiving ECMO support [4, 5], which is rather lower than other ECMO respiratory indications. Recent report based on data from ELSO registry and expanded dataset from individual institutions demonstrated that younger age, vasoactive use, PHT and a rapidly progressive course were independently and significantly associated with higher mortality [3]. The patient with pertussis is characterized by increased mass of leukocytes and high level of pertussis toxin. Pertussis toxin can cause the occlusion of the pulmonary vessels by the increased mass of leukocytes, which leads to PHT, and even includes acute pulmonary vasoconstriction. The refractory airway spasm is the most common clinical manifestation. Until now, there has no report about the effect of recurrent pertussis toxins-induced airway spasm on the management of ECMO in infantile fetal pertussis.

We report the successful outcome of a 6-month-old infant diagnosed as severe pertussis treated by early initiation of ECMO. Both prone position ventilation and care

* Correspondence: zhangyc@shchildren.com.cn; zyucai2018@163.com
[1]Department of Critical Care Medicine, Shanghai Children's Hospital, Shanghai Jiao Tong University, No.355 Luding Road, Putuo District, Shanghai 200062, China
[2]Institute of Pediatric Critical Care, Shanghai Jiao Tong University, No.355 Luding Road, Putuo District, Shanghai 200062, China

bundle might be considered as key factors of the lifesaving support under ECMO in infant with severe pertussis complicated with recurrent airway spasm.

Case presentation

A 6-month old, 7.5 kg, male baby born at 31 weeks of gestation was admitted to a local hospital with a 20-day history of cough, wheezing, 5-day history of fever and with pleural effusion indicated by chest X-ray. Detection of *Bordetella pertussis* by polymerase chain reaction was positive with the nasopharyngeal specimen. The child was admitted to Pediatric Intensive care unit (PICU) in Shanghai Children's Hospital with breathless with a temperature of 37.1 °C and heart rate 170 to 190 beats/min, who developed respiratory failure requiring intubated and mechanical ventilation [positive end-expiratory pressure (PEEP) of 6 cmH2O; a pressure support of 18 cmH2O; a respiratory rate (RR) of 25 /min; and a fraction of inspired oxygen of 0.6; Peak inspiratory pressures (PIPs) were between 27 and 29 cmH_2O]. Meanwhile, laboratory studies revealed the presence of leukocytosis [26,780 white blood cells (WBCs)/μL] with 1 mg/L C-reactive protein (CRP). A chest X-radiograph showed dense opacification of the right upper and right middle lobe and patchy opacification of the left upper lobe (Fig. 1a). Over the next 48 h, despite application of lung protective strategies and a restrictive fluid strategy, the patient deteriorated with worsening lung compliance and hypoxemia, as well as the dense opacification of the right upper and right middle lobe enlarged (Fig.1b). At the same time, the tidal volume decreased from 6 mL/kg to 2.5 mL/kg, and Cdyn (Pulmonary dynamic compliance) decreased from 3.3 (0.44/kg) to 1.2 (0.16/kg). The patient's PIPs continued to rise to 40 cmH_2O with a plateau pressure of 31 cmH_2O, PaO_2/FiO_2 dropped to 60 mmHg and oxygen index (OI) raised to 30 lasting for 6 h. Importantly, the echocardiography (performed 3rd day after admission) demonstrated PHT (46 mmHg) with a normal left ventricular function. The diameter of the pulmonary artery was 1 cm, pulmonary artery blood flow was 1.0 m/s, the tricuspid regurgitation flow was 1.5 m/s, the tricuspid annulus was 1.5 cm, and TAPSE was 18. Furthermore, septic shock occurred, norepinephrine (0.3μg/kg.min) and dobutamine (10μg/kg.min) were needed to maintain his blood pressure.

Considering in anticipation of a rapid hemodynamic collapse resulting from severe PHT in pertussis, the initiation of ECMO was performed with an arterial blood gas noted as pH 7.20, $PaCO_2$ 77.9 mmHg and PaO_2 60 mmHg. The ECMO support was equipped with a centrifugal pump and an artificial lung was used (Medtronic Bio-Medicus, Minneapolis, MN, USA). The patient inserted cannula through right neck vessels, and was placed on veno-arterial (VA) ECMO support with a

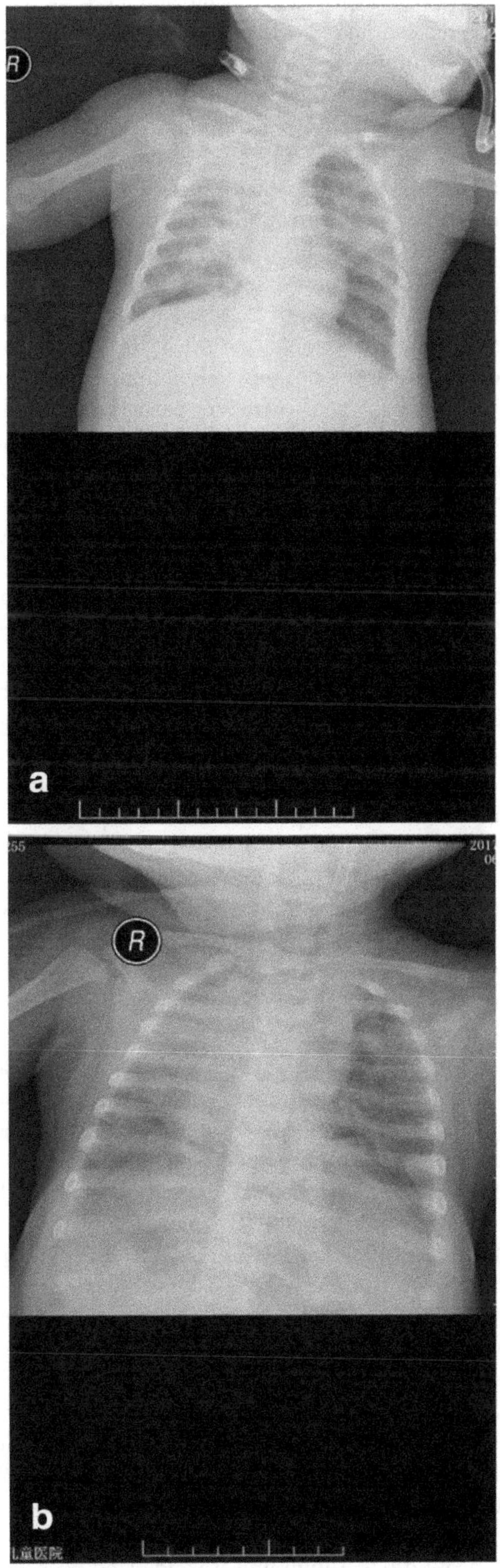

Fig. 1 The chest radiograph. (**a**) on admission, (**b**) at 48 h after admission

pump flow of 500 to 600 mL/min and FiO_2 of 1.0. The 12-Fr arterial cannula (Bio-Medicus) was placed in the right common carotid artery and the 14-Fr venous cannula (Bio-Medicus) in the right internal jugular vein. (Fig. 2a). During ECMO support, the ventilator setting was mode with SIMV+PS, FiO_2 0.4, PIP 25–26 cmH_2O, PEEP 8-9cmH_2O, RR 25 rpm, which ensured a 3-5 ml/kg tidal volume. During prone position ventilation, the setting was mode with SIMV+PS, FiO_2 0.4, PIP 24-25cmH_2O, PEEP 8cmH_2O, RR 20–25 rpm.

During the first 3 days of ECMO support, the tidal volume of this patient was only 2.5 mL/kg, and lung compliance was poor. Prone position ventilation was conducted. A team requires 5 staff members participated. A doctor positioned up to the patient's head and fixed the catheters, one nurse positioned on each side of the bed to manage the lines and tubes. We firstly placed a blanket around the patient's arms and turned the patient toward the ventilator. Then, the doctor held the patient's head and fixed the catheters, while two nurses turned the patient prone. Lastly, we straightened the blanket and adjusted lines and tubes, and placed the patient's arms in the swimmers position (the arms were positioned up toward the baby's shoulders). During this process, another doctor was responsible for monitoring the ECMO and a third nurse was responsible for administering drugs. To supine the patient, the process was performed reversely.

There was no change in cannula position shown by X-ray when changing position (Fig. 2a, b), and there was no malfunction of blood access due to bending or dislodgement of the cannula when changing position. At day 4 after ECMO initiation, exhaled tidal volumes were increased to 6 mL/kg and effusion in lung were improved indicated by chest radiographs (Figs. 2c).

During the first 5 days of ECMO support, the patient was characterized by recurrent attacks of airway spasm lasting for 20s to 2 min each time. Consequently, the airway spasm resulted in sudden declined ECMO flow (0.15 L/min), decreased blood oxygen saturation (80%), and decreased ventilator tidal volume (2 mL/kg). Except for prone position, magnesium sulfate was given and care bundles including hand washing, heightened focus on oral hygiene, closed endotracheal suctioning, prone position ventilation, appropriate sedation, reducing unnecessary stimulus (eg. assess the state of consciousness when put the position), following the nursing sequence of sputum aspiration, diapering and feeding, using full-barrier precautions during the insertion of all catheters were performed to help improving lung compliance and reduce airway spasm. The ECMO flow started around 0.55 L/min and was adjusted according to the hemodynamic status (maintained mean airway pressure [MAP] at 50–60 mmHg). The target blood flow was 80 mL/kg/min, and coagulation profile was monitored

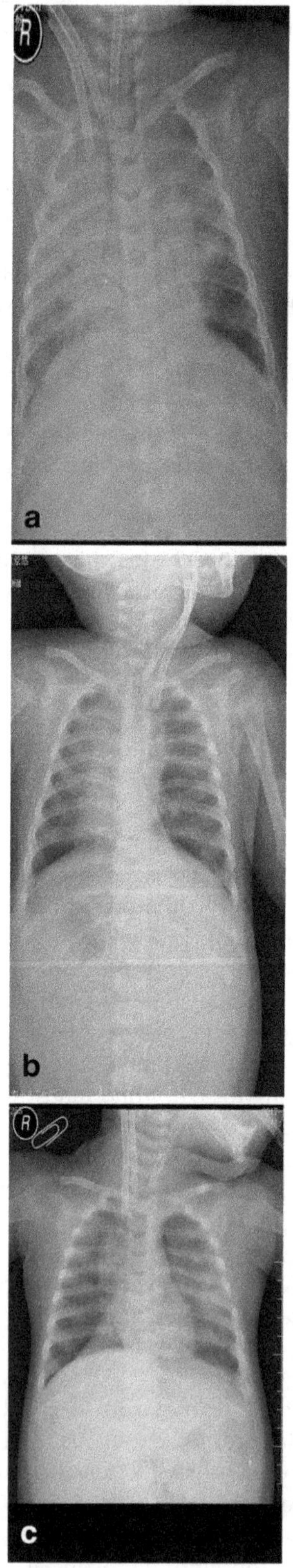

Fig. 2 The chest radiograph. (**a**) at the onset of ECMO therapy, (**b**) during prone position ventilation, (**c**) on the 4th day of ECMO support

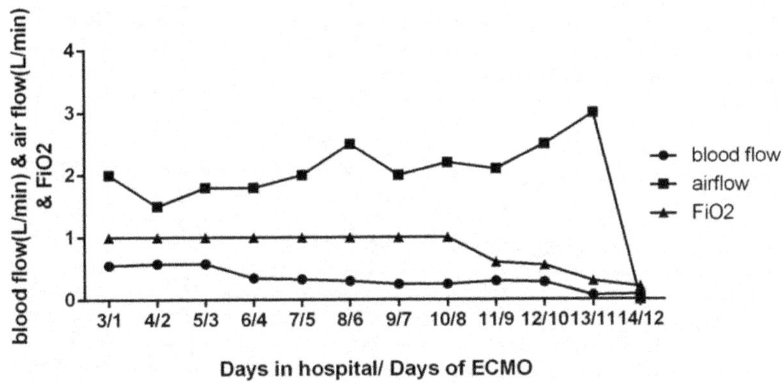

Fig. 3 Time course of initiation of ECMO therapy and the ventilator setting

through detecting the levels of activated coagulation time (ACT) and activated partial thromboplastin time (aPTT). The values of ACT were detected once 3–4 h and aPTT were detected once per 4–6 h. According to the results of ACT and aPTT, the dose of heparin was regulated to maintain an ACT of 180–220 s or APTT with 1.5–2 fold of normal value. During ECMO therapy, ECMO flow was adjusted to keep the serum $ScVO_2 > 60\%$ and lactate level < 2 mmol/L. The target oxygenation was a normal arterial partial pressure of carbon dioxide ($PaCO_2$) and partial pressure of oxygen (PaO_2) (Fig. 3).

From the 6th day of ECMO therapy, the clinical feature of airway spasm was improved. And ventilator setting was gradually reduced. After 297-h of ECMO support, the patient was weaned off V-A ECMO. During the period of ECMO therapy, respiratory mechanical parameters were monitored as shown in Fig. 4. And the ECMO flow dropped with the occurrence of airway spasm, the relationship between tidal volume and ECMO flow were shown in Fig. 5, which represented the onset and impact of airway spasm, as well as the duration of prone position. The enteral nutrition (Infatrini, Nutricia) was conducted through nasogastric tube which provided 80-100 kcal/kg.d.

One week later, the child was successfully extubated. After a 7-day high flow nasal cannula oxygen therapy, he was transferred to the escort ward on 26 days after PICU admission, and eventually discharged with a near normal neurologic examination. The time line of this case can be consulted in the Additional file 1.

Discussion and conclusions

Patients infected Bordetella pertussis were characterized by cough-associated apnea, cyanosis, PHT and encephalopathy [6]. When these infants with severe respiratory failure is poorly responsive to conventional and alternative therapies, ECMO can be considered as a promising rescue therapy [7], even if pertussis itself implies worse outcome among the indications for ECMO initiation for pediatric respiratory failure [8]. Based on ELSO Registry data, younger age, lower PaO_2/FiO_2 ratio, vasoactive use, PHT, and a rapidly progressive course were associated with increased mortality [3].

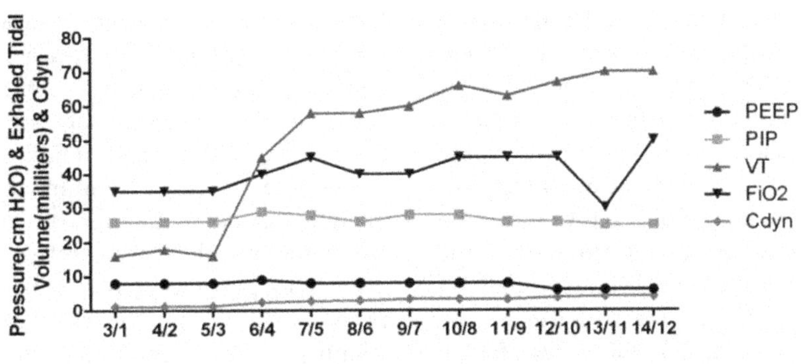

Fig. 4 Time course of initiation of ECMO therapy and its effects on pulmonary compliance. After initiation of ECMO therapy, there was sustained recruitment of alveoli evidenced by an increase in the amount of exhaled tidal volume. PEEP, positive end-expiratory pressure; PIP, peak inspiratory pressure, VT, tidal volume; Cdyn, Pulmonary dynamic compliance

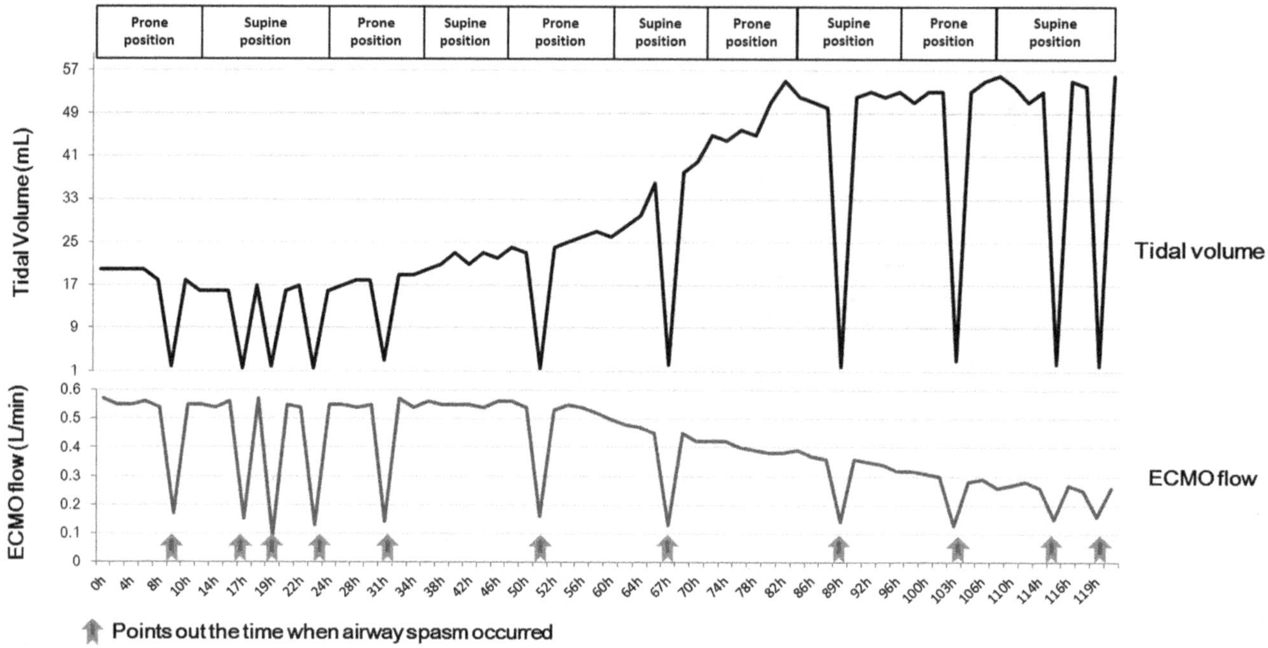

Fig. 5 Schematic diagram of timing for the onset and impact of airway spasm on ECMO flow and tidal volume after ECMO initiated, as well as the duration of prone position

In this case report, the male child of 6-month-old was successfully recovered by V-A ECMO supporting. Prone position ventilation and care bundle played crucial role in the management of ECMO flow influenced by pertussis toxin-induced airway spasm. Pertussis toxin produces lymphocyte proliferation and results in a hyper viscosity, is thought to be responsible for the leukocytosis observed with pertussis infection [9], and results in a hyper viscosity syndrome that leads to obstruction of the pulmonary arterioles [10]. Here, we describe a 6-month-old boy who developed respiratory failure and septic shock induced by *B. pertussis* infection. The WBC count was 26,780/μL, which was lower than the reported hyperleucocytosis (> 100,000/μL) [11, 12]. It was also reported that young infants infected with *B. pertussis* exhibit prolonged apneic pauses [13]. According to the previous report [14], increased airway pressure decreases the transmural pressure of the right atrium and superior vena cava through lung-heart interaction. Airway spasm causes airway pressure shoot up, then intrathoracic pressure increases and affect the venous return, thus decrease the preload of heart. Another hypothesis is that by previous point of view B. pertussis pneumonia triggers acute pulmonary vasoconstriction resulting in the increased afterload of right heart [15]. Given that ECMO flow is affected by the preload and afterload of heart, we speculate that B. pertussis-induced bronchospasm might contribute to a sharp increase of intrathoracic pressure which reduce the venous return, as well as acute pulmonary vasoconstriction reduced ECMO flow through influencing both the preload and afterload of right heart. Importantly, pertussis toxin-induced recurrent airway spasm brought the challenging for the ECMO flow management during EMCO support, which was the specific clinical feature in this case. During the first 5 days of ECMO therapy, recurrent airway spasm resulted in a sudden decline in ECMO flow, decreased blood oxygen saturation, and decreased ventilator tidal volume. It is the first report about the clinical features about pertussis during EMCO supporting according to our knowledge. Magnesium sulfate was used to relieve bronchial spasm, and had some auxiliary functions. Magnesium has an effect on smooth muscle cells, with hypomagnesemia causing contraction and hypermagnesemia causing relaxation. It has been reported that intravenous magnesium sulfate benifit patients with acute severe asthma who do not respond to standard therapeutic medications [16]. In addition, a strict following of nursing sequence of sputum aspiration, diapering and feeding, along with appropriate sedative, benefited. Anti-pressure ulcer pads were put under chest and abdomen to preventing possible pressure injury while in prone position. The greatest contribution of care bundle in this patient was minimization of unnecessary stimulus thus gain the time to waiting and recovering from airway spasm. What we concerned most is that frequently sudden drop of ECMO blood flow will cause blood clotting in ECMO circulation, so we monitor both activated clotting time and activated partial thromboplastin time (aPTT) [17]. In our study, the values of ACT and aPTT were correlated well during ECMO therapy. Based on our clinical experience from this case, there was no correlation between the drop of ECMO flow or the shorten of ACT or aPTT, which need further investigation in the future.

Pertussis toxin-induced recurrent airway spasm resulted in decreased arterial oxygen saturation and the increased circulating leukocyte caused by pertussis toxin may restrict pulmonary blood flow, which cause cardiac failure, shock, and acute respiratory distress [15]. Prone position ventilation is an effective method for improving oxygenation in patients with acute respiratory distress syndrome (ARDS) [18, 19]. Importantly, prone positioning can be safely performed and managed among critically ill pediatric patients with ARDS [20–22]. It has been proved that when changed from a supine to prone position, ARDS patients demonstrate a dramatic redistribution of CT lung densities because of re-expansion of previously atelectatic posterior regions. After perfusion improves in these previously hypoxic, vasoconstricted posterior lung regions when turn to prone position, ventilation/ perfusion improves [23]. When the patient ventilated prone position, the central blood volume increased by shift of splanchnic blood volume to the thorax, which could induce pulmonary vascular recruitment, then airway spasm relief, thus help to prevent reductions in ECMO flow. On the other hand, prone position may facilitate sputum drainage. So we assume that prone position ventilation does not directly relief airway spasm, but it improves ventilation/ perfusion, facilitate sputum drainage, thus improves lung compliance. The effect of prone position on oxygenation-lung compliance of pediatric ARDS patients may be in doubt. From the research in adult ARDS patients, both low tidal volumes and increased proning duration contribute to a lower mortality in ARDS patients, and the effects were marked in the subgroup in which the duration of prone positioning was more than 10 h/session [24–26]. Recent study indicated that prone positioning was performed for 4 h, every 8 h, for 10 days in a 17-day-old infant with severe pertussis under ECMO support [10]. Thus, for pediatric ARDS patients, the duration and efficacy of prone position need to be verified through more clinical trials. In this case, prone ventilation proved to be effective for improving compliance indicated by significantly increased low Cdyn after supine to prone and then prone to supine position. And cannula-related complications such as accidental removal or dislodgement of a central venous catheter, tracheal tube and cannula for extracorporeal circulation did not happened during prone positioning. These results suggested that prone positioning is a safe and effective procedure in patients with severe pertussis receiving extracorporeal circulation.

There were some limitation in this case report. We did not continuously detect the WBC counts during ECMO support. Since the patient was born premature, we are now unable to report on the long-term outcome of the patient's neurodevelopment. These need further investigation in cased with severe pertussis treated by ECMO supporting.

From this case review, we speculated that ECMO management is challenging in patients with pertussis contributing to the high mortality of these patients under ECMO support. Prone position ventilation contributes to better oxygenation and lung compliance. And detailed care bundle is essential for patients with pertussis challenged by recurrent airway spasm.

Abbreviations

ACT: Activated clotting time; aPTT: Activated partial thromboplastin time; ARDS: Acute respiratory distress syndrome; Cdyn: Pulmonary dynamic compliance; CRP: C-reactive protein; ECMO: Extracorporeal membrane oxygenation; ELSO: Extracorporeal Life Support Organization; MAP: Mean airway pressure; OI: Oxygen index; $PaCO_2$: Arterial partial pressure of carbon dioxide; PaO_2: Partial pressure of oxygen; PEEP: Positive end-expiratory pressure; PHT: PHT; PICU: Pediatric Intensive care unit; PIP: Peak inspiratory pressure; RR: Respiratory rate; $ScVO_2$: Central venous oxygen saturation; WBC: White blood cells

Acknowledgements

Not applicable.

Fundings

This study was supported by Science and Technology Commission of Shanghai Municipality (18411951000), Shanghai Municipal Education Commission-Gaofeng Clinical Medicine Grant support (DLY201618, 20171928), New Advanced Technology Project at the Shanghai City Hospital Development Center (SHDC12014116)

Authors' contributions

Y Cui and YC Zhang were the main administrators of ECMO management. JY Shi and CX Wang analyzed and interpreted the patient data, and are major contributors in writing the manuscript. All authors read and approved the final manuscript.

Competing interests

The authors declare that they have no competing interests.

References

1. Yeung KHT, Duclos P, Nelson EAS, Hutubessy RCW. An update of the global burden of pertussis in children younger than 5 years: a modelling study. Lancet Infect Dis. 2017;17(9):974–80.
2. Ulloa-Gutierrez R, Boza R, Carvajal-Riggioni D, Baltodano A. Pertussis: should we improve intensive care management or vaccination strategies? Expert Rev Vaccines. 2011;10(1):49–53.
3. Domico M, Ridout D, MacLaren G, Barbaro R, Annich G, Schlapbach LJ, et al. Extracorporeal membrane oxygenation for pertussis: predictors of outcome including PHT and leukodepletion. Pediatr Crit Care Med. 2018;19(3):254–61.
4. Halasa NB, Barr FE, Johnson JE, Edwards KM. Fatal PHT associated with pertussis in infants: does extracorporeal membrane oxygenation have a role? Pediatrics. 2003;112(6 Pt 1):1274–8.

5. Rowlands HE, Goldman AP, Harrington K, Karimova A, Brierley J, Cross N, et al. Impact of rapid leukodepletion on the outcome of severe clinical pertussis in young infants. Pediatrics. 2010;126(4):e816–27.
6. Straney L, Schibler A, Ganeshalingham A, Alexander J, Festa M, Slater A, et al. Burden and outcomes of severe pertussis infection in critically ill infants. Pediatr Crit Care Med. 2016;17(8):735–42.
7. Pooboni S, Roberts N, Westrope C, Jenkins DR, Killer H, Pandya HC, et al. Extracorporeal life support in pertussis. Pediatr Pulmonol. 2003; 36(4):310–5.
8. Bailly DK, Reeder RW, Zabrocki LA, Hubbard AM, Wilkes J, Bratton SL, et al. Development and validation of a score to predict mortality in children undergoing extracorporeal membrane oxygenation for respiratory failure: pediatric pulmonary rescue with extracorporeal membrane oxygenation prediction score. Crit Care Med. 2017;45(1):e58–66.
9. Kerr JR, Matthews RC. Bordetella pertussis infection: pathogenesis, diagnosis, management, and the role of protective immunity. Eur J Clin Microbiol Infect Dis. 2000;19(2):77–88.
10. Assy J, Seguela PE, Guillet E, Mauriat P. Severe neonatal pertussis treated by leukodepletion and early extra corporeal membrane oxygenation. Pediatr Infect Dis J. 2015;34(9):1029–30.
11. Pierce C, Klein N, Peters M. Is leukocytosis a predictor of mortality in severe pertussis infection? Intensive Care Med. 2000;26(10):1512–4.
12. Asadollahi K, Beeching NJ, Gill GV. Leukocytosis as a predictor for non-infective mortality and morbidity. QJM. 2010;103(5):285–92.
13. Nieves D, Bradley JS, Gargas J, Mason WH, Lehman D, Lehman SM, et al. Exchange blood transfusion in the management of severe pertussis in young infants. Pediatr Infect Dis J. 2013;32(6):698–9.
14. Lansdorp B, Hofhuizen C, van Lavieren M, van Swieten H, Lemson J, van Putten MJ, et al. Mechanical ventilation-induced intrathoracic pressure distribution and heart-lung interactions*. Crit Care Med. 2014;42(9):1983–90.
15. Paddock CD, Sanden GN, Cherry JD, Gal AA, Langston C, Tatti KM, et al. Pathology and pathogenesis of fatal Bordetella pertussis infection in infants. Clin Infect Dis. 2008;47(3):328–38.
16. Devi PR, Kumar L, Singhi SC, Prasad R, Singh M. Intravenous magnesium sulfate in acute severe asthma not responding to conventional therapy. Indian Pediatr. 1997;34(5):389–97.
17. Oliver WC. Anticoagulation and coagulation management for ECMO. Semin Cardiothorac Vasc Anesth. 2009;13(3):154–75.
18. Alsaghir AH, Martin CM. Effect of prone positioning in patients with acute respiratory distress syndrome: a meta-analysis. Crit Care Med. 2008;36(2):603–9.
19. Gattinoni L, Tognoni G, Pesenti A, Taccone P, Mascheroni D, Labarta V, et al. Effect of prone positioning on the survival of patients with acute respiratory failure. N Engl J Med. 2001;345(8):568–73.
20. Gainnier M, Michelet P, Thirion X, Arnal JM, Sainty JM, Papazian L. Prone position and positive end-expiratory pressure in acute respiratory distress syndrome. Crit Care Med. 2003;31(12):2719–26.
21. Fineman LD, LaBrecque MA, Shih MC, Curley MA. Prone positioning can be safely performed in critically ill infants and children. Pediatr Crit Care Med. 2006;7(5):413–22.
22. Masuda Y, Tatsumi H, Imaizumi H, Gotoh K, Yoshida S, Chihara S, et al. Effect of prone positioning on cannula function and impaired oxygenation during extracorporeal circulation. J Artif Organs. 2014;17(1):106–9.
23. Mok YH, Lee JH, Rehder KJ, Turner DA. Adjunctive treatments in pediatric acute respiratory distress syndrome. Expert Rev Respir Med. 2014;8(6):703–16.
24. Kallet RH. A comprehensive review of prone position in ARDS. Respir Care. 2015;60(11):1660–87.
25. Beitler JR, Shaefi S, Montesi SB, Devlin A, Loring SH, Talmor D, et al. Prone positioning reduces mortality from acute respiratory distress syndrome in the low tidal volume era: a meta-analysis. Intensive Care Med. 2014;40(3):332–41.
26. Malhotra A, Ayas N, Kacmarek R. Prone positioning of patients in acute respiratory failure. N Engl J Med. 2002;346(4):295–7.

Tobacco use among Latinx adolescents: exploring the immigrant paradox

Anna E. Epperson[1*], Jan L. Wallander[2], Marc N. Elliott[3] and Mark A. Schuster[4,5,6]

Abstract

Background: Research suggests that an immigrant paradox exists where those who were not born in the United States (1st generation) have significantly better health than those who were born in the U.S. (2nd generation or more). The aim of the current study was to examine the immigrant paradox with respect to tobacco-related perceptions and parenting influences in smoking initiation among Latinx adolescents.

Methods: Data came from the 7th and 10th grade Healthy Passages™ assessments of Latinx participants in three U. S. urban areas ($N = 1536$) who were first (18%), second (60%), and third (22%) generation. In addition to demographics, measures included perceived cigarette availability and peer smoking, intentions and willingness to smoke, and general monitoring by parents. Parents reported on generational status and their own tobacco use. The primary outcome was participant's reported use of cigarettes.

Results: By 10th grade, 31% of Latinx youth had tried a cigarette, compared to 8% in 7th grade. After controlling for age, gender, and socioeconomic status, regression analyses indicated that there were no significant differences related to generational status in cigarette smoking initiation in either 7th or 10th grade. Youth tobacco-related perceptions, general parental monitoring, and parental tobacco use predicted Latinx adolescent cigarette use initiation by 10th grade.

Conclusions: Latinx adolescents might not have deferential smoking rates based on generation status, suggesting that the immigrant paradox concept may not hold for smoking initiation among Latinx adolescents. Rather, factors influencing cigarette initiation generally in adolescents as a group appear to apply to Latinxs as well.

Keywords: Latinxs, Immigrant paradox, Generational status, Tobacco use, Adolescent

Background

Over 37 million adults in the U.S. are current smokers [1] and most (80%) of these smokers began smoking cigarettes before the age of 17 [2]. Despite significant public health efforts to reduce the prevalence of smoking in the U.S., tobacco use continues to be the leading cause of preventable death and is associated with numerous negative health outcomes, including respiratory problems, lung cancer, and cardiovascular disease [3]. National health data suggest that time of smoking initiation varies by race/ethnicity [4], with Latinxs initiating much earlier than (non-Latinx) Whites. With thousands of youth beginning to smoke each day [2] and more male Latinx youth initiating cigarette smoking before age 13 years (13%) compared to their White (10%) and Black (10.5%) peers [4], there is a need to understand factors associated with smoking initiation during adolescence. Such information may help with the development of prevention efforts, especially those targeted at Latinx youth.

Previous research has indicated that immigrants to the U.S. and children of immigrants may be less likely to engage in behaviors that are harmful to health and may have a morbidity and mortality advantage compared to those without a recent immigration history, regardless of level of socioeconomic status or race/ethnicity [5]. This finding has been reported for a variety of health risk behaviors, including substance use and sexual risk behaviors [6–8], and health conditions [9, 10], such as mental health disorders and certain types of cancers and cancer outcomes. This phenomenon of engaging less frequently

* Correspondence: aepper@stanford.edu
[1]Stanford Prevention Research Center, Department of Medicine, Stanford University, 1265 Welch Road, Suite 300, Palo Alto, CA 94305, USA

in risk behaviors and having better overall health in the current and recent immigrant generation is referred to as the *immigrant paradox* [11, 12]. Moreover, for adults, there is an overall mortality advantage, where 1st and 2nd generation Latinxs have a longer life expectancy compared to 3rd generation Latinxs, defined as those born in the U.S. to parents born in the U.S. [13].

Despite studies documenting the immigrant paradox for a broad range of health issues, we are aware of only two studies that have examined the role of immigrant generational status on smoking among Latinx youth. Both studies used data from the National Longitudinal Study of Adolescent Health (Add Health), a national, longitudinal study following youth from 7th grade into young adulthood. One study found evidence to support the paradox [14] after controlling for demographic covariates (age, gender, parental education, and household composition), whereas the other found no significant difference by generational status after controlling for other covariates, including parental control and parental smoking [15]. Consequently, conclusions regarding the existence of the paradox in relation to Latinx adolescent smoking are unclear. Findings for Latinx adults have also been mixed, with two studies reporting that 1st [16, 17] and 2nd [18] generation Latinxs were less likely to be smokers compared to 3rd generation and that 3rd generation have the highest overall tobacco use, but another study reporting no difference by generational status [19].

Previous research has shown that initiation of tobacco use among youth is associated with many sociodemographic factors and tobacco-related perceptions and attitudes. The theory of planned behavior is a widely used theoretical framework for understanding factors associated with smoking initiation among youth [20, 21] and links behavior with intentions and perceptions about external influences [22]. Adolescent tobacco use initiation has been shown to be strongly associated with availability of cigarettes [23], peer smoking [24, 25], parent smoking [26], parental monitoring [27], and intentions and willingness to smoke [28–30], with at least one previous study finding that intentions to smoke are associated with smoking among Latinx adolescents [30]. Further, having friends who smoke cigarettes [25] is associated with increased smoking intentions, willingness, and future initiation. Being closely monitored by a parent has also been found to be related to decreased smoking willingness and initiation [24]. Few studies, however, have examined the extent to which these influences are significant for Latinx adolescents specifically, and we know of none that considers immigrant generational status together with tobacco-related perceptions (intentions and willingness to smoke).

The current study updates previous work and examines tobacco use among Latinx adolescents beginning in middle school (7th grade). We also examine the immigrant paradox together with demographic and parent and perceptual factors in cigarette smoking initiation. We hypothesized that among Latinx adolescents, (1) more recent immigrant generations (1st vs. 3rd and 2nd vs. 3rd) evidence lower prevalence of smoking initiation by 7th and 10th grade and tobacco-related perceptions of willingness and intent to use in 7th grade compared to 10th grade. Based on past findings, we further hypothesized (2) that tobacco-related perceptions and parenting influences in 7th grade predict, beyond generational status differences, smoking initiation by 10th grade. Specifically, we examined as predictors perceptions of tobacco availability and peer smoking, future smoking intentions and willingness to smoke, and parental tobacco use and general monitoring.

Methods

Data came from the Healthy Passages™ study, a longitudinal (2004–2011), multi-site cohort study of health and health behaviors in youth in 5th, 7th, and 10th grades [31, 32].

Participants

Fifth-grade students were recruited from public school classrooms in three locations (Birmingham, Alabama; Los Angeles, California; Houston, Texas) to participate in the Healthy Passages™ study. Using a two-stage probability sampling procedure, participants were selected. To ensure adequate sample sizes of students who identified as Black, Latinx, and White, schools within Birmingham, Los Angeles, and Houston were randomly selected with probabilities proportionate to a weighted measure of the scarcity of a school's students relative to targets of these three racial/ethnic groups. Within these selected schools, all 5th grade students were invited to participate [32]. Among the participants (and their parents/caregivers) that granted permission to be contacted and completed interviews in 5th grade ($N = 5147$; 51% female; 35% Latinx), 4773 (93%) and 4521 (89%) completed follow-up assessments at the second (2 years later) and third (3 years later) wave, corresponding to when the participants generally were in 7th and 10th grade.

The analysis sample ($n = 1536$) contained participants who had reported no tobacco use at baseline (5th grade), identified as Hispanic/Latinx based on their parent's report, completed all three waves, and could be classified as first- (18.4%), second- (59.9%), or third (21.7%) generation (see below for definition). The sample (51% female) had a mean age of 11.13 ($SD = 0.58$) at 5th grade, 13.10 ($SD = 0.63$) at 7th grade, and 16.12 ($SD = 0.64$) at 10th grade. Selected sample characteristics are shown in Table 1 (see [32] for further details).

Table 1 Sample characteristics ($N = 1536$)

	N	Wtd %
Female	774	50.5
Generational Status		
1st Generation	272	18.4
2nd Generation	883	59.9
3rd Generation	381	21.7
Parental level of education		
Some HS or less	631	44.9
HS diploma/GED	360	23.6
Some college/2 year degree	351	21.8
4 year degree or higher	186	9.8
Parent household composition		
Single parent household	532	33.2
Two- parent household	1002	66.8

Wtd Weighted, % is calculated with weights to reflect sampling, *HS* High School, *GED* General Equivalence Diploma

Procedure

Following standard procedures approved by the Institutional Review Boards at all study sites, two trained interviewers completed the Healthy Passages™ assessment protocol with the adolescent and one parent/caregiver at their home or another agreed upon location at each assessment. Written informed consent was provided by the parent, and the adolescent provided written assent. The interviews were conducted using both computer-assisted personal and self-interview procedures with the adolescent and parent separated in private spaces [31]. A Spanish version could be chosen by either at each assessment, except for youth at 10th grade (applied partly or fully at 5th grade: 8% of youth, 23% of parents; 7th grade: 4% of youth, 30% of parents; 10th grade: 30% of parents). Third-generation adolescent participants were the largest group to complete the interview mainly or entirely in English (98%), followed by second- (81%), and first- (50%) generation.

Measures

The outcome of focus was **cigarette smoking initiation**, measured at 7th and 10th grade with the question, "Have you ever tried cigarette smoking, even one or two puffs?" (0 = *no;* 1 = *yes).*

Generational Status. During enrollment in the study, each parent was asked whether they had been born inside or outside the U.S. Parents were also asked whether their child was born inside or outside the U.S. Based on a classification scheme described by Coll and Marks [11], the child was classified as one of the following: 1) *first-generation,* if both the participant (child) and the parent were born outside the U.S.; 2) *second-generation,* if the participant (child) was born in the U.S. but the parent was born outside the U.S.; and 3) *third-generation,* if both the participant (child) and the parent were born inside the U.S.

Perceived peer smoking was measured in 7th grade with one question, "How many of your closest friends do you think have smoked cigarettes?" (1 = *none,* 3 = *many*). This was dichotomized into 0 = *no peer use* or 1 = *peer use.*

Perceived cigarette availability was assessed in 7th grade with one question, "Has anyone ever offered you a cigarette?" (0 = *no* or 1 = *yes).*

Intentions to smoke were measured in 7th grade with one question, "Do you think you will smoke cigarettes at any time during the next year?" with responses ranging from 0 = *no,* 1 = *maybe*, or 2 = *yes.* This was recoded into a dichotomized variable with 0 = *no* and 1 = *maybe/yes.*

Willingness to smoke was measured in 7th grade with one question, "If one of your closest friends offered you a cigarette, would you smoke it?" with responses ranging from 0 = *no,* 1 = *maybe*, or 2 = *yes.* This was recoded into a dichotomized variable with 0 = *no* and 1 = *maybe/yes.*

Monitoring was measured in 7th grade using five questions from a previous study [31] in which the adolescent was asked to indicate on a four-point scale (1 = *do not know much,* 4 = *know a lot*) how much his or her parent knew generally about what he or she did with free time (e.g., "How much do your parents know about where you are most afternoons after school?") and who his or her friends were (e.g., "How much do your parents know about who your friends really are?"). The five items were summed with scores ranging from 5 to 20 ($\alpha = .80$).

Parent tobacco use was measured in 7th grade with two questions posed to the parent, "During the past 12 months, how many cigarettes did you smoke per day?" (*0 = none; 7 = more than 30 per day*) and, "During the past 12 months, did you use chewing tobacco, snuff, or dip, or smoke cigars or a pipe? (1 = *Yes*; 2 = *No*"). These were combined to create a dichotomized variable, where "None" (0) or "No" (2) on both questions was recoded as a "No" (0) and all other response combinations were coded as "Yes" (1).

Control Variables. Several covariates were included in the analysis including age, gender (male/female), highest level of education in household, and household composition. Highest level of education reported for either parent was classified into four categories ranging from less than high school graduation (1) to completion of a four-year college degree or higher (4). Household composition was coded based on parent report as either "two-parent" household or "other" (i.e., "single" parent).

Data analysis

All analyses were conducted with design weights to account for differential probabilities of selection of students according to their school and a cluster variable to account for clustering of students within schools using IBM SPSS Statistics™ Complex Sampling module. Weighting also accounted for non-participation (by school, race/ethnicity, gender, and combinations thereof) initially, dropout, and differences between the retained sample (10th grade) and the original sample (5th grade), producing unbiased estimates among respondents if the characteristics used in the weights account for all nonresponse bias. Sensitivity analyses indicated that participants who completed all three waves (analytic sample) did not differ on any of the demographic or tobacco-related factors from participants who did not complete the second or third (final) wave except on highest level of education in household and household composition. For highest level of education in household, participants who did not complete all waves were more likely to have some high school education or less (49.7%) and not be from a two-parent household (48.3%) versus those who completed all waves (40.4 and 56.7%, respectively; p's < .05). Two variables had missing data present [education (0.5%) and cigarette smoking initiation (8.1%)]; therefore, participants with missing data on these variables were excluded from the analysis. Analyses indicated they did not significantly differ from the analysis sample on any demographic variables. To further test the potential role of missing data, the multiple imputation method was used to estimate these missing values. This approach produced substantively identical results (available upon request).

Descriptive statistics and tests for group differences in tobacco use initiation, tobacco-related perceptions, and parental influences by generational status were conducted first using one-way ANOVA and chi-square tests. Logistic regression analyses followed to examine associations between tobacco-related perceptions and parental influences with tobacco use initiation in 7th grade and to predict initiation in 10th grade, starting with generational status (Model 1) and then adding in turn, tobacco-related perceptions (Model 2) and then parental tobacco use and general monitoring (Model 3). All models controlled for the covariates of age, gender, and household education and composition. Two-way interactions between generational status and other predictors (e.g., monitoring, perceived peer smoking) were tested in the model; interaction results are not presented as none were significant.

Results

Descriptive statistics are presented in Table 1. As shown in Fig. 1, approximately 8% of the overall sample of Latinx adolescents reported having tried cigarette smoking by 7th and 31% by 10th grade. For smoking-related perceptions reported in the 7th grade, 34% reported that they believed their friends smoked cigarettes, 16% reported having been offered a cigarette, 9% reported that they had future intentions to smoke and 8% that they would be willing to smoke in the future if offered cigarettes (Table 2). Seventeen percent of parents reported using tobacco.

Generational status

Results (Tables 2 & 3) indicated that there were no significant differences in cigarette smoking initiation

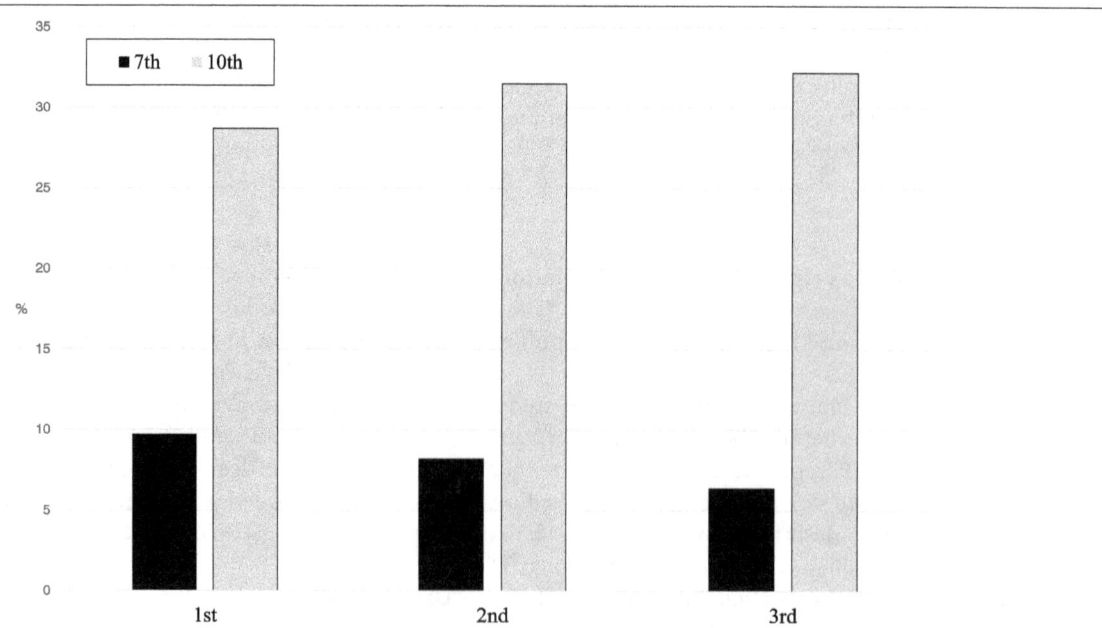

Fig. 1 Prevalence of cigarette smoking initiation in 7th and 10th grade by immigration generation status

Table 2 Tobacco-related variables by generational status ($N = 1536$)

	Overall		1st Generation	2nd Generation	3rd Generation	
	N	Wtd.%	Wtd.%	Wtd. %	Wtd. %	χ^2
Total	1536	–	18.4	59.9	21.7	
7th grade Cigarette Smoking Initiation	118	8.1	9.7	8.2	6.4	2.34
10th grade Cigarette Smoking Initiation	430	31.2	28.7	31.5	32.2	0.92
Perceived Cigarette Availability	243	16.1	18.1	15.5	16.3	1.14
Perceived Peer Smoking	513	33.8	28.9	34.1	37.4	4.95
Intentions to Smoke	134	8.7	7.7	9.1	8.4	0.58
Willingness to Smoke	123	8.4	7.4	8.3	9.5	0.93
Parent Tobacco Use	256	16.8	13.9[a]	15.8[b]	22.2[c]	**9.15**
	M (SE)					*F*
Monitoring	16.81 (0.11)		16.87(0.14)[a,b]	16.68(0.13)[a]	17.12(0.17)[b]	**2.38**

Wtd Weighted, % is calculated with weights to reflect sampling, *HS* High School
[a,b,c]Different superscripts within generational status subgroups for row variable indicates statistically significant difference as per $\chi 2$ or *F* tests. Boldface indicates statistical significance ($p < .05$)

among Latinx youth of varying generational status in 7th (χ^2 [2, $N = 1536$] = 2.34, $p = .39$) or 10th grade (χ^2 [2, $N =$ 1536] = 0.92, $p = .73$). There were no significant differences among generational status groups in tobacco-related perceptions or general parental monitoring or tobacco use (p's > .05).

Adolescent tobacco-related perceptions

As shown in Table 3, Model 2 for cigarette smoking, Latinx adolescents who reported cigarette availability in the 7th grade were at least twice as likely to report initiating cigarette smoking in both the 7th and 10th grades compared to those who did not report being offered cigarettes ($p = .004$, $p = .001$, respectively). Believing that friends smoked cigarettes was associated with a higher likelihood of having initiated cigarette smoking by 7th grade ($p < .001$), and was predictive of cigarette smoking initiation by 10th grade ($p = .001$). Both intentions to smoke in the next year and willingness to smoke if offered cigarettes were associated with a higher likelihood of initiating smoking by 7th grade (p's < .05), and Latinx adolescents reporting intentions and willingness were twice as likely to smoke by 10th grade ($p < .001$ and $p = .012$, respectively).

Parental influences

As shown in Table 3, Model 3, when added to the regressions predicting tobacco use in 7th and 10th grade, having increased general parental monitoring was associated with a decreased odds of cigarette smoking initiation in 7th grade ($p = .001$) and predicted a lower likelihood of trying cigarettes in the 10th grade ($p < .001$). Finally, parental tobacco use was predictive of cigarette smoking in the 10th grade ($p = .021$), but was not associated with cigarette smoking in the 7th grade ($p = .208$). Perceptual variables generally remained significant predictors of tobacco use when parental variables were added to the regression model.

Demographic influences

Increased age was associated with an increased odds of cigarette smoking initiation in 10th grade ($p = .005$) but was not associated with cigarette smoking in the 7th grade ($p = .544$). Gender, level of education, and household composition were not significantly associated with cigarette smoking in the 7th or 10th grades (p's > .05).

Discussion

Cigarette smoking among Latinx adolescents increased almost four-fold between 7th (ages 12–13) and 10th (15–16) grade, from 8 to 31%. However, there is little evidence for the immigrant paradox accounting for this pattern, at least when based on the adolescents' generational status. Smoking in Latinx youth in 10th grade was predicted, as expected, by tobacco-related cognitive processes present in 7th grade pertaining to peer norms, cigarette availability, and intentions and willingness to try cigarettes, as well as by a parent who uses tobacco and provides less general monitoring.

Our finding that there were not significant differences between Latinx adolescents of varying generational status for smoking initiation is consistent with one previous study that controlled for demographic, behavioral, and parental factors [15], but is in contrast with the second study that found that 3rd generation adolescents were more likely to smoke cigarettes compared to 2nd and 1st generation [14]. Our findings may have differed as our study was conducted in three specific metropolitan areas in the U.S, while previous work used national data from Add Health. Although not previously examined, we also found that there were no differences in tobacco-related

Table 3 Logistic Regression Model for Tobacco Use Initiation by 7th and 10th Grade

	Cigarette Smoking					
	7th Grade			10th Grade		
OR (95% CI)	Model 1	Model 2	Model 3	Model 1	Model 2	Model 3
Generational Status						
1st generation	Ref.	Ref.	Ref.	Ref.	Ref.	Ref.
2nd generation	0.93 (0.48, 1.78)	0.73 (0.32, 1.64)	0.69 (0.30, 1.57)	1.29 (0.85, 1.95)	1.18 (0.77, 1.81)	1.15 (0.75, 1.77)
3rd generation	0.70 (0.36, 1.34)	0.48 (0.21, 1.07)	0.46 (0.20, 1.03)	1.26 (0.77, 2.07)	1.21 (0.72, 2.04)	1.17 (0.70, 1.97)
Age	**1.80 (1.25, 2.59)**	1.12 (0.81, 1.55)	1.11 (0.79, 1.55)	1.61 (1.37, 1.90)	**1.29 (1.09, 1.52)**	**1.28 (1.08, 1.52)**
Female (referent: male)	0.79 (0.51, 1.24)	0.71 (0.44, 1.13)	0.78 (0.49, 1.24)	0.98 (0.74, 1.31)	0.98 (0.70, 1.36)	1.03 (0.74, 1.45)
Parental level of education						
Some HS or less	Ref.	Ref.	Ref.	Ref.	Ref.	Ref.
HS diploma/GED	1.49 (0.72, 3.07)	1.21 (0.55, 2.68)	1.15 (0.52, 2.55)	1.30 (0.84, 2.02)	1.25 (0.80, 1.94)	1.24 (0.79, 1.93)
Some college	1.27 (0.59, 2.71)	0.92 (0.36, 2.36)	0.91 (0.36, 2.35)	1.29 (0.84, 1.98)	1.15 (0.74, 1.81)	1.12 (0.70, 1.78)
4 year degree or higher	1.63 (0.73, 3.64)	1.37 (0.55, 3.41)	1.23 (0.49, 3.04)	1.39 (0.95, 2.02)	1.26 (0.86, 1.87)	1.18 (0.79, 1.76)
Single parent household (referent: two-parent)	**1.66 (1.13, 2.42)**	1.18 (0.75, 1.85)	1.18 (0.75, 1.85)	**1.30 (1.01, 1.68)**	1.12 (.85, 1.49)	1.08 (0.82, 1.42)
Perceptions /Attitudes						
Cigarette availability	**2.36 (1.34, 4.13)**		**2.21 (1.25, 3.90)**		**2.00 (1.40, 2.87)**	**1.91 (1.33, 2.74)**
Peer smoking	**3.05 (1.88, 4.94)**		**3.08 (1.89, 5.04)**		**1.74 (1.26, 2.40)**	**1.72 (1.25, 2.37)**
Future smoking intentions	**3.72 (2.23, 6.21)**		**3.62 (2.18, 6.00)**		**2.62 (1.70, 4.04)**	**2.53 (1.67, 3.83)**
Smoking willingness	**4.25 (2.64, 6.83)**		**3.54 (2.14, 5.86)**		**2.25 (1.33, 3.80)**	**1.92 (1.16, 3.18)**
Family Influences						
Monitoring			**0.90 (0.84, 0.96)**			**0.92 (0.88, 0.96)**
Parental Tobacco Use			1.44 (0.81, 2.55)			**1.59 (1.08, 2.34)**

All models controlled for: gender, child age in years at 7th grade, parent household composition, and parent education. *OR* odds ratio, *CI* confidence interval.
Model 1: Generation status and covariates only; Model 2: Tobacco use attitudes and perceptions added; Model 3: Parental influences added
Boldface indicates statistical significance ($p < .05$)

perceptions (intentions and willingness) due to generational status. The association between these tobacco-related cognitive processes reported in middle school (7th grade) and smoking initiation in high school (10th grade) supports previous findings that youth who report intentions and willingness to smoke in the future are more likely to initiate smoking [27, 28]. Finally, results indicating that perceptions about cigarette availability, peer and parental smoking, and parental general monitoring predicted smoking initiation also supported previous findings among Black, Latinx, and White adolescents [29, 30].

Several limitations in this research should be noted. The longitudinal cohort design hinders causal inferences based on these findings. As noted previously, this study was conducted in three specific metropolitan areas in the U.S, and caution should be exercised in generalizing to other populations. Further, Latinx youth in this study predominantly have Mexican and Central America heritage, also raising caution about generalizing to Latinx groups with other origins. Immigration status was only recorded for one parent. Further, generational status is often used as a proxy for acculturation which may have limitations. Acculturation is a complex psychological and sociological process that has multiple dimensions and may be better assessed with both psychometric measures and specific age of migration for youth and both parents. Tobacco use and all covariates, except generational status, were measured by youth self-report.

Despite these limitations, this is one of the first studies to examine longitudinally how generational status measured in middle school is associated with tobacco use in high school. It is the first study we know of to examine generational status together with sociodemographic and tobacco-related perceptions and attitudes. The current study differs from previously published work by examining both smoking-related future intentions and willingness to smoke and actual initiation of smoking among Latinx adolescents from primary school (5th grade) to middle school (7th grade). Our results add to previous findings suggesting that the immigrant paradox may not apply specifically for cigarette smoking among Latinx youth. Although findings from this study do not support the concept of the immigrant paradox, results suggest that believing that cigarettes were available and having family or friends who smoked increased the likelihood that Latinxs would try cigarette smoking by 10th grade. This has implications for smoking prevention efforts with this population, where interventions should aim to address these social and perceptual influences. The association with perceived cigarette availability may be due to increased access to tobacco for school age youth, as previous research has shown that tobacco retailers are often clustered in higher concentrations near schools [33]. Strong policies banning the sale of tobacco and enforcement of these policies for neighborhoods with schools and large school-aged populations could protect youth from tobacco products.

Conclusion

Finding no significant differences in tobacco initiation and related perceptions due to generational status and finding that predictors of tobacco initiation for Latinx youth are highly similar to those demonstrated repeatedly in general samples of youth suggest that there is little basis for substantially different prevention approaches. Therefore, current tobacco use prevention efforts mainly implemented through public schools are likely to be applicable to Latinx youth with varying personal and family migration histories. Nonetheless, there may be benefits to certain cultural adaptations of generally applicable prevention programs, such as those used for HIV-prevention and alcohol abuse programs among Latinxs [34, 35]. Our findings raise questions about the immigrant paradox as it applies to tobacco use for Latinx adolescents. It is hoped that these findings and this line of research may help practitioners and researchers further determine effective components of prevention and intervention efforts.

Abbreviations

Add Health: National Longitudinal Study of Adolescent Health; HIV: Human immunodeficiency virus

Acknowledgments

The contributions made to this research by study participants, other Healthy Passages investigators, field teams at each site, and the CDC Division of Adolescent and School Health are gratefully acknowledged.

Funding

This work was supported by the Centers for Disease Control and Prevention (Cooperative Agreements CCU409679, CCU609653, CCU915773, U48DP000046, U48DP000057, U48DP000056, U19DP002663, U19DP002664, and U19DP002665). The findings and conclusions in this report are those of the authors and do not necessarily represent the official position of the Centers for Disease Control and Prevention. The Centers for Disease Control and Prevention contributed collaboratively with the research team to the design of the study, however, they had no involvement in the collection, analysis, and interpretation of data and in writing the manuscript. A postdoctoral training grant T32 (HL007034) from the National Heart, Lung and Blood Institute (NHLBI) supported Dr. Epperson. NHLBI had no involvement in the study design, the collection, analysis, and interpretation of data and in the writing of the manuscript.

Authors' contributions

AEE analyzed data and co-drafted the initial manuscript. JLW supervised the statistical analysis and co-drafted the initial manuscript. JLW, MNE, and MAS made substantial contributions to the conception and design of the study and acquisition of data. All authors have read the manuscript, have been involved in revising it critically for important intellectual content, and have approved the final version.

Competing interests

The authors declare that they have no competing interests to disclose.

Author details

[1]Stanford Prevention Research Center, Department of Medicine, Stanford University, 1265 Welch Road, Suite 300, Palo Alto, CA 94305, USA. [2]Psychological Sciences and Health Sciences Research Institute, University of California, Merced, 5200 Lake Rd, Merced, CA 95340, USA. [3]RAND Corporation, 1776 Main Street, Santa Monica, CA 90401, USA. [4]Division of General Pediatrics, Boston Children's Hospital, 300 Longwood Ave, Boston, MA 02115, USA. [5]Department of Pediatrics, Harvard Medical School, 25 Shattuck St, Boston, MA 02115, USA. [6]Kaiser Permanente School of Medicine, 100 S. Los Robles Avenue, Pasadena, CA 91101, USA.

References

1. Jamal A, Phillips E, Gentzke AS, et al. Current cigarette smoking among adults-United States, 2016. MMWR Morb Mortal Wkly Rep. 2018;67(2):53–9.
2. U.S. Surgeon General. Preventing tobacco use among youth and young adults: a report of the surgeon general. Washington D.C.: U.S. Dept of Health and Human Services; 2012.
3. U.S. Surgeon General. The Health Consequences of Smoking—50 Years of Progress. Atlanta, GA: U.S. Department of Health and Human Services; 2014.
4. Kann L, McManus T, Harris WA, et al. Youth risk behavior Survelliance – United States, 2017. MMWR Surveill Summ. 2018;67(8):1–114 Available from: https://www.cdc.gov/mmwr/volumes/67/ss/pdfs/ss6708a1-H.pdf

5. Franzini L, Ribble JC, Keddie AM. Understanding the Hispanic paradox. Ethn Dis. 2001;11:496–518.
6. Salas-Wright CP, Vaughn MG, Clark Goings TT, Cordova D, Schwartz SJ. Substance use disorders among immigrants in the United States: a research update. Addict Behav. 2018;76:169–73. https://doi.org/10.1016/j.addbeh.2017.08.014.
7. Bacio GA, Mays VM, Lau AS. Drinking initiation and problematic drinking among Latino adolescents: explanations of the immigrant paradox. Psychol Addict Behav. 2013;27:14–22.
8. Guarini TE, Marks AK, Patton F, Coll CG. The immigrant paradox in sexual risk behavior among Latino adolescents: impact of immigrant generation and gender. Appl Dev Sci. 2011;15:201–9.
9. Salas-Wright CP, Kagotho N, Vaughn MG. Mood, anxiety, and personality disorders among first and second generation immigrants to the United States. Psychiatry Res. 2014;220:1028–36.
10. Gomez SL, Quach T, Horn-Ross PL, et al. Hidden breast Cancer disparities in Asian women: disaggregating incidence rates by ethnicity and migrant status. Am J Public Health. 2010;100(Suppl 1):S125–31. https://doi.org/10.2105/AJPH.2009.163931.
11. Coll CG, Marks AK. The immigrant paradox in children and adolescents: is becoming American a developmental risk? Washington DC: American Psychological Association; 2012.
12. Marks AK, Ejesi K, Coll CG. Understanding the U.S. immigrant paradox in childhood and adolescence. Child Dev Perspect. 2014;8:59–64.
13. Shor E, Roelfs D, Vang ZM. The "Hispanic mortality paradox" revisited: meta-analysis and meta-regression of life-course differentials in Latin American and Caribbean immigrants' mortality. Soc Sci Med. 2017;186:20–33.
14. Kopak HM. The relative importance of immigrant generation for Mexican Americans' alcohol and tobacco use from adolescence to early adulthood. J Immigr Minor Health. 2013;15:569–76.
15. Bui HN. Racial and ethnic differences in the immigrant paradox in substance use. J Immigr Minor Health. 2013;15:866–81.
16. Acevedo-Garcia D, Pan J, Jun H, Osypuk TL, Emmons KM. The effect of immigrant generation on smoking. Soc Sci Med. 2005;61:1223–42.
17. Echeverria SE, Gundersen DA, Manderski MTB, Delnevo CD. Social norms and its correlates as a pathway to smoking among young Latino adults. Soc Sci Med. 2015;124:187–95.
18. Lariscy JT, Hummer RA, Rath JM, Villanti AC, Hayward MD, Vallone DM. Race/ethnicity, nativity, and tobacco use among U.S. young adults: results from a nationally representative survey. Nicotine Tob Res. 2013;15(8):1417–26.
19. Fenelon A. Revisiting the Hispanic mortality advantage in the United States: the role of smoking. Soc Sci Med. 2013;82:1–9.
20. Hill AJ, Boudreau F, Amyot E, Dery D, Godin G. Predicting the stages of smoking acquisition according to the theory of planned behavior. J Adolesc Health. 1997;21:107–15.
21. McMillan B, Conner M. Using the theory of planned behaviour to understand alcohol and tobacco use in students. Psychol Health Med. 2003;8:317–28.
22. Ajzen I. The theory of planned behavior. Org Behav Hum Decis Process. 1991;50:179–211.
23. Stock ML, Gibbons FX, Gerrard M, et al. Racial identification, racial composition, and substance use vulnerability among African American adolescents and young adults. Health Psychol. 2013;32:237–47.
24. Gerrard M, Gibbons FX, Stock ML, Lune LS, Cleveland MJ. Images of smokers and willingness to smoke among African American pre-adolescents: an application of the prototype/willingness model of adolescent health risk behavior to smoking initiation. J Pediatr Psychol. 2005;30:305–18.
25. Olvera N, Poston WSC, Rodriguez A. Parental socialization of smoking initiation in Latino youth. J Adolesc Health. 2006;39:758–60.
26. Chuang Y, Ennett ST, Bauman KE, Foshee VA. Neighborhood influences on adolescent cigarette and alcohol use: mediating effects through parent and peer behaviors. J Health Soc Behav. 2005;46:187–204.
27. Gibbons FX, Gerrard M, Blanton H, Russell DW. Reasoned action and social reaction: willingness and intention as independent predictors of health risk. J Pers Soc Psychol. 1998;74:1164–80.
28. Andrews JA, Hampson SE, Barckley M, Gerrard M, Gibbons FX. The effect of early cognitions on cigarette and alcohol use during adolescence. Psychol Addict Behav. 2008;22:96–106.
29. van den Eijnden RJ, Spijkerman R, Engels RC. Relative contribution of smoker prototypes in predicting smoking among adolescents: a comparison with factors from the theory of planned behavior. Eur Addict Res. 2006;12:113–20.
30. Guilamo-Ramos V, Dittus P, Holloway I, Bouris A, Crossett L. An integrated framework for the analysis of adolescent cigarette smoking in middle school Latino youth. Youth Soc. 2011;43(1):193–224.
31. Windle M, Grunbaum JA, Elliott M, et al. Healthy passages: a multi-level, multimethod longitudinal study of adolescent health. Am J Prev Med. 2004;27:164–72.
32. Schuster MA, Elliott MN, Kanouse D, et al. Racial and ethnic health disparities among fifth graders in three cities. N Engl J Med. 2012;367:735–45.
33. Henriksen L, Feighery EC, Schleicher NC, Cowling DW, Kline RS, Fortmann SP. Is adolescent smoking related to the density and proximity of tobacco outlets and retail cigarette advertising near schools? Prev Med. 2008;47:210–4.
34. Davidson T, Lopez C, Danielson C, et al. Development and preliminary evaluation of a behavioural HIV-prevention programme for teenage girls of Latino descent in the USA. Cult Health Sex. 2014;16(5):533–46.
35. Field CA, Cabriales JA, Woolard RH, Tyroch AH, Caetano R, Castro Y. Cultural adaptation of a brief motivational intervention for heavy drinking among Hispanics in a medical setting. BMC Public Health. 2015;15:724.

21

Adaptation of pain scales for parent observation: are pain scales and symptoms useful in detecting pain of young children with the suspicion of acute otitis media?

Johanna M. Uitti[1,2*], Sanna Salanterä[3,4], Miia K. Laine[5], Paula A. Tähtinen[1,2] and Aino Ruohola[1,2]

Abstract

Background: The assessment of ear pain is challenging in young, mostly preverbal children. Our aim was to investigate whether pain scales are useful tools for parents to detect pain in their young children with the suspicion of acute otitis media (AOM), and to assess associations between 16 symptoms and the severity of pain.

Methods: This cross-sectional study included 426 children (6–35 months) with symptoms suggestive of AOM. We surveyed symptoms and pain via parental interview. As part of the interview, parents assessed their child's pain by using two pain scales: The Faces Pain Scale-Revised (FPS-R) and the Face, Legs, Activity, Cry, Consolability (FLACC) Scale. The outcome of interest was moderate/severe pain. We used the χ^2 test or Fisher's test as applicable to compare the severity of pain between three parental pain assessment methods (the parental interview, the FPS-R and the FLACC Scale). We also used multivariable logistic regression models to study the association between the severity of pain and AOM and to study the association between symptoms and the severity of pain.

Results: In children with AOM ($n = 201$), pain was assessed by parents as moderate/severe in 65% via interview; 90% with the FPS-R; and 91% with the FLACC Scale ($P < 0.001$). In children without AOM ($n = 225$), the percentages were 56, 83 and 88%, respectively ($P < 0.001$). Between children with and without AOM, the occurrence of moderate/severe pain did not differ with any of the pain evaluation methods. Of symptoms, ear pain reported by child and restless sleep were significantly associated with moderate/severe pain, regardless of the pain evaluation method.

Conclusions: It seems that nearly all the children with respiratory tract infection, either with or without AOM, might suffer from moderate/severe pain. Without pain scales, parents may underestimate their child's pain. Of symptoms, ear pain reported by child and restless sleep might indicate pain in children with respiratory tract infection. We suggest that the adaptation of pain scales for parent observation is a possibility in children with respiratory tract infection which, however, requires further studies.

Keywords: Child, Otitis media, Pain scales, Parents, Respiratory tract infection

* Correspondence: johanna.uitti@utu.fi
[1]Department of Paediatrics and Adolescent Medicine, Turku University Hospital, Turku, Finland
[2]Department of Paediatrics and Adolescent Medicine, University of Turku, Turku, Finland

Background

Acute otitis media (AOM) is one of the most common diseases in early childhood, causing variety of symptoms. Ear pain is considered as the most important and specific symptom of AOM and parents perceive it as one of the greatest burden in young children with AOM [1]. Furthermore, ear pain is used as one of the key criteria when defining the severity of AOM, which, in turn, guides the management of AOM [2]. Consequently, it is crucial to be able to reliably assess whether young children have any ear pain.

The assessment of ear pain is challenging in young, mostly preverbal children. First, they cannot provide self-reports which are often considered a primary source for estimates of pain intensity [3]. Therefore, the pain assessment is based on the opinion of parents and health care professionals. Ear pain of preverbal children is suggested to emerge as various non-specific symptoms, according to The American Academy of Pediatrics AOM guideline [2]. Nevertheless, the guideline does not give any instructions how to further convert the non-specific symptoms as mild, moderate or severe pain behavior. The study of Shaikh et al. [4] suggested ear rubbing and fussiness to be the most important symptoms in influencing parental perception of ear pain in preverbal children with AOM. However, as they stated, their results are preliminary and are based on hypothetical patient scenarios. To our knowledge, the adaptation of pain scales for parental use to assess acute, non-procedural pain in young children in an outpatient setting has not been investigated.

We adapted two well-established pain scales for parent observation. Our primary aim was to investigate whether pain scales are useful tools for parents to detect pain in their young, mostly preverbal children with the parental suspicion of AOM. Furthermore, we investigated which symptoms are associated with moderate/severe pain in young children.

Methods

Study population

This study was part of a project examining diagnostics and treatment of AOM at the primary care level (www.clinicaltrials.gov, identifier NCT00299455) between 2006 and 2008 in Turku, Finland [5]. Written informed consent was obtained from a parent of all children before they could participate in the study. All visits were free of charge, and no compensation for participation was given. The study protocol was approved by The Ethics Committee of the Hospital District of Southwest Finland (reference number: Dnro 4/2016).

Children 6 to 35 months of age were eligible when they had acute symptoms and parental suspicion of AOM. The exclusion criteria have been previously described in detail [5]. The focus of the study is on the child's symptoms and clinical findings at the time of an enrolment, on day 1. In this cross-sectional study, we used the same cohorts as in our previous reports regarding symptoms, nasopharyngeal bacteria, and respiratory viruses [6–8].

Symptom questionnaire

Before examining the child the study physician interviewed the parents about the occurrence of 17 symptoms of their child by using a standardized, structured symptom questionnaire, which is described in detail below. We defined fever as temperature ≥ 38 °C within the preceding 24 h, but we also accepted if parents reported that their child had been febrile even though temperature had not been measured with a thermometer. We asked about three *ear-related symptoms*: parentally reported ear pain, ear pain reported by child (the child verbally expressed of having ear pain), and ear rubbing. Parents also assessed the severity of their child's ear pain classified as mild, moderate or severe. Furthermore, we asked parents to assess their child's pain with the pain scales (described in detail below). Apart from this, we interviewed the parents about *non-specific symptoms*: irritability, excessive crying, restless sleep, decreased activity, poor appetite; *respiratory symptoms*: rhinitis, nasal congestion, cough, hoarse voice, conjunctivitis, mucus vomiting; and *gastrointestinal symptoms*: vomiting, and diarrhea. Finally, the study physician asked about the duration of the parental suspicion of AOM.

Pain scales

Due to the shortage of validated pain scales to obtain parent measures of acute and nonsurgical pain of their young child, we performed a preliminary study and used two pain scales and adapted them for parent observation in children with the suspicion of AOM. First, we used The Faces Pain Scale-Revised (FPS-R) (Fig. 1) [9], which is a validated self-report tool for children measuring the pain intensity, but it has likewise been previously adapted for parental use as an observational pain measurement tool [10, 11]. The FPS-R consists of 6 horizontally positioned faces, representing increasing levels of pain from left ("no pain") to right ("very much pain"), scored as 0–2–4-6-8-10 [9]. The parents pointed out the face which best reflected their child's pain at its worst within the preceding 24 h. The FPS-R was chosen since it is easy to comprehend and does not require a lot of time or special skills [12, 13]. However, FPS-R is not a behaviorally anchored rating scale [14] and hence another scale was added to the study. Second, we used The Face, Legs, Activity, Cry, Consolability (FLACC) Scale, which is an observational pain measurement tool (Table 1) [15]. The FLACC Scale includes 5 behavioral

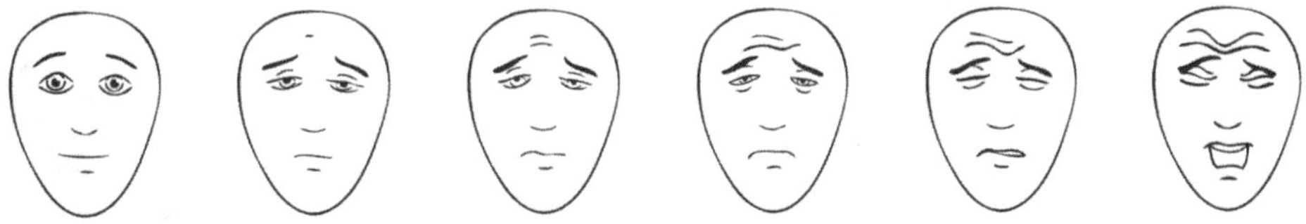

Fig. 1 "Faces Pain Scale - Revised (FPS-R)". www.iasp-pain.org/fpsr. Copyright ©2001, International Association for the Study of Pain®. Reproduced with permission

categories: facial expression, leg movement, bodily activity, cry or verbalization, and consolability. The parents rated their child's pain at its worst within the preceding 24 h in each category on a scale of 0 to 2, thus an overall pain score ranging from 0 to 10. The FLACC Scale has previously been translated into Finnish. The FLACC Scale was chosen since it is a well-established and validated tool, suitable for children from 0 to 18 years of age [14, 16]. Furthermore, the FLACC Scale has low burden, it has excellent inter-rater reliability, and moderate concurrent validity and it is recommended for evaluating pain in brief painful events [14].

We had three conventionally used clinical pain categories: with the FPS-R, the scores 0 and 2 were classified as "none or mild", 4 and 6 as "moderate" and 8 and 10 as "severe" pain. With the FLACC scale, the scores from 0 to 3 were classified as "none or mild", from 4 to 6 as "moderate" and from 7 to 10 as "severe" pain or discomfort, respectively [12, 17–19].

After the symptom questionnaire, the study physician performed clinical examination on the child, including tympanometry, pneumatic otoscopy, and video otoscopy, as described in detail elsewhere [5]. The diagnosis of AOM was based on the following three criteria. First, middle ear effusion had to be detected by pneumatic otoscopy (at least two of the following signs on tympanic membrane: bulging position, decreased or absent mobility, abnormal color or opacity not due to scarring, or air-fluid interfaces). Second, at least one acute inflammatory sign of tympanic membrane had to be identified (distinct erythematous patches/streaks, or increased vascularity over full/bulging/yellow convexity). Third, there had to be symptoms and signs of acute infection.

Statistical analysis

The outcome of interest was moderate/severe pain. We compared the proportions with χ^2 test or Fisher's test as applicable. We compared the medians with the Mann-Whitney *U* test. Absolute percentage-point differences in rates and 95% confidence intervals (CI) were calculated. We used multivariable logistic regression models for two purposes: first, to study the association between the severity of pain and AOM. We calculated the odds ratios (ORs) with 95% confidence intervals (CI) for AOM and adjusted the models by age (1 month as a unit), use of analgesics (yes vs. no) and the duration of the parental suspicion of AOM (1 h as a unit); and second, to study the association between symptoms and the severity of pain. We calculated the ORs (with 95% CI) for moderate/severe pain and adjusted the models by age (1 month as a unit), diagnosis of AOM (yes vs. no), and use of analgesics (yes vs. no). We performed statistical analyses by using SPSS version 22.0 (IBM SPSS Statistics, IBM Corporation, Armonk, NY).

Results

Children were enrolled to the study between March 16, 2006 and December 5, 2008, excluding June and July of each year. The study population consisted of 426 children (6–35 months). Of those, 201 (47%) had AOM

Table 1 The FLACC scale. Each of the five categories Face; Legs; Activity; Cry; Consolability is scored from 0 to 2, which results in a total score between 0 and 10

Categories	Scoring		
	0	1	2
Face	No particular expression or smile	Occasional grimace or frown, withdrawn, disinterested	Frequent to constant quivering chin, clenched jaw
Legs	Normal position or relaxed	Uneasy, restless, tense	Kicking, or legs drawn up
Activity	Lying quietly, normal position, moves easily	Squirming, shifting back and forth, tense	Arched, rigid or jerking
Cry	No cry (awake or asleep)	Moans or whimpers; occasional complaint	Crying steadily, screams or sobs, frequent complaints
Consolability	Content, relaxed	Reassured by occasional touching, hugging or being talked to, distractable	Difficult to console or comfort

From Merkel SI, Voepel-Lewis T, Shayevitz JR, Malviya S. The FLACC: A behavioral scale for scoring postoperative pain in young children. Pediatr Nurs. 1997;23:293–297 [15]

(AOM group) and 225 (53%) did not have AOM (non-AOM group). The patient characteristics are shown in Table 2. Children with AOM had used analgesics more often than children without AOM (60% [121/201] vs. 48% [109/225], $P = 0.02$).

The distributions of the FPS-R and FLACC Scale scores in the AOM group and in the non-AOM group are presented in Fig. 2 and Fig. 3.

Severity of pain in the AOM group and in the non-AOM group

Figure 4a and Fig. 4b show the occurrence of none/mild and moderate/severe pain in the AOM group and in the non-AOM group, respectively. In the AOM group (Fig. 4a), parents assessed their child's pain significantly more often as moderate/severe with the FPS-R and with the FLACC Scale, compared with the parental interview ($P < 0.001$). The rate difference for moderate/severe pain between the FPS-R and parental interview was 25% (95% CI, 17 to 34%), and between the FLACC Scale and parental interview 26% (95% CI, 18 to 35%), respectively.

Table 2 Characteristics of 426 children with and without acute otitis media

	AOM (*N* = 201)	Non-AOM (*N* = 225)	*P*
Median (range) age, mo	15 (6–35)	13 (6–35)	0.37
Age, n (%)			0.75
6–11 mo	76 (38)	91 (40)	
12–23 mo	85 (42)	95 (42)	
24–35 mo	40 (20)	39 (17)	
Male gender, n (%)	109 (54)	118 (52)	0.71
Symptom interview answered by			0.25
Mother, n (%)	144 (72)	174 (77)	
Father, n (%)	22 (11)	24 (11)	
Both parents, n (%)	33 (16)	27 (12)	
Other guardian, n (%)	2 (1)	0 (0)	
Median (Q1, Q3)[a] duration (h) of the parental suspicion of AOM	21 (12, 38)	24 (16, 48)	0.04
The use of analgesics ≤24 h, n (%)	121 (60)	109 (48)	0.02
Number of previous AOM episodes, n (%)[b]			0.25
0 episodes, n (%)	62 (31)	70 (32)	
1–3 episodes, n (%)	108 (54)	105 (47)	
> 3 episodes, n (%)	31 (15)	47 (21)	
Median (range) age at first AOM episode, mo[c]	9 (0–27)	9 (0–29)	0.47

[a]Q1, the 25th quartile; Q3, the 75th quartile
[b]Data were missing in 3/225 children without AOM
[c]Among those who had had at least one episode of AOM. Data were missing in 8/139 and 18/152 children with AOM and non-AOM

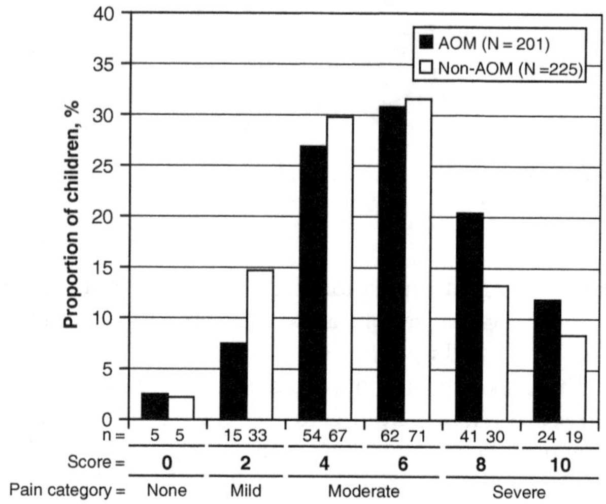

Fig. 2 Distribution of the Faces Pain Scale-Revised (FPS-R) scores in children in the AOM group and in children in the non-AOM group. The numbers below the bars show the number of children with the score, indicating the numerator (n)

In the non-AOM group (Fig. 4b), parents likewise assessed their child's pain significantly more often as moderate /severe with the FPS-R and with the FLACC Scale, compared with the parental interview ($P < 0.001$). The rate difference for moderate/severe pain between the FPS-R and parental interview was 27% (95% CI, 19 to 36%), and between the FLACC Scale and parental interview 32% (95% CI, 23 to 40%), respectively.

Comparison of pain between AOM group and non-AOM group

First, via parental interview, moderate/severe pain was reported in 130/201 (65%) children in the AOM group, compared with 126/225 (56%) children in the non-AOM group ($P = 0.07$). When parents had assessed their child to have moderate/severe pain via parental interview, the adjusted OR for AOM was 1.32 (95% CI, 0.88–1.98). Second, the parental pain assessment with the FPS-R showed moderate/severe pain in 181/201 (90%) children in the AOM group, compared with 187/225 (83%) children in the non-AOM group ($P = 0.04$). When parents had assessed their child to have moderate/severe pain with the FPS-R, the adjusted OR for AOM was 1.75 (95% CI, 0.97–3.15). Third, the parental pain assessment with the FLACC Scale showed moderate/severe pain in 183/201 (91%) children in the AOM group, compared with 197/225 (88%) children in the non-AOM group ($P = 0.25$). When parents had assessed their child to have moderate/severe pain with the FLACC Scale, the adjusted OR for AOM was 1.46 (95% CI, 0.77–2.75).

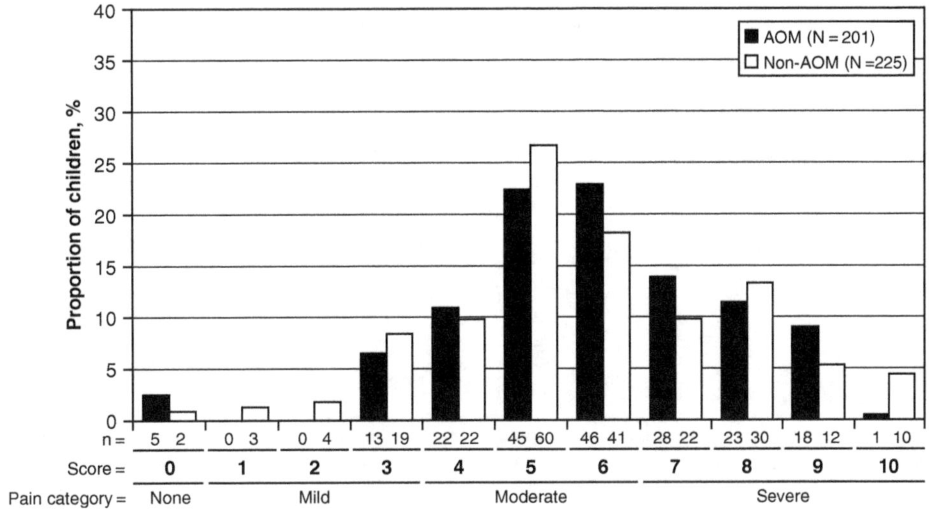

Fig. 3 Distribution of the Face, Legs, Activity, Cry, Consolability (FLACC) Scale scores in children in the AOM group and in children in the non-AOM group. The numbers below the bars show the number of children with the score, indicating the numerator (n)

Association of individual symptoms with moderate/severe pain

Among all the 426 children with the parental suspicion of AOM, the associations between individual symptoms and moderate/severe pain are presented in Fig. 5a, b and c. As parents assessed their child's pain via interview (Fig. 5a), ear pain reported by child and restless sleep had significant associations with moderate/severe pain. As parents assessed their child's pain with the FPS-R (Fig. 5b), following symptoms had significant associations with moderate/severe pain: ear pain reported by child, excessive crying, restless sleep and poor appetite. Finally, as parents assessed their child's pain with the FLACC Scale (Fig. 5c), following symptoms had significant associations with moderate/severe pain: ear pain reported by child, restless sleep and nasal congestion.

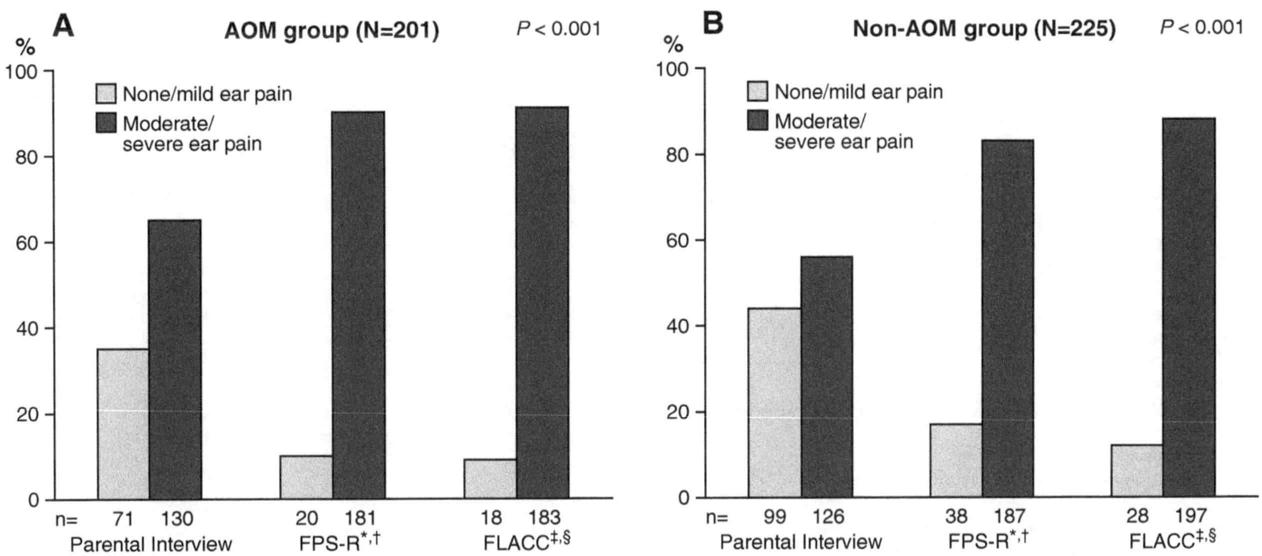

Fig. 4 a, b The occurrence of none/mild and moderate/severe pain in the AOM group (**a**) and in the non-AOM group (**b**), assessed by parents via interview, with the Faces Pain Scale-Revised (FPS-R) and with the Face, Legs, Activity, Cry, Consolability (FLACC) Scale. Footnote: * Scores 0 and 2 were classified as none/mild pain, and scores 4, 6, 8 and 10 as moderate/severe pain, respectively. † $P < 0.001$ for the comparison between none/mild pain and moderate/severe pain, assessed by parents with the FPS-R and via interview. ‡ Scores from 0 to 3 were classified as none/mild pain, and scores from 4 to 10 as moderate/severe pain, respectively. § $P < 0.001$ for the comparison between none/mild pain and moderate/severe pain, assessed by parents with the FLACC Scale and via interview

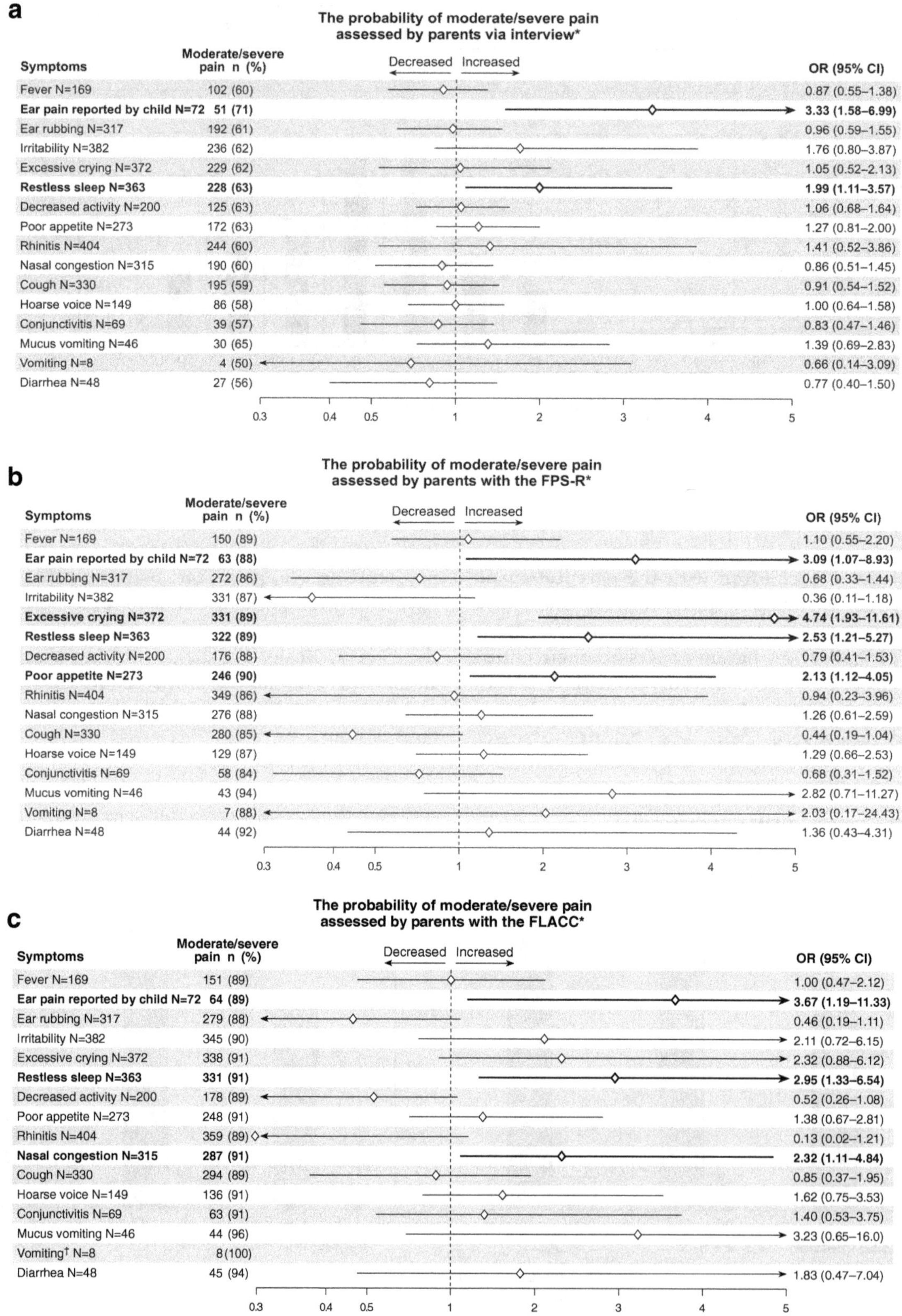

Fig. 5 (See legend on next page.)

(See figure on previous page.)

Fig. 5 The occurrence and the probability of moderate/severe pain, assessed by parents via interview (**a**), with the Faces Pain Scale-Revised (FPS-R) (**b**) and with the Face, Legs, Activity, Cry, Consolability (FLACC) Scale (**c**), in relation to the presence of 15 parentally reported symptoms and ear pain reported by children in 426 children with the suspicion of AOM, analysed with multivariable logistic regression model and adjusted for age, diagnosis of AOM and use of analgesics. Footnote: * Diamonds indicate odds ratio (OR), lines 95% confidence intervals (CI), arrows are added when CI is beyond the scale. †The association of moderate/severe pain with the symptom was 100%

Discussion

Our main finding is that pain scales, namely the FPS-R and the FLACC Scale, might be useful for detecting pain by parents in young children with respiratory tract infection (RTI), either with or without AOM. What is more, without the pain scales, parents may underestimate pain in young children with RTI. Furthermore, nearly all children might suffer from moderate/severe pain or distress during RTI, regardless of the diagnosis of AOM.

Parental pain assessment with the FPS-R and the FLACC Scale indicated that the great majority of the children with RTI, either with or without AOM, seem to suffer from moderate/severe pain. In contrast, when parents were being interviewed about their child's pain, moderate/severe pain was reported only in two thirds of the children with RTI. The difference in the results between the pain assessment methods is obvious and thus requires further attention. Since the pain results cannot be compared with children's self-reports of pain, the most reliable pain evaluation method cannot be stated for absolute certainty. It can be debated that in our study, children were conventionally classified as having moderate pain with the FPS-R scores of 4 or 6. On the contrary, the study of Tsze et al. proposes that only children with the FPS-R scores of 6 would be classified as having moderate pain, although considerable overlap of scores associated with mild and moderate pain could be seen in their study [20]. In our study, however, moderate/severe pain was detected at the similar rate with both the FPS-R and with the FLACC Scale, thus suggesting the reliability of our pain category classification for moderate pain with the FPS-R.

Worth noting, the FPS-R was originally designed and validated to be a self-report measure to assess the intensity of children's acute pain from age 4 or 5 onward [9], and it is not validated for the observational use, although faces scales have also been adapted for global observational ratings by parents and nurses [10, 11, 14, 21]. On the contrary, the FLACC Scale, which was initially developed for evaluating postoperative pain in young children [15], has further been established as a valid observational measure for all kinds of pain in preverbal children by nurses [22], although its clinical utility has recently been challenged [23]. Thus, it should be acknowledged that neither of the pain scales are validated to assess acute, non-surgical pain of young children by parents. Therefore, we can only present preliminary results. For instance, parents may overestimate their child's pain with faces scales and with the FLACC Scale [24, 25] although underestimation with the faces scale, as well as with the parental interview have likewise been reported [11, 26]. However, parents are considered as most reliable proxy for assessing young children's possible pain, if the self-report is not possible, because children are often more expressive in the presence of parents than strangers, such as health care professionals [27]. Parents are likewise familiar with the child's normal behavior and thus they are more able to discriminate child's pain behavior from other aberrant behavior [14, 28].

Overall, there seems to be relatively pervasive and systematic tendency for proxy judgments to underestimate the pain experience of others [29]. However, direct observations of pain behavior and self-reports of pain intensity are more likely to be significantly related to each other, if the individual being studied has acute pain, instead of chronic pain, because nociception plays a greater role in the display of observable behavior among persons with acute pain [30]. In fact, acute pain of young children has recently been shown to be reliably assessed with the FLACC Scale by nurses [31]. Taken these findings together, we cautiously suggest that the FLACC Scale might also be used by parents in children with RTI. Since the pain results of the FLACC Scale and the FPS-R were highly similar, this implies that the FPS-R could possibly be applied as the parental pain observation tool as well. Consequently, we suggest that the parental assessment with the FLACC Scale and with the FPS-R might be more useful for detecting pain in young children with RTI, than the parental interview about their child's pain, because pain scales might better freezeframe a moment for the parents to ponder their child's pain, than the parental interview.

The occurrence of moderate/severe pain did not significantly differ between AOM and non-AOM groups with any of the three pain evaluation methods. At first sight, this may seem conflicting. However, symptoms of RTI may likewise cause severe distress to young children. In fact, when parents assessed their child's pain with the FLACC Scale, which is validated to measure distress behavior, nasal congestion had a significant association with moderate/severe pain. Furthermore, ear-related pain may likewise accompany children with RTI due to the blocked ear and dysfunction of the Eustachian tube. Our current results also support our previous findings that symptoms of AOM and RTI are overlapping [6]. Our study illustrates the difficulties that the parents of young children are facing, when interpreting, which of the child's symptoms are due to ear pain, or due to distress from RTI. Based on our preliminary results, we suggest that young children with RTI, without AOM, might suffer from equal amount of distress or discomfort as do children with AOM. Thus, when parents suspect their child with RTI to have AOM, we recommend that clinicians would actively offer pain medication, although AOM was not diagnosed. All in all, further studies are needed to investigate the severity of pain and its assessment in outpatient children with RTI.

The key symptoms associating with the parental assessment of their child to suffer from moderate/severe pain were ear pain reported by child and restless sleep. These two symptoms stood out, regardless of the pain evalution method. Indeed, restless sleep or fussiness has also previously been related as suggestive of ear pain in preverbal children [2, 4]. On the other hand, restless sleep has not been shown to resolve significantly faster with the antimicrobial treatment in children with AOM, compared to the treatment with the placebo [5]. Thus, this suggests that restless sleep may reflect the general pain and distress due to RTI, for example headache, sore throat or nasal congestion, rather than ear pain specifically. Interestingly, when pain was assessed by parents with the FPS-R, poor appetite seemed to be the sign for moderate/severe pain, although it has more commonly been held as a sign for child's impaired overall condition. Hence, we suggest that if the validated pain scales are not available in the clinical practice, the clinician could ask about these specific symptoms (such as ear pain reported by child, restless sleep, poor appetite) to interpret whether a child with RTI suffers from moderate/severe pain.

Our study implies that the undertreatment of pain might be prevented in young children with the use of pain scales, such as the FPS-R and the FLACC Scale. This would have consequential impact on young children's life, because pain experiences in early childhood may induce long-term alterations in pain sensitivity [32, 33]. Hence, our study might offer a valuable new perspective for clinicians who treat young children with RTI. Pain scales might be used as a simple tool at the primary care to explore the possible need for pain medication. However, more studies are mandatory before implementing pain scales for parental use in clinical practice.

Our study is not without limitations. First, due to the tight schedule at the study visit, we explained the pain scales to the parents very briefly, leaving parents a possibility of misunderstanding of matching the child's facial expression to the faces in the FPS-R figure, despite the instructions. On the other hand, this reflects the real life in clinical practice and was thus also a strenght. However, it may be argued that the FPS-R is a relatively coarse scale with six categories for adult observers and that they would be capable of finer distinctions, for example with a finer-grained numerical rating scale. Second, to our experience, parents considered the FLACC Scale as challenging, because they had to recall their child's behavior in each of the five behavioral categories, possibly causing recall bias. Third, the data about parental education level or occupation is missing, which may be seen as a limitation because higher level of parental education has been shown to be associated with higher reported pain levels [4]. However, our study population came from all the postal code regions of Turku area which shows the sosioeconomic heterogeneity of the population. Nonetheless, our study has also several strenghts. First, the standardized, structured symptom questionnaire allowed us to investigate the symptoms rigorously. Second, parents were surveyed about the symptoms via interview conducted by study physician. This represents well the actual real life situation in the primary care, reflecting generalisability of our results. Third, the diagnosis of AOM is firm due to our careful diagnostics [5]. This strenghtens our findings that children with RTI seem to suffer from moderate/severe pain, regardless of the diagnosis of AOM.

Conclusions

The pain scales, such as the FPS-R and the FLACC Scale, might be more useful for parents to detect pain of young children with RTI, than the parental interview about pain. Equally important, the FPS-R and the FLACC Scale seem to indicate that the majority of children with RTI, either with or without AOM, might suffer from moderate/severe pain. Hence, we suggest that pain scales, such as the FPS-R and the FLACC Scale, might be used by parents in clinical practice. However, this is the first study to use the FPS-R and the FLACC Scale for parent observation in children with RTI. Hence, more studies are needed.

Abbreviations

AOM: Acute otitis media; CI: Confidence interval; FLACC Scale: Face, Legs, Activity, Cry, Consolability Scale; FPS-R: Faces Pain Scale-Revised; OR: Odds ratio; RTI: Respiratory tract infection

Acknowledgments

We thank all the families who participated in this study; Raakel Luoto, MD, PhD and Elina Lahti, MD, PhD for their help with data collection; and Professor Olli Ruuskanen for giving Dr. Uitti the opportunity to draft the manucript in the Research Unit of the Turku University Hospital Research Foundation.

Funding
This work was supported by the Fellowship Award of the European Society for Paediatric Infectious Diseases (to Dr. Ruohola) and by grants from Research Funds from Specified Government Transfers; the Foundation for Paediatric Research; the Jenny and Antti Wihuri Foundation; The Finnish Medical Foundation; University of Turku Graduate School and Doctoral Programme of Clinical Investigation; The Maud Kuistila Memorial Foundation; The Emil Aaltonen Foundation; University of Turku; The Finnish Cultural Foundation, Varsinais-Suomi Regional Fund; The Turku University Hospital Research Foundation; The Finnish-Norwegian Medical Foundation; The Turku University Foundation, The Paulo Foundation; and The Outpatient Care Research Foundation.

Authors' contributions
Conceptualization: SS AR. Data curation: JU MKL PAT AR Formal Analysis: JMU. Funding Acquisition: JMU MKL PAT AR. Investigation: MKL PAT AR. Methodology: JMU SS AR. Project Administration: JMU AR. Resources: SS AR. Software: -. Supervision: SS AR. Validation: JMU AR. Visualization: JMU AR. Writing – Original Draft preparation: JMU. Writing – Review & Editing: SS MKL PAT AR. All the authors have read and approved the final version of the submitted manuscript.

Competing interests
The authors declare that they have no competing interests.

Author details
[1]Department of Paediatrics and Adolescent Medicine, Turku University Hospital, Turku, Finland. [2]Department of Paediatrics and Adolescent Medicine, University of Turku, Turku, Finland. [3]Department of Nursing Science, University of Turku, Turku, Finland. [4]Hospital District of Southwest Finland, Turku, Finland. [5]Department of Clinical Microbiology, Turku University Hospital, Turku, Finland.

References
1. Barber C, Ille S, Vergison A, Coates H. Acute otitis media in young children – what do parents say? Int J Pediatr Otorhinolaryngol. 2014;78:300–6.
2. Lieberthal AS, Carroll AE, Chonmaitree T, Ganiats TG, Hoberman A, Jackson MA, et al. The diagnosis and management of acute otitis media. Pediatrics. 2013;131:e964–99.
3. Twycross A, Voepel-Lewis T, Vincent C, Franck LS, von Baeyer CL. A debate on the proposition that self-report is the gold standard in assessment of pediatric pain intensity. Clin J Pain. 2015;31:707–12.
4. Shaikh N, Kearney DH, Colborn DK, Balentine T, Feng W, Lin Y, et al. How do parents of preverbal children with acute otitis media determine how much ear pain their child is having? J Pain. 2010;11:1291–4.
5. Tähtinen PA, Laine MK, Huovinen P, Jalava J, Ruuskanen O, Ruohola A. A placebo-controlled trial of antimicrobial treatment for acute otitis media. N Engl J Med. 2011;364:116–26.
6. Laine MK, Tähtinen PA, Ruuskanen O, Huovinen P, Ruohola A. Symptoms or symptom-based scores cannot predict acute otitis media at otitis-prone age. Pediatrics. 2010;125:e1154–61.
7. Ruohola A, Pettigrew MM, Lindholm L, Jalava J, Räisänen KS, Vainionpää R, et al. Bacterial and viral interactions within the nasopharynx contribute to the risk of acute otitis media. J Inf Secur. 2013;66:247–54.
8. Uitti JM, Tähtinen PA, Laine MK, Huovinen P, Ruuskanen O, Ruohola A. Role of nasopharyngeal Bacteria and respiratory viruses in acute symptoms of young children. Pediatr Infect Dis J. 2015;34:1056–62.
9. Hicks CL, von Baeyer CL, Spafford PA, van Korlaar I, Goodenough B. The faces pain scale-revised: toward a common metric in pediatric pain measurement. Pain. 2001;93:173–83.
10. Berberich FR, Landman Z. Reducing immunization discomfort in 4- to 6-year-old children: a randomized clinical trial. Pediatrics. 2009;124:e203–9.
11. Chambers CT, Reid GJ, Craig KD, McGrath PJ, Finley GA. Agreement between child and parent reports of pain. Clin J Pain. 1998;14:336–42.
12. Tsze DS, von Baeyer CL, Bulloch B, Dayan PS. Validation of self-report pain scales in children. Pediatrics. 2013;132:e971–9.
13. Herr KA, Spratt K, Mobily PR, Richardson G. Pain intensity assessment in older adults: use of experimental pain to compare psychometric properties and usability of selected pain scales with younger adults. Clin J Pain. 2004; 20:207–19.
14. von Baeyer CL, Spagrud LJ. Systematic review of observational (behavioral) measures of pain for children and adolescents aged 3 to 18 years. Pain. 2007;127:140–50.
15. Merkel SI, Voepel-Lewis T, Shayevitz JR, Malviya S. The FLACC: a behavioral scale for scoring postoperative pain in young children. Pediatr Nurs. 1997; 23:293–7.
16. Manworren RC, Stinson J. Pediatric pain measurement, assessment, and evaluation. Semin Pediatr Neurol. 2016;23:189–200.
17. Malviya S, Voepel-Lewis T, Burke C, Merkel S, Tait AR. The revised FLACC observational pain tool: improved reliability and validity for pain assessment in children with cognitive impairment. Paediatr Anaesth. 2006;16:258–65.
18. Breivik H, Borchgrevink PC, Allen SM, Rosseland LA, Romundstad L, Hals EK, et al. Assessment of pain. Br J Anaesth. 2008;101:17–24.
19. McConahay T, Bryson M, Bulloch B. Defining mild, moderate, and severe pain by using the color analogue scale with children presenting to a pediatric emergency department. Acad Emerg Med. 2006;13:341–4.
20. Tsze DS, Hirschfeld G, Dayan PS, Bulloch B, von Baeyer CL. Defining no pain, mild, moderate, and severe pain based on the faces pain scale-revised and color analog scale in children with acute pain. Pediatr Emerg Care. 2016; Published ahead of print. https://doi.org/10.1097/PEC.0000000000000791.
21. Manne SL, Jacobsen PB, Redd WH. Assessment of acute pediatric pain: do child self-report, parent ratings, and nurse ratings measure the same phenomenon? Pain. 1992;48:45–52.
22. Manworren RC, Hynan LS. Clinical validation of FLACC: preverbal patient pain scale. Pediatr Nurs. 2003;29:140–6.
23. Crellin DJ, Harrison D, Santamaria N, Babl FE. Systematic review of the face, legs, activity, cry and Consolability scale for assessing pain in infants and children: is it reliable, valid, and feasible for use? Pain. 2015;156:2132–51.
24. Chambers CT, Giesbrecht K, Craig KD, Bennett SM, Huntsman E. A comparison of faces scales for the measurement of pediatric pain: children's and parents' ratings. Pain. 1999;83:25–35.
25. Voepel-Lewis T, Malviya S, Tait AR. Validity of parent ratings as proxy measures of pain in children with cognitive impairment. Pain Manag Nurs. 2005;6:168–74.
26. Bellman MH, Paley CE. Pain control in children. Parents underestimate children's pain. BMJ. 1993;307:1563.
27. von Baeyer CL, Spagrud LJ. Social development and pain in children. In: McGrath PJFG, editor. The context of pediatric pain: biology, family, culture. Seattle, WA: IASP Press; 2003. p. 8–97.
28. Schechter NL, Berde CB, Yaster M. Pain in Infants, Children, and Adolescents. 2nd ed. Philadelphia, PA: LWW (PE); 2002.
29. American Academy of Pediatrics. Committee on psychosocial aspects of child and family health, task force on pain in infants, children, and adolescents. The assessment and management of acute pain in infants, children, and adolescents. Pediatrics. 2001;108:793–7.
30. Labus JS, Keefe FJ, Jensen MP. Self-reports of pain intensity and direct observations of pain behavior: when are they correlated? Pain. 2003; 102:109–24.

31. Kochman A, Howell J, Sheridan M, Kou M, Shelton Ryan EE, Lee S, et al. Reliability of the faces, legs, activity, cry, and Consolability scale in assessing acute pain in the pediatric emergency department. Pediatr Emerg Care. 2017;33:14–7.
32. Hermann C, Hohmeister J, Demirakca S, Zohsel K, Flor H. Long-term alteration of pain sensitivity in school-aged children with early pain experiences. Pain. 2006;125:278–85.
33. Wollgarten-Hadamek I, Hohmeister J, Zohsel K, Flor H, Hermann C. Do school-aged children with burn injuries during infancy show stress-induced activation of pain inhibitory mechanisms? Eur J Pain. 2011;15: 423 e1–423.10.

22

Complementary feeding and effect of spontaneous fermentation on anti-nutritional factors of selected cereal-based complementary foods

Degnet Teferi Asres*, Amanuel Nana and Girma Nega

Abstract

Background: Malnutrition has been responsible directly or indirectly for 10.9 million deaths worldwide annually among children under five. Childhood malnutrition is highly related to poor nutritional quality diet in developing countries where there is limited access to animal based foods. Most foods consumed by young children are cereal based which contain high amounts of anti-nutritional factors. Fermentation is thought to significantly lower the content of anti-nutrients in cereal grains. This study therefore, aimed to determine complementary feeding practices and effect of spontaneous fermentation on anti-nutritional factors and mineral contents of selected cereals.

Methods: Cross sectional survey was conducted in Ebinat district to determine complementary feeding practices among 324 lactating mothers. Laboratory analysis was carried out for teff and wheat cereal grains to determine the effect of spontaneous fermentation on anti-nutrients as well as mineral contents.

Results: Prevalence of appropriate complementary feeding practice was 1.5%. Fermentation of the sampled cereals for 12 h significantly ($p < 0.05$) reduced total phytate and total tannin. The reduction continued and most of the reduction of phytate and tannin contents occurred during the 72 h of fermentation for both cereal samples. However, the reduction for some fermentation times was not statistically significant. A significant ($p < 0.05$) variation was also noticed in the total amounts of calcium, iron and zinc in both sampled cereals within the 72 h of fermentation.

Conclusion: Prevalence of appropriate complementary feeding practice was very low. There were significant reductions of phytate and tannin contents with concomitant increments of minerals after fermentation of cereals. Phytate: mineral ratios were significantly decreased after fermentation for all the parameters examined. It is recommended to ferment cereals while preparing complementary foods for children so as to enhance their micronutrient uptake.

Keywords: Fermentation, Complementary feeding, Antinutritional factors, Minerals contents

Background

Childhood malnutrition continues to be one of the most stubborn public health problems throughout the developing world including Ethiopia. Demographic and Health surveys data from twenty-one developing countries indicated that poor complementary feeding of children aged 6–23 months contributes to negative growth trends [1]. In sub-Saharan African countries, suboptimal infant feeding practices including poor nutritional quality of complementary foods, micronutrient deficiencies accompanied by frequent infections contribute to high mortality rates among infants and young children [2].

Inappropriate complementary feeding practices remain one of the most determinant factors which prone children susceptible to irreversible outcomes of stunting, poor cognitive development and increased risk of infectious diseases [3]. For instance, malnutrition has been responsible directly or indirectly for 10.9 million (60%) of the annual children under five deaths worldwide [4].

* Correspondence: degnet2006@gmail.com
Department of Applied Human Nutrition, Biotechnology Research Institute, Bahir Dar Institute of Technology, Bahir Dar University, Bahir Dar, Ethiopia

Malnutrition is particularly a significant public health problem for infants and young children in Ethiopia. The Ethiopian mini demographic and health survey (DHS, 2014) shows that national rates of stunting, underweight and wasting among under 5 years children were 40, 25 and 9% respectively [5], have declined only slightly in the last decade and remained serious public health problems.

It is strongly evident that promotion of appropriate complementary feeding practices reduces the rates of stunting and contributes to better child health and growth outcomes [6]. For this reason, WHO and UNICEF recommend introduction of adequate complementary foods at 6th month and improving the quantity and quality of foods children consume while maintaining breastfeeding [7]. It is believed that practicing exclusive breastfeeding for the first six months, introduction of adequate complementary foods at 6th month and continued breastfeeding for 2 years of age or beyond have a potential role to improve the nutritional status of children in developing countries [8]. However, in Ethiopia, only 4% of young children at the age of 6–23 months are fed in accordance with recommended IYCF practices [5].

In developing countries there is limited access to animal products such as meat, egg, fish, milk and milk products even though they provide high concentrations of micronutrients including heme iron, calcium and zinc. The main dietary sources of iron, calcium and zinc in these countries are therefore cereals and legumes [9]. Nevertheless, cereal based foods contain high amounts of anti-nutritional factors which strongly bind minerals like iron, calcium and zinc [10] lead to poor bioavailability. On the other hand, large amounts of these nutrients are required during early life due to accelerated physical and mental growth [11], so ensuring their bioavailability is critical.

The selected district for the survey which is found in south Gondar administrative zone, Northwest Ethiopia is one of the most food insecure districts. It is also long known for its high level of vulnerability to food insecurity with more than one-third of the total population being undernourished [12]. As a result, it is more likely that children should have limited access to animal products and their diet should be cereal based that contain high amounts of anti-nutrients.

Fermentation is an important process which helps to lower the content of anti-nutrients (phytates, tannins, and polyphenols) of cereal grains [13]. It activates several endogenous enzymes and results in products with reduced anti-nutritional factors [14]. It also improves other nutrients and sanitary qualities of foods [15]. Fermentation of cereals generally leads to improvement in nutritional value, digestibility, shelf life, texture, taste and aroma of cereal products [16]. This study therefore, aimed to evaluate the effect of spontaneous fermentation on contents of anti-nutrients and bioavailability of minerals.

Methods and materials

Survey

A community-based cross-sectional survey was conducted in Ebinat district from May to July, 2016. It is one of the 12 districts of South Gondar administrative zone of Amhara region with an estimated area of 2494.27 km^2 having 35 rural and 2 urban Kebeles administrations. The sample size for the survey was determined using a single population proportion formula considering the following assumptions: Proportion of appropriate complementary feeding (p = 10.75%) in Tigray region, Northern Ethiopia [17]; 95% level of confidence (Z = 1.96); marginal error (d = 5%)

$$n = \frac{\mathrm{Z}\,\alpha/2)\ 2\mathrm{p}\ (1-\mathrm{p})}{\mathrm{d2}}$$

From above formula, the calculated sample size was 147. By considering design effect of 2 and non-response rate of 10%, the final sample size was estimated to be 324.

The district was purposively selected due to its high level of vulnerability to food insecurity and has a very long history of aid [12]. In the district there are 37 kebeles of which 20% were randomly selected. Proportional to size allocation method was used to take appropriate sample from each kebele. Finally, systematic random sampling method was used to select respondent households. When more than one, mother-infant/child pairs were randomly selected.

Data for the survey were collected using a validated questionnaire adapted from the Ethiopian Health and Demographic Survey and WHO and LINKAGE project which were designed to assess infant and young child feeding practices in developing countries [4, 18, 19]. A structured questionnaire was used to collect data on maternal complementary feeding practices using four indicators; timely introduction of complementary feeding, minimum dietary diversity, minimum meal frequency and minimum acceptable diet. The indicators were operationalized as follows [20].

Timely introduction of complementary feeding: proportion of children at the age of 6–23 months who started complementary foods at 6th month.

Minimum dietary diversity: proportion of children at the age of 6–23 months who consumed foods from four or more food groups during the previous day. The seven food groups used for formulation of this indicator were: grains, roots and tubers; legumes and nuts; dairy products (milk, yogurt, cheese); flesh foods (meat, chicken and liver/organ meats); eggs; vitamin A rich fruits and vegetables; and other fruits and vegetables.

Minimum meal frequency: proportion of breastfed and non-breastfed children at the age of 6–23 months who got solid, semi-solid or soft foods the minimum number of times or more (2 times for breastfed infants 6–8 months; 3 times for breastfed children 9–23 months and 4 times for non-breastfed children 6–23 months) in the preceding day of the survey.

Minimum acceptable diet: proportion of breastfed children at the age of 6–23 months who had at least the minimum dietary diversity and the minimum meal frequency during the preceding day of the survey.

Appropriate complementary feeding practice: If the mother responds correctly all the above four indicators and if at least one indicator was not fulfilled, it was assumed to be inappropriate.

The data quality for the survey was ensured through training of data collectors, supervision and pre-test on 10% of the sample size. The questionnaire was prepared in English, translated in to Amharic and contextualized to the local situation. Pre-test was done before actual data collection. The completeness and consistency of the collected data have been checked before the study participants leave. The survey data were entered in to Epi Info version 6, checked for missing values and outliers and analyzed using SPSS (SPSS version 20).

Laboratory analysis

Most commonly used cereals for complementary feeding were Teff (Kuncho) and wheat (LOGAWSHIBO; TT14) and collected from Amhara seed enterprise. In all the treatments (sample preparation, laboratory determination and data analysis), the cereals were processed separately.

Sample materials were cleaned manually to remove husks, damaged grains, stones, dust, light materials, glumes, stalks, undersized and immature grains and other extraneous materials.

The cleaned grains of each cereal were dried in drying oven at 55 C for about 2 h to facilitate and make the milling process conducive. The dried cereals were milled into flour to pass through a 1 mm aperture size test sieve to obtain a fine powder. The milled samples were then packed in airtight polythene plastic bags until further analysis.

Suspensions of cereals flour in de-ionized water were prepared in plastic containers at a concentration of 1:3 dilutions (*w*/*v*). The cereals flour slurries were allowed to ferment spontaneously at room temperature (20–23 C) for 0, 12, 24, 36, 48 and 72 h in 12 plastic containers. The supernatant was decanted and samples were withdrawn. The fermented samples were transferred to aluminum dishes after each fermentation time and dried in a hot air oven-drier at 70 °C for 36 h. All samples were analyzed for Phytate, tannin and minerals (Ca, Fe, and Zn).

Phytate was determined by the method of Latta and Eskin [21] which was later modified by Vantraub and Lapteva [22]. About 0.1000 g of fresh samples were extracted with 10 ml 2.4% HCl in a mechanical shaker for 1 h at an ambient temperature and centrifuged at 3000 rpm for 30 min. The clear supernatant was used for phytate estimation. A 2 ml of Wade reagent (containing 0.03% solution of $FeCl_3.6H_2O$ and 0.3% of sulfosalicilic acid in water) was added to 3 ml of each sample solution and the mixture was mixed on a Vortex for 5 s. The absorbances of the sample solutions were measured at 500 nm using UV-VIS spectrophotometer. A series of standard solutions of phytic acid were prepared in 0.2 N HCl. A 3 ml of standard was added into 15 ml of centrifuge tubes with 3 ml of water which was used as a blank. A 1 ml of the Wade reagent was added to each test tube and the solution was mixed on a Vortex mixer for 5 s. Then mixtures were centrifuged for 10 min and the absorbances' of the solutions (both the sample and standard) were measured at 500 nm by using de-ionized water as a blank. Standard curves were made from absorbance versus concentration and the slope and intercept was used for calculation. Phytate: mineral molar ratios were calculated using the molecular weight of IP6 = 660.

Tannin content was determined by the method of Burns [23] latter modified by Maxson and Rooney [24]. About 2.0 g of the samples were weighed in a screw cap test tube. The samples were extracted with 10 ml of 1% HCl in methanol for 24 h at room temperature with mechanical shaking and the solutions were centrifuged at 1000 rpm for 5 min after 24 h shaking. A 1 ml of supernatant was taken and mixed with 5 ml of vanillin-HCl reagent (prepared by mixing equal volume of 8% HCl in methanol and 4% vanillin in methanol). D-catechin was used as standard for condensed tannin determination. A 40 mg of D-catechin was weighed and dissolved in 1000 ml of 1% HCl in methanol and used as stock solution. A 0, 0.2, 0.4, 0.6, 0.8 and 1 ml of stock solutions were taken in test tube and the volume of each test tube was accustomed to 1 ml with 1% HCl in methanol. A 5 ml of vanillin-HCl reagent was added into each test tube. After 20 min, the absorbance of sample solutions and the standard solutions were measured at 500 nm by using water to zero the spectrophotometer. The calibration curves were made from the series of standard solutions using SPSS-20. Standard curves were prepared from absorbance versus concentration and the slopes and intercepts were used for calculation.

The mineral contents (calcium, iron, and zinc) were determined by the procedure of AOAC (1984) using an Atomic Absorption Spectrophotometer. After removal of organic material by dry ashing, the residue was dissolved in dilute acid. The solution was sprayed into the flame of Atomic Absorption Spectrophotometer and the absorption of the metal to be analyzed was measured at a specific wavelength. The stock standard solutions of minerals (iron, zinc and calcium) were diluted with 0.3 N HCl to concentrations that fall within the working range (0, 0.6, 1.0, 1.4, 1.8, μg/ml for zinc analysis; 1.0, 1.5, 2.5, and 3.0 μg/ml for calcium analysis and 0, 2.0, 6.0, 10.0 12.0 μg/ml for iron analysis). The ash obtained from dry ashing was mixed with 5 ml of 6 N HCl and dried on a low temperature hot plate. A 7 ml of 3 N HCl was added to the dried ash and heated on the hot plate until the solution just boils. The ash solution was cooled to room temperature at open air in a hood and filtered through a filter paper into a 50 ml graduated flask. A 5 ml of 3 N HCl was added into each crucible dishes and heated until the solution just boiled, cooled, and filtered into the flask. The crucible dishes were again washed three times with de-ionized water and the washings were filtered into the flask. A 2.5 mL of 10% Lanthanum chloride solution was added into each graduated flask. Then the solution was cooled and diluted to the mark (50 ml) with de-ionized water. A blank was prepared by taking the same procedure as the sample.

For all experiments, determinations were made in triplicates. Errors were calculated as standard deviations of the mean (SD) and SAS 9.1.3 service pack 4 was used to analyze the results. Means were separated using Duncan's Multiple Range Test. Significance was accepted at 0.05 level of probability.

Results

Complementary feeding practices

Majority (70.1%) of the mothers initiated complementary feeding at 6 months. However, only 1.5% of mothers practiced appropriate complementary feeding (Table 1).

Household level food processing

During the preparation of family foods, mothers/care takers perform various household level food processing techniques. Out of all respondents, 196 (60.5%) reported that they usually ferment grains during the preparation of family foods (Table 2). However, they hardly do for complementary foods.

Production and marketing of complementary foods

Almost all (97.2%) of the respondents reported that they are willing to use complementary foods produced at community level if they got opportunity in their locality. The huge majority (86.1%) of them responded in favor of involvement in the production and marketing of complementary foods (Table 2).

Effect of spontaneous fermentation on anti-nutrients and mineral contents

Phytate (mg/100 g) and tannin (mg/100 g) contents of teff and wheat samples (expressed as plus or minus of the standard deviations) are shown in Table 3 as affected by different periods of fermentation (0, 12, 24, 36, 48 and 72 h).

Phytate contents of unfermented samples were 541.45 ± 13.40 and 464.10 ± 0.00 mg/100 g for teff and wheat, respectively while the tannin contents were 0.87 ± 0.00 and 0.58 ± 0.00 mg/100 g for the sample cereals respectively. Fermentation of the cereals for 12 h significantly ($p < 0.05$) reduced total phytate from 541.45 to 471.84 and 464.10 to 417.69 mg/100 g for teff and wheat, respectively (Table 3). The reduction rate continued (though some are not significant) and reached its minimum value of 440.89 mg/100 g and 371.28 mg/100 g for teff and wheat respectively when the flours were fermented for 72 h.

Fermentation of the sampled cereals for 12 h also significantly ($p < 0.05$) reduced total tannin from 0.87 to 0.79 and 0.58 to 0.56 mg/100 g for teff and wheat, respectively (Table 3). The reduction continued and reached its minimum value of 0.74 mg and 0.47 mg/100 g for teff and wheat cereals respectively when the flours were fermented for 72 h.

Furthermore, correlation analysis also showed that phytate and tannin contents are inversely related with period of fermentation with Pearson correlation coefficient (r) values of 0.771 and 0.858 for Phytate and tannin respectively for the teff sample. Phytate and tannin contents of wheat also inversely correlated with fermentation time with Pearson correlation coefficient (r) values of 0.816 and 0.948 for phytate and tannin respectively.

The regression model that estimates the relationship between phytate content with respect to period of fermentation was also $Y = 504.10 - 1.17x$ and $Y = 445.65 - 0.99x$ for teff and wheat, while the curve fit that relates fermentation time with tannin content in this study was $Y = 0.83 - 0.02x$ and $Y = 0.57 - 0.01x$ for these cereals respectively.

The mineral contents of the two sampled cereals (teff and wheat) are shown in Table 4. The values of the unfermented flour in both sampled cereals were significantly different ($p < 0.05$) from fermented samples in all the parameters along with period of fermentation time. The total mineral values of both spontaneously fermented sampled cereals were higher as compared to the unfermented samples of the cereals.

The contents of calcium, iron and zinc in unfermented cereals were 160, 6.19 and 1.93 for teff and 80.0, 3.10 and 1.15, for wheat in mg/100 g respectively and increased in to 320, 15.94 and 2.63 for teff and 110.0, 13.10 and 1.51 for wheat after 72 h of fermentation.

Table 1 Complementary feeding practice of mothers for their children, Ebinat district, Northwestern Ethiopia, 2016

Variables		Frequency (N)	Percentage (%)
Timely introduction of complementary feeding		227	70.1
Dietary diversity from 24 h recall	Grains, roots and tubers	172	53.1
	Legumes and nuts	107	33.0
	Dairy products	116	35.8
	Vitamin A-rich fruits	80	24.7
	Flesh foods	40	12.3
	Eggs	100	30.9
	Other fruits & vegetables	158	48.8
Minimum dietary diversity (≥4 food groups)		15	4.6
Minimum meal frequency		155	47.84
Minimum acceptable diet		10	3.08
Appropriate complementary feeding		5	1.5

Furthermore, the phytate to mineral molar ratios in the two sampled cereals (teff and wheat) are shown in Table 5. The phytate: calcium molar ratios were below 0.24 (critical molar ratio) in all the fermented and unfermented samples of teff and 72 h fermented wheat. The phytate: iron molar ratios were above > 0.15 (critical point) in both samples of cereals examined. Phytate: zinc molar ratios were also above 15 in both samples of cereals analyzed.

Discussion

In this study, the overall prevalence of appropriate complementary feeding practice and the effect of spontaneous fermentation on anti-nutrients and mineral contents were assessed. The phytate to mineral molar ratios were also presented.

Complementary feeding practices

Timely introduction of complementary feeding was determined and possible provisions of most common non-human milk alternative liquids including water, milk, butter and fenugreek before the age of 6 months were also assessed. The result indicated that majority (70.1%) of the mothers initiated complementary feeding at 6 months though low compared to WHO cut-off point (80 to 94%) for good practice of complementary feeding [19] and reports in India, 77.5% [25] and Abyi-Adi, Ethiopia, 79.7% [17], while it is consistent with a study from Bangladesh, 71% [26] and Benishangul Gumuz Regional State, Northwest, Ethiopia, 73.9% [27]. However, it was higher than the findings (65.7%) reported by a review in Southern Ethiopia [28], 63% in Lalibela district, Northeast Ethiopia [29] and 56.4% in Enemay district, Northwest Ethiopia [30]. The discrepancies might be attributed to differences in status of institutional delivery, health care settings and utilization of antenatal care (ANC) and postnatal care (PNC) services as nutrition education and counseling are components of these services that would bring an added benefit to improve mothers' awareness on appropriate child feeding practices [17]. In this study, many women met the criteria for introduction of complementary foods at 6 months and this might be attributed to the effort of health extension workers as mothers who had sufficient knowledge on complementary feeding practices are more likely to introduce timely as compared to mothers who had not sufficient knowledge [30].

Table 2 Proportion of mothers/care takers considered household food processing techniques and willing in the production and marketing of complementary foods, Ebinat district, Northwest Ethiopia, 2016

Household food processing	Frequency(n)	Percentage (%)
Fermentation	196	60.5
Roasting	241	74.4
Soaking	191	59.0
Germination	171	52.8
Removal of bran	229	70.7
Willingness to use complementary foods produced at community level	315	97.2
Interest to be a member of women's groups for production and marketing of complementary foods	279	86.1

Proportion of mothers offered four or more food groups to their children was far low (4.6%) compared to similar studies in India, 15.2% [31], Kenya, 17.9% [32], Zambia, 12% [33],and Ethiopian national report, 10.8% [34], northern Ethiopia, 17.8% [17], Arsi Negele district, southeastern Ethiopia [35] that reported 18.8% and Dangila, Northwest, Ethiopia which reported 12.6% [36]. The discrepancies might be attributed to differences in agroecological characteristics as the study district is

Table 3 Phytate and tannin content of teff and wheat samples during spontaneous fermentation, Ebinat district, Northwestern Ethiopia, 2016

Fermentation time	Parameters			
	Phytate(mg/100 g)		Tannin(mg/100 g)	
	Teff	Wheat	Teff	Wheat
0 h	541.45 ± 13.40a	464.10 ± 0.00a	0.87 ± 0.00a	0.58 ± 0.00a
12 h	471.84 ± 13.39b	417.69 ± 0.00b	0.79 ± 0.00b	0.56 ± 0.00b
24 h	448.63 ± 26.79c	394.49 ± 0.00c	0.78 ± 0.00c	0.54 ± 0.00c
36 h	464.10 ± 0.00bc	394.49 ± 0.00c	0.77 ± 0.00d	0.49 ± 0.00d
48 h	433.16 ± 26.79c	417.69 ± 0.00b	0.76 ± 0.00e	0.48 ± 0.00e
72 h	440.89 ± 23.20bc	371.28 ± 0.00d	0.74 ± 0.00f	0.47 ± 0.00f

Values are means of triplicate samples (± SD). Means not sharing a common letter in a column are significantly different at p < 0.05 as assessed by Duncan's Multiple Range Test

drought prone area that might result in low accessibility to diversified foods. The most frequently consumed food groups were grains, roots and tubers (53.1%) while the least frequently consumed were animal source foods such as meat and fish (12.3%). Only 30.9% of children consumed eggs and 35.8% got dairy products. This might be an indication that the area has limited access to animal source foods and children might be more likely to suffer from micronutrient deficiencies.

Proportion of mothers who met the minimum meal frequency is lower (47.8%) compared to other reports such as Paskistan, 56.4% [37], northern Ghana, 57.3% [38] and other similar studies like Arsi Negele district, southeastern Ethiopia, 67.3% [35] and Dabat District, northwest Ethiopia, 72.2% [39]. However, it is similar with a study from Dangila, Northwest, Ethiopia, 50.4% [28]. The discrepancies might be due to differences in literacy level, awareness of mothers on IYCF and other socioeconomic statuses as this study was in remote district area.

Over all practice of appropriate complementary feeding is very low (1.5%) compared with other similar studies including a review report from five Asian counties [40], Tanzania [41], Ethiopian national average [18], Enemay district, Northwest Ethiopia, [30] and Arsi Negele district, southeastern Ethiopia [35]. These differences might be attributed to the district's vulnerability to drought that would result in limited access to diversified foods which is implicated in very low diet diversity.

Effect of spontaneous fermentation on anti-nutrients and mineral contents

Fermentation of the sampled cereals for 12 h significantly ($p < 0.05$) reduced total phytate in both teff and wheat sample cereals. The results of this study are in agreement with other similar studies [42, 43], which reported significantly low concentration of phytate sorghum produces compared to unfermented one. A study from Nigeria also concluded that fermentation is the most effective processing technique that reduced phytic acid in the cereal flours [44].

It has been suggested that the loss of phytate during fermentation could be a result of the activity of native phytase and the fermentative microflora as reported by different researchers [42, 45, 46]. In this study, most of the reduction in phytate occurred during the 72 h of fermentation. This might be due to the prevailing pH which is considered to be an optimum for microbial phytase activity since all enzymes have a specific pH in which they function most capably [42]. However, for

Table 4 Mineral contents of teff and wheat samples during spontaneous fermentation, Ebinat district, Northwestern Ethiopia, 2016

Fermentation time	Parameters					
	Ca (mg/100 g)		Fe(mg/100 g)		Zn(mg/100 g)	
	Teff	Wheat	Teff	Wheat	Teff	Wheat
0 h	160.00 ± 6.67^{e}	80.00 ± 0.00^{d}	6.19 ± 0.48^{d}	3.10 ± 0.24^{e}	1.93 ± 0.02^{f}	1.15 ± 0.02^{d}
12 h	266.67 ± 6.67^{d}	86.67 ± 0.00^{c}	10.79 ± 0.55^{b}	4.92 ± 0.27^{d}	2.01 ± 0.02^{e}	1.26 ± 0.02^{c}
24 h	282.22 ± 3.85^{c}	86.67 ± 0.00^{c}	10.95 ± 0.95^{b}	5.24 ± 0.95^{d}	2.11 ± 0.02^{d}	1.41 ± 0.02^{b}
36 h	291.11 ± 3.85^{c}	86.67 ± 0.00^{c}	9.68 ± 0.73^{c}	6.51 ± 0.27c	2.28 ± 0.02^{c}	1.22 ± 0.02^{c}
48 h	304.44 ± 3.85^{b}	97.78 ± 3.85^{b}	11.43 ± 0.48^{b}	8.33 ± 0.24 ^{b}	2.48 ± 0.02^{b}	1.37 ± 0.04^{b}
72 h	320.00 ± 6.67^{a}	110.00 ± 3.33^{a}	15.94 ± 0.24^{a}	13.10 ± 0.24^{a}	2.63 ± 0.04^{a}	1.51 ± 0.02^{a}

Values are means of triplicate samples (± SD). Means not sharing a common letter in a column are significantly different at $p < 0.05$ as assessed by Duncan's Multiple Range Test

Table 5 Effect of spontaneous fermentation on molar ratios of phytate and minerals in teff and wheat samples, Ebinat district, Northwest Ethiopia, 2016

Fermentation time	Parameters					
	phytate: calcium		phytate: iron		phytate: zinc	
	Teff	Wheat	Teff	Wheat	Teff	Wheat
0 h	0.21 ± 0.01a	0.35 ± 0.00a	7.44 ± 0.43a	12.77 ± 0.99a	27.68 ± 0.87a	39.87 ± 0.70a
12 h	0.11 ± 0.00b	0.29 ± 0.00b	3.72 ± 0.25b	7.22 ± 0.39b	22.72 ± 0.56b	32.53 ± 0.53b
24 h	0.10 ± 0.01c	0.28 ± 0.00c	3.49 ± 0.38cb	6.54 ± 1.21cb	20.89 ± 1.36c	27.62 ± 0.41b
36 h	0.09 ± 0.00c	0.28 ± 0.00c	4.08 ± 0.30cb	2.56 ± 0.04c	20.04 ± 0.18c	31.76 ± 0.46c
48 h	0.09 ± 0.01 dc	0.26 ± 0.01d	3.22 ± 0.33c	5.45 ± 0.24d	17.27 ± 1.00d	30.01 ± 0.88d
72 h	0.08 ± 0.01d	0.21 ± 0.01e	2.35 ± 0.11d	3.78 ± 0.11e	16.48 ± 0.89d	24.17 ± 0.33e

Values are means of triplicate samples (± SD). Means not sharing a common letter in a column are significantly different at $p < 0.05$ as assessed by Duncan's Multiple Range Test

some of the fermentation times reductions in phytate content for both cereals were not significant. These fluctuations in values of phytate content could be attributed to the metabolic activities of the microorganisms.

Fermentation of the cereals for 12 h also significantly ($p < 0.05$) reduced total tannin in both cereals. The reduction continued and reached its minimum value when the flours were fermented for 72 h. Overall reduction in tannin content of fermented samples is significant ($p < 0.05$) compared to unfermented samples in all fermentation times. It is in agreement with a study where reduction in tannin content of fermented samples of sorghum was highly significant ($P < 0.05$) compared to unfermented samples [42]. Reduction in tannin contents due to fermentation might have been caused by the activity of polyphenoloxidase or tanniase of fermenting microflora [44]. However, this result is in contrary to other study that reported fermentation for 36 h at room temperature was found to cause no changes in tannin content of fermented dough for millet cultivars [45]. Other study also reported that, tannin content of pearl millet sample showed significant increase after fermentation [47]. This might be attributed to differences in room temperature where microorganisms could suitably grow and produce tannin degrading enzymes.

The mineral contents of the unfermented flours in both teff and wheat sampled cereals were significantly different ($p < 0.05$) from fermented samples along with period of fermentation time. Overall, a significant ($p < 0.05$) variation was noticed in the total amounts of calcium, iron and zinc in both sampled cereals within the 72 h of fermentation. This is in agreement with a study conducted on soymilk where there was increase in calcium, magnesium, zinc and iron contents during natural fermentation of soymilk [48]. The increase in the mineral contents of fermented samples may be due to the fact that minerals (bound to anti-nutrients) were released from chelated complex compound through the activities of microorganisms responsible for the fermentation [49]. However, there were reductions in the mineral contents during fermentation times of 24 h and 36 h. The reduction of total minerals in those fermentation times might be ascribed due to the microorganisms could have utilized some of the hydrolyzed elements for their metabolic activities as the time might be comfortable for their metabolic actives [50]. On the other hand, the results of the present study contradict with the observation made on maize that fermentation does not have effect on the contents of total minerals [51].

Furthermore, the phytate to mineral molar ratios in the two cereals (teff and wheat) were also assessed. The phytate:calcium molar ratio was below the critical molar ratio [52] in all the fermented and unfermented samples of teff and 72 h fermented wheat. Thus, the result indicates favorable Ca absorption in teff and 72 h fermented wheat.

The bioavailability of iron was low since phytate:iron molar ratios were above the critical value [53] in both fermented and unfermented cereals examined which is regarded as indicative of poor iron bioavailability. This might be because of the high levels of phytic acid in both the samples of cereals examined.

Phytate:zinc molar ratios were also > 15 in both the sample cereals analyzed which it is an indicative of poor zinc bioavailability [53–55].

In general, phytate: mineral ratios were significantly decreased after fermentation for all the parameters examined even if the critical values were not achieved for iron and zinc. This study is in agreement with those of fermented rice-dehulled black gram blends [56] and fermented cereal based complementary foods [57, 58]. The lower phytate: mineral ratios for the fermented teff and wheat cereal grains might be partly ascribed to the decreased content of phytic acid during fermentation. Thus, fermentation enhances bioavailability of minerals by degrading phytate with microbial and native phytases that entangle macro- and trace elements. Above mentioned studies also indicated that fermentation hydrolyzed anti-nutrients from their organic bonds to increase mineral bioavailability.

Limitations of the study

Due to limitations in finance and long distance of the survey area from the laboratory, sensory analysis of fermented products had not been carried out with survey participants.

Conclusions

Prevalence of appropriate complementary feeding practice was very low which indicated the need of immediate support and follow up. There were significant reductions of phytate and tannin contents with concomitant increments of minerals after fermentation of cereals. Phytate: mineral ratios were significantly decreased after fermentation for all the parameters examined. Besides of spontaneous fermentation lowers phytic acid and tannin contents and improve the extractability of minerals, it is a promising and simple method as it doesn't require even fuel. Therefore, spontaneous fermentation should be promoted with community awareness interventions through existing health and agriculture system of the government so as to enhance micronutrient uptake of young children. Health and agriculture extension workers should be trained so as to include it in their package. Community and religious leaders should also be educated so as to get better acceptance by the community. To this effect, the information should be disseminated to the regional bureaus as well as district offices.

Abbreviations

AOAC: Association of Official Analytical Chemists; DHS: Demographic and Health Survey; IYCF: Infant and Young Child Feeding; SAS: Statistical Analysis System; SD: Standard Deviation; SPSS: Statistical Package for Social Sciences; UNICEF: United Nations for Children's Fund; WHO: World Health Organization

Acknowledgments

The authors acknowledge Biotechnology Research Institute, Bahir Dar University for funding the research. We would like to thank data collectors and women for their willingness to participate. We also thank Amhara regional health bureau, South Gondar zone and Ebinat district health offices and Amhara seed enterprise for their support and cooperation.

Funding

Biotechnology Research Institute, Bahir Dar University was source of fund for the research. However, the Institute had no role in designing the study, data collection and analysis, interpretation of the data and preparation of the manuscript or decision to publish.

Authors' contributions

DT initiated and designed the study, coordinated the data collection, performed the analysis and interpretation of data. GN and AN assisted with the design of the study, worked on data collection, data entry and analysis. DT also wrote the report and drafted the manuscript. All authors read and approved the final manuscript.

Competing interest

The authors declare that they have no competing interests.

References

1. Dewey K. Guiding principles for complementary feeding of the breastfed child; 2002.
2. Black RE, Allen LH, Bhutta ZA, Caulfield LE, De Onis M, Ezzati M, et al. Maternal and child undernutrition: global and regional exposures and health consequences. Lancet. 2008;371(9608):243–60.
3. Brown K, Dewey K, Allen L. Complementary feeding of young children in developing countries: a review of current scientific knowledge; 1998.
4. WHO and UNICEF. Global strategy for infant and young child feeding: World Health Organization; 2003.
5. EDHS. Ethiopia Mini Demographic and Health Survey. Ethiopia: Central Statistical Agency Addis Ababa; 2014.
6. Bhutta ZA, Das JK, Rizvi A, Gaffey MF, Walker N, Horton S, et al. Evidence-based interventions for improvement of maternal and child nutrition: what can be done and at what cost? Lancet. 2013;382(9890):452–77.
7. WHO. Indicators for assessing infant and young child feeding practices: part 2: measurement. 2010.
8. Lassi ZS, Das JK, Zahid G, Imdad A, Bhutta ZA. Impact of education and provision of complementary feeding on growth and morbidity in children less than 2 years of age in developing countries: a systematic review. BMC Public Health. 2013;13(3):1.
9. Samia M, AbdelRahaman EEB, Abdullahi H. Effect of fermentation on antinutritional factors and HCl extractability of minerals of pearl millet cultivars. J Food Technol. 2005;3(4):516–22.
10. Lopez HW, Leenhardt F, Coudray C, Remesy C. Minerals and phytic acid interactions: is it a real problem for human nutrition? Int J Food Sci Technol. 2002;37(7):727–39.
11. Neumann C, Harris DM, Rogers LM. Contribution of animal source foods in improving diet quality and function in children in the developing world. Nutr Res. 2002;22(1–2):193–220.
12. Siyoum AD, Hilhorst D, Van Uffelen G-J. Food aid and dependency syndrome in Ethiopia: local perceptions. J Hum Assistance 2012;20.
13. Sindhu SC, Khetarpaul N. Probiotic fermentation of indigenous food mixture: effect on antinutrients and digestibility of starch and protein. J Food Compos Anal. 2001;14(6):601–9.
14. Greiner R, Konietzny U. Phytase for food application. Food Technol Biotechnol. 2006;44(2).
15. Nout MR. Rich nutrition from the poorest–cereal fermentations in Africa and Asia. Food Microbiol. 2009;26(7):685–92.
16. ZK-J K. Fermentation of cereals for specific purpose. J Food Nutri Res. 2007; 46(2):51–7.
17. Mekbib E, Shumey A, Ferede S, Haile F. Magnitude and factors associated with appropriate complementary feeding among mothers having children 6–23 months-of-age in northern Ethiopia; a community-based cross-sectional study. J Food Nutr Sci. 2014;(2, 2):36.
18. EDHS, Ethiopian Demographic and Health survey 2011, central statistical agency, Addis Ababa. Ethiopia, ICF International Calverton, Maryland, USA. 2012.
19. WHO. Infant and young child feeding: a tool for assessing national practices, policies and programmes. 2003.
20. WHO. Indicators for assessing infant and young child feeding practices: conclusions of a consensus meeting held 6–8 November 2007 in Washington DC, USA: World Health Organization (WHO); 2008.
21. Latta M, Eskin M. A simple and rapid colorimetric method for phytate determination. J Agric Food Chem. 1980;28(6):1313–5.

22. Vaintraub IA, Lapteva NA. Colorimetric determination of phytate in unpurified extracts of seeds and the products of their processing. Anal Biochem. 1988;175(1):227–30.
23. Burns RE. Method for estimation of tannin in grain sorghum 1. Agron J. 1971;63(3):511–2.
24. Maxson E, Rooney L. Evaluation of methods for tannin analysis in sorghum grain. Cereal Chem. 1972;49(6):719.
25. Rao S, Swathi P, Unnikrishnan B, Hegde A. Study of complementary feeding practices among mothers of children aged six months to two years-a study from coastal South India. Australas Med J. 2011;4(5):252.
26. Kabir I, Khanam M, Agho KE, Mihrshahi S, Dibley MJ, Roy SK. Determinants of inappropriate complementary feeding practices in infant and young children in Bangladesh: secondary data analysis of demographic health survey 2007. Matern Child Nutr. 2012;8(s1):11–27.
27. Guracho YD, Amentie MA. Infant and young child feeding practices and associated factors in Benishangul Gumuz regional state, north West, Ethiopia.
28. Henry CJ, Whiting SJ, Regassa N. Complementary feeding practices among infant and young children in southern Ethiopia: review of the findings from a Canada-Ethiopia project. J Agric Sci. 2015;7(10):29.
29. Sisay W, Edris M, Tariku A. Determinants of timely initiation of complementary feeding among mothers with children aged 6–23 months in Lalibela District, Northeast Ethiopia, 2015. BMC public health. 2016;16(1):884.
30. Gessese D, Bolka H, Alemu Abajobir A, Tegabu D. The practice of complementary feeding and associated factors among mothers of children 6-23 months of age in Enemay district, Northwest Ethiopia. Nutr Food Sci. 2014;44(3):230–40.
31. Patel A, Pusdekar Y, Badhoniya N, Borkar J, Agho KE, Dibley MJ. Determinants of inappropriate complementary feeding practices in young children in India: secondary analysis of National Family Health Survey 2005–2006. Matern Child Nutr. 2012;8(s1):28–44.
32. Gichana MB. Nutritional knowledge of mothers and nutritional status of their children 6–59 months under Malezi bora Programme in Kawangware sub location. Dagoretti, Nairobi County: University of Nairobi. 2013.
33. Mallard SR, Houghton LA, Filteau S, Mullen A, Nieuwelink J, Chisenga M, et al. Dietary Diversity at 6 Months of Age Is Associated with Subsequent Growth and Mediates the Effect of Maternal Education on Infant Growth in Urban Zambia, 2. J Nutr. 2014;144(11):1818–25.
34. Aemro M, Mesele M, Birhanu Z, Atenafu A. Dietary diversity and meal frequency practices among infant and young children aged 6–23 months in Ethiopia: a secondary analysis of Ethiopian demographic and health survey 2011. Journal of nutrition and metabolism. 2013;2013.
35. Kassa T, Meshesha B, Haji Y, Ebrahim J. Appropriate complementary feeding practices and associated factors among mothers of children age 6–23 months in southern Ethiopia, 2015. BMC Pediatr. 2016;16(1):131.
36. Beyene M, Worku AG, Wassie MM. Dietary diversity, meal frequency and associated factors among infant and young children in Northwest Ethiopia: a cross-sectional study. BMC Public Health. 2015;15(1):1007.
37. Bhutta ZA, Soofi SB, Zaidi SSH, Habib A. Pakistan National Nutrition Survey, 2011; 2011.
38. Saaka M, Larbi A, Mutaru S, Hoeschle-Zeledon I. Magnitude and factors associated with appropriate complementary feeding among children 6–23 months in northern Ghana. BMC Nutrition. 2016;2(1):2.
39. Belew AK, Ali BM, Abebe Z, Dachew BA. Dietary diversity and meal frequency among infant and young children: a community based study. Ital J Pediatr. 2017;43(1):73.
40. Senarath U, Agho KE, Akram DeS, Godakandage SS, Hazir T, Jayawickrama H, et al. comparisons of complementary feeding indicators and associated factors in children aged 6–23 months across five south Asian countries. Matern Child Nutr 2012;8(s1):89–106.
41. Victor R, Baines SK, Agho KE, Dibley MJ. Factors associated with inappropriate complementary feeding practices among children aged 6–23 months in Tanzania. Matern Child Nutr. 2014;10(4):545–61.
42. Wedad HA, El Tinay AH, Mustafa AI, Babiker EE. Effect of fermentation, malt-pretreatment and cooking on antinutritional factors and protein digestibility of sorghum cultivars. Pak J Nutr. 2008;7(2):335–41.
43. Makokha A, Oniang'o R, Njoroge S, Kamar O. Effect of traditional fermentation and malting on phytic acid and mineral availability from sorghum (Sorghum bicolor) and finger millet (Eleusine coracana) grain varieties grown in Kenya. Food Nutr Bull. 2002;23(3 Suppl):241–5.
44. Fagbemi T, Oshodi A, Ipinmoroti K. Processing effects on some antinutritional factors and in vitro multienzyme protein digestibility (IVPD) of three tropical seeds: breadnut (Artocarpus altilis), cashewnut (Anacardium occidentale) and fluted pumpkin (Telfairia occidentalis). Pak J Nutr. 2005;4(4): 250–6.
45. Elyas SH, El Tinay AH, Yousif NE, Elsheikh EA. Effect of natural fermentation on nutritive value and in vitro protein digestibility of pearl millet. Food Chem. 2002;78(1):75–9.
46. Shimelis EA, Rakshit SK. Influence of natural and controlled fermentations on α-galactosides, antinutrients and protein digestibility of beans (Phaseolus vulgaris L.). Int J Food Sci Technol. 2008;43(4):658–65.
47. Osman MA. Effect of traditional fermentation process on the nutrient and antinutrient contents of pearl millet during preparation of Lohoh. J Saudi Soc Agric Sci. 2011;10(1):1–6.
48. Obadina A, Akinola O, Shittu T, Bakare H. Effect of natural fermentation on the chemical and nutritional composition of fermented soymilk nono. Nigerian Food J. 2013;31(2):91–7.
49. Gabriel, R.A.O. Effect of fermentation on the nutritional and antinutritional content of Jack beans, *Canavalia ensiformis L.* MSc Thesis, The Federal University Technology, Akure, Nigeria. 2002.
50. Hassan AB, Osman GA, Babiker EE. Effect of domestic processing on antinutrients and availability of protein and minerals of Lupin (*Lupinus termis*) seeds. J Food Technol. 2005;3:255–62.
51. Ejigui J, Savoie L, Marin J, Desrosiers T. Beneficial changes and drawbacks of a traditional fermentation process on chemical composition and antinutritional factors of yellow maize (Zea mays). J Biol Sci. 2005;5(5):590–6.
52. Frontela C, Scarino ML, Ferruzza S, Ros G, Martínez C. Effect of dephytinization on bioavailability of iron, calcium and zinc from infant cereals assessed in the Caco-2 cell model. World J Gastroenterol: WJG. 2009; 15(16):1977.
53. Umeta M, West CE, Fufa H. Content of zinc, iron, calcium and their absorption inhibitors in foods commonly consumed in Ethiopia. J Food Compos Anal. 2005;18(8):803–17.
54. Adeyeye E, Arogundade L, Akintayo E, Aisida O, Alao P. Calcium, zinc and phytate interrelationships in some foods of major consumption in Nigeria. Food Chem. 2000;71(4):435–41.
55. Walingo MK. Indigenous food processing methods that improve zinc absorption and bioavailability of plant diets consumed by the Kenyan population. Afr J Food Agric Nutr Dev. 2009;9(1):523–35.
56. Sharma A, Khetarpaul N. Effect of fermentation with whey on the HCl extractability of minerals from rice-dehulled blackgram blends. J Agric Food Chem. 1997;45(6):2258–61.
57. Urga K, Narasimha H. Phytate: zinc and phytate x calcium: zinc molar ratios in selected diets of Ethiopians. Bull Chem Soc Ethiop. 1998;12(1):1–8.
58. Odumodu C. Optimum fermentation period for micronutrients content of cereal based complementary food. Pak J Nutr. 2007;6(6):518–23.

23

Availability, affordability and costs of pediatric medicines in Mongolia

Gereltuya Dorj[1*], Bruce Sunderland[2], Tsetsegmaa Sanjjav[1], Gantuya Dorj[3] and Byambatsogt Gendenragchaa[1]

Abstract

Background: The Essential Medicines List for Children (EMLc) was developed by the World Health Organization (WHO) to assist member countries to achieve Millennium Development Goals (MDG). The Government of Mongolia has adopted a National Essential Drug List (NEDL) with the seventh update published in 2014. The objective of this study was to determine the accessibility, availability and costs of essential pediatric medicines in Mongolia.

Methods: A standardized methodology developed by the WHO and Health Action International (HAI) was employed to conduct a study on the availability, costs and affordability of pediatric medicines in Mongolia. A data collection tool collected information in regards to retail and wholesale availability and costs of essential pediatric medicines at pharmacy outlets during January and August of 2016.

Results: Availability of individual essential pediatric medicines varied across the country. The average availability of medicines was 72.6% in the public sector (9.1–100%). Correspondingly, average availability of all selected medicines in the private sector was 76.7% (26.7–100%). Lowest price medicines were 2.45 times higher than the international reference price (IRP) in the private sector and was 1.95 times higher in the public sector. The lowest cost medicines in the public sector were more affordable for all conditions. The least affordable treatment was estimated to be for respiratory tract infections, or otitis media using amoxicillin clavulanic acid, suspension costing up to 1.03 days wages.

Conclusion: Procurement, supply and distribution of essential pediatric medicines needs to be regularly investigated in order to identify the availability and costs of pediatric formulations in Mongolia.

Keywords: Essential medicines, Pediatric, Availability, Cost, Mongolia

Background

Mongolia is a country with a vast land of 1.56 million km^2 with a population of three million. The country is divided into 21 provinces (aimags) and a metropolitan city (Ulaanbaatar). Ulaanbaatar city has 9 districts and they are sub-divided into 152 khoroos. Most of the population lives in urban areas and approximately 20% is nomadic. Unemployment was about 10.6% and the inflation rate was 0.9% in 2016 [1]. According to the World Bank, Mongolia is a lower middle income country with an estimated Gross Domestic Product (GDP) of United States Dollar (USD) 11.76 billion in 2015. About 14% of the population lives on less than USD 1 per day [2]. The infant mortality rate was 15.3 per 1000 live births in 2014 [3].

* Correspondence: gereltuya@gmail.com
[1]School of Pharmacy and Biomedicine, Mongolian National University of Medical Sciences, S.Zorig Street, Ulaanbaatar 14210, Mongolia

Pharmaceutical sector

The Drugs Act of Mongolia was approved in 1998 with an aim of ensuring good quality, effective and safe drugs [4]. The Government subsequently promulgated the National Drug Policy of Mongolia (NDPM) in 2000 which was updated in 2014 [5]. Currently, 1496 pharmacies are operating in Mongolia of which 75% had one or two branches. There were 306 pharmacies working under the drug revolving fund (DRF) initiative [6].

The Essential Medicines List for Children (EMLc) [7] was developed by the World Health Organization (WHO) to assist member countries to achieve Millennium Development Goals(MDG) [8]. In December 2007, the WHO has also initiated the "Make Medicines Child Size" with a purpose of improving the accessibility of safe, effective and quality medicines for children by promoting awareness and action through research, regulatory measures and changes in government policy [9]. In accordance with

WHO recommendations [10], the Government has adopted a National Essential Drug List since 1991 with regular updates, the seventh being completed in 2014 (7thEML). The NEDL contains 419 unique formulations, including 181 pediatric drugs [11]. There were 591 new drugs (salts or doses), 48 raw materials registered and the registration period was extended for a total of 428 drugs in 2014 [12].

In order to overcome barriers in supplying pediatric medicines and increase the accessibility to appropriate pediatric formulations, it is necessary to evaluate the availability and costs of essential medicines in pharmacy outlets and national medicines lists. Based on evidence and reliable scientific data, governments can apply necessary policy decisions and undertake interventions. Previous findings suggest that the availability and affordability of essential medicines needs to be improved in order to ensure accessibility to essential medicines in Mongolia [13]. However, no study has assessed the situation of essential pediatric medicines in Mongolia.

Therefore this study aimed to investigate the accessibility, availability and costs of essential pediatric medicines in Mongolia.

Methods

A standardized methodology developed by the WHO and Health Action International (HAI) [14] was applied to conduct the study. The validation of the WHO/HAI methodology has been reported in several studies previously [15, 16]. A data collection tool was employed to collect availability information and retail and wholesale costs of essential pediatric medicines at pharmacy outlets during January and August of 2016. This timeline was selected due to the seasonal variables and high incidences of diseases in winter (January).

Selection of pharmacy outlets

Data collection included six aimags/regions/provinces, Ulaanbaatar city, Erdenet city, Khuvsgul aimag, Dornod aimag, Govi-Altai aimag and Selenge aimag. The capital city Ulaanbaatar was selected as the major urban centre of Mongolia and an additional five districts were selected randomly from those which could be reached within a day's travel from Ulaanbaatar city. The selection of study sites consistently included both urban and rural areas in all districts.

In each study area, five to ten pharmacy outlets were randomly selected from the list provided by the Health Development Centre, Ministry of Health and Sports of Mongolia.

The private sector sample included a total of 45 pharmacy outlets. Of those 11 private pharmacy outlets were located in public hospitals. Pharmacy outlets were selected based on active registration status and market volume size [17].

Selection of medicines

As specified in the "Better Medicines for Children Project", a core list of EMLc's representative of commonly used medicines for treatment of various pediatric conditions prevalent in low middle/income countries was adopted for the study. The core list included pediatric dosage forms for 23 formulations plus one device [18].

The study included all formulations on the core- list but excluded Artemether+lumefantrine as it is used for treatment of malaria which is not prevalent in Mongolia. Alternative formulations were registered in Mongolia were added into the list of core medicines and were investigated. A total of 30 medicines and one device were surveyed in this study (Table 1).

The highest and lowest costs for each medicine were surveyed and brand or generic medicines were recorded. Medicines provided at public hospitals were procured by a general procurement (tender) process, therefore only the availability was recorded.

Data collection

Trained data collectors visited pharmacy outlets and collected information regarding the cost, availability using a standardized data collection form and data were entered into a pre-programmed MS Excel Workbook provided as a part of the WHO/ HAI methodology. Data collectors provided the pharmacy outlets with written documentation describing the requirements for participation in the study. It was made clear that they could refuse to take part or terminate participation at any time. A verbal consent from the study participants was obtained prior to data collection.

Availability of medicines

Availability of medicines was recorded on the day of data collection by the data collector and checked by the supervisor. Data collectors worked in pairs, visited selected medicine outlets, collected data and completed the Medicine Prices Data Collection Forms. A data entry person entered data from the hard copy Medicine Price Data Collection Forms into the electronic survey, and was responsible for data validation by running the double entry program to ensure accuracy. The Workbook's auto checker was also used to assist in the verification process.

Cross-country and international comparisons

Reference prices, developed by the Management Sciences for Health (MSH), were used to facilitate national and international comparisons as these were found to be the most useful standard [19].

Cost comparison was completed across the country and internationally, median prices were expressed as ratios relative to a standard set of international reference prices (Eq. 1):

Table 1 List of pediatric medicines surveyed in Mongolia

No.	Disease	Medicine	Formulation	Strength	Target size pack
1	Intestinal parasite	Albendazole	tablet	200 mg	2
2	Infectious disease	Amoxicillin	capsule	250 mg	10
	Infectious disease	Amoxicillin	suspension	125 mg	100 ml
3		Aminophyllin	injection	25 mg/ml	1 vial
4	Infectious disease	Amoxicillin_Clavulanic acid	tablet	125 mg + 125 mg, tab	10
	Infectious disease	Amoxicillin_Clavulanic acid	suspension	125 mg + 31.25 mg	100 ml
	Infectious disease	Amoxicillin_Clavulanic acid	suspension	250 mg + 62.50 mg	100 ml
5	Infectious disease	Azithromycin	capsule	250 mg	6
	Infectious disease	Azithromycin	suspension	200 mg/5 ml	100 ml
6	Asthma	Beclomethason	inhaler	50 mg/day	1 inhaler (200 doses)
7	Infectious disease	Benzylpenicillin	injection	600 mg = 1 million IU	1 vial
8	Seizure Disorder	Carbamazepine	tablet	100 mg	20
	Seizure Disorder	Carbamazepine	suspension	100 mg/5 ml	100 ml
9	Infectious disease	Cefazolin	injection	1 g, vial	1 vial
10	Infectious disease	Ceftriaxone	injection	500 mg vial	1 vial
11	Infectious disease	Chloramphenicol	tablet	250 mg	10
	Infectious disease	Chloramphenicol	injection	1 g, vial	1 vial
12	Infectious disease	Chlorpheniramine	tablet	4 mg	24
13	Infectious disease	Clarithromycin	suspension	125 mg/ 5 ml	100 ml
	Infectious disease	Clarithromycin	tablet	125 mg	10
14	Infectious disease	Cotrimoxazole	tablet	100 mg + 20 mg (also expressed as 400 mg + 80 mg)	10
	Infectious disease	Cotrimoxazole	suspension		100 ml
15	Seizure Disorder	Diazepam	tablet	5 mg	10
16	Anemia	Ferrous salt	suspension	30 mg/5 ml	100 ml
17	Fungal infection	Fluconazole	capsule	150 mg	6
18	Infectious disease	Gentamycin	injection	10 mg/ml	1 vial
19	Pain/inflammation	Ibuprofen	tablet	2 mg	24
	Pain/inflammation	Ibuprofen	suspension		100 ml
20	Tuberculosis	Isoniazide	tablet	100 mg	56
21	Pain	Morphine	tablet	10 mg	56
	Pain	Morphine	oral solution	10 mg/5 ml	100 ml
22	Dehydration	ORS	sachet	500 ml	1 sachet
23	Pain/inflammation	Paracetamol	tablet	250 mg	10
	Pain/inflammation	Paracetamol	suppository	125 mg	10
	Pain/inflammation	Paracetamol	suppository	250 mg	10
	Pain/inflammation	Paracetamol	suspension	125 mg	100 ml
24	Seizure Disorder	Phenobarbital	tablet	30 mg	10
	Seizure Disorder	Phenobarbital	injection	100 mg/ml	1 vial
25	Seizure Disorder	Phenytoin	tablet	50 mg,	90
	Seizure Disorder	Phenytoin	suspension	25 mg, 30 mg/5 ml	500 ml
26	Infectious disease	Procain penicillin	injection	1 g, vial	1 vial
27	Asthma	Salbutamol	inhaler	100mcg	1 inhaler (200 doses)
28	Xerophthalmia	Vitamin A	capsule	100.000 IU	50
29	Anemia	Vitamin B6	injection	50 mg/ml	1 vial
30	Dehydration	Zinc	tablet	20 mg	14
31	Spacer	Device			

$$\textit{Median Price Ratio} = \textit{median local unit price} / \textit{international reference unit price} \quad (1)$$

The exchange rate used to calculate MPRs was 1 USD = 1988.5 Mongolian tugrigs as of the first day of data collection [20].

Affordability

As defined by the WHO, affordability is estimated using the daily wage of the lowest-paid unskilled government worker by determining the number of days' wages required to purchase selected courses of treatment for various conditions [18]. For the study, a total of seven conditions causing high pediatric mortality and morbidity in Mongolia and commonly used medicines were selected. These were; respiratory infections, urinary tract infections, otitis media, infections due to susceptible organisms, pneumonia, asthma, dehydration, pain and inflammation, seizure disorder and xerophthalmia. Treatment duration was defined as a full course of therapy for acute conditions whereas a supply of 30 days treatment duration was considered for chronic diseases [21].

Results

Availability of medicines on the day of data collection

There was a variation in availability of specific drugs however, a similar result was observed between the public and private sectors. The average availability of medicines was 72.6% in the public sector (range (9.1–100%). Correspondingly, the average availability of all selected medicines in the private sector was 76.7% (range 26.7–100%) (Fig. 1).

Public and private sector patient coats

The lowest cost medicines were investigated and they were 1.95 times higher than the international reference price in the public sector. Generally, the lowest cost medicines were sold at 2.45 times higher than the international reference cost in the private sector. About one third of the medicines were costed at 1.85 (25 percentile) to 2.52 (75 percentile) times the international reference cost in the private sector with moderate cost variations existing across the sector (Table 2).

Affordability of standard treatment regimens

Affordability of standard treatment regimens recommended by the WHO were analyzed for selected pediatric medicines. Lowest cost medicines in the private sector were less affordable than in the public sector for most conditions. As indicated in Table 3, lowest cost medicines in the public sector were more affordable for all conditions, with standard treatment costing a day's wage or more. The least affordable treatment was estimated to be for respiratory tract infections or otitis media requiring amoxicillin clavulanic acid, suspension costing up to 1. 03 days wages (Table 3).

Discussion

The study has evaluated the availability and affordability of essential pediatric medicines in Mongolia. The average availability of essential pediatric medicines was relatively good being on average over 70% in both sectors. Inconsistent and higher costs and lower affordability of medicines was found in the private sector. Pediatric formulations recommended in the WHO EMLc, including beclomethasone- inhaler [1], carbamazepine- suspension [1], diazepam-rectal solution [1], chloramphenicol –

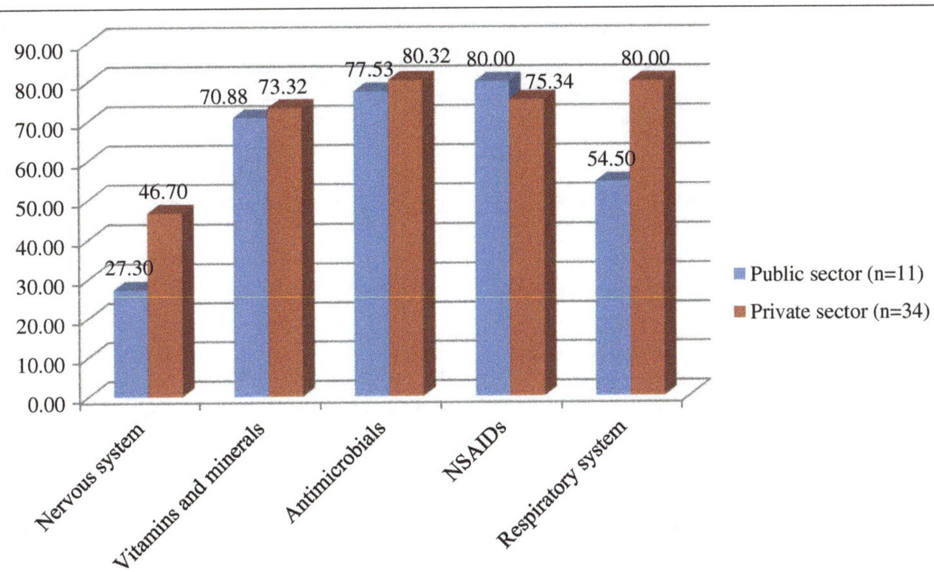

Fig. 1 Average availability of the lowest cost medicines in the public and private sectors

Table 2 Public and private sector patient prices

Medicine	Formulation	Target size pack	Lowest price medicines MPR (25th -75th percentile)	
			Public sector	Private sector
Albendazole	Tablet, 200 mg	2	3.83 (3.83–5.74)	3.83 (3.83–31.91)
Amoxicillin	Capsule, 250 mg	10	0.18 (0.17–0.34)	0.17(0.17–0.18)
Amoxicillin	Suspension, 125 mg	100 ml	2.51 (2.51–3.56)	4.19 (2.51–4.47)
Aminophyllin	Injection, 25 mg/ml	1 vial	–	–
Amoxicillin_Clavulanic acid	Tablet, 125 mg + 125 mg, tab	10	3.18 (3.01–3.26)	5.65 (3.51–5.65)
Amoxicillin_Clavulanic acid	Suspension, 125 mg + 31.25 mg	100 ml	2.03 (1.85–2.40)	4.59 (1.85–4.59)
Amoxicillin_Clavulanic acid	Suspension, 250 mg + 62.50 mg	100 ml	3.75 (3.28–4.37)	3.28 (3.16–3.30)
Azithromycin	Capsule, 250 mg	6	1.81 (1.63–1.90)	1.41 (0.80–1.86)
Azithromycin	Suspension, 200 mg/5 ml	100 ml	2.84 (2.63–2.84)	3.13 (2.84–3.13)
Beclomethason	Inhaler, 50 mg/ day	1 inhaler (200 doses)	–	–
Benzylpenicillin	Injection, 600 mg = 1 million IU	1 vial	0.89 (0.82–0.93)	1.41 (0.80–1.90)
Carbamazepin	Tablet, 100 mg	20	2.26 (2.03–3.59)	3.61 (2.03–3.61)
Carbamazepin	Suspension, 100 mg/5 ml	100 ml		
Cefazolin	Injection, 1 g, vial	1 vial	1.37 (1.31–1.54)	1.31 (1.31–1.43)
Ceftriaxone	Injection, 500 mg vial	1 vial	1.14 (1.05–1.31)	1.32 (1.32–1.58)
Chloramphenicol	Tablet, 250 mg	10	2.10 (1.99–2.21)	2.10 (1.99–2.21)
Chloramphenicol	Injection,1 g, vial	1 vial		
Chlorpheniramine	Tablet, 4 mg	24	17.01 (17.01–17.75)	17.38 (17.01–19.23)
Clarithromycin	Suspension, 125 mg/ 5 ml	100 ml	1.14 (1.05–1.33)	1.33 (1.33–1.39)
Clarithromycin	Tablet, 125 mg	10	1.51 (1.34–2.51)	2.35 (2.22–2.51)
Cotrimexazol	Tablet, 100 mg + 20 mg or 400 mg + 80 mg	10	3.56 (3.56–3.86)	3.96 (3.56–11.48)
Cotrimexazol	Suspension, 40 mg/5 ml	100 ml	0.41 (0.38–0.42)	0.42 (0.38–0.42)
Diazepam	Tablet, 5 mg	10	2.25 (2.14–3.05)	3.21 (3.10–4.28)
Ferrous salt	Suspension, 30 mg/5 ml	100 ml	0.53 (0.51–0.55)	0.65 (0.59–0.69)
Fluconazole	Capsule, 150 mg	6	0.70 (0.70–0.73)	3.02 (0.70–3.91)
Gentamycin	Injection, 10 mg/ml	1 vial	0.59 (0.59–0.64)	0.59 (0.59–0.80)
Ibuprofen	Tablet, 2 mg	24	12.38 (11.73–12.38)	12.38 (10.42–14.66)
Ibuprofen	Suspension, 100 mg/5 ml	100 ml	3.75 (3.76–4.46)	4.46 (4.46–4.64)
Isoniazide	Tablet, 100 mg	56	–	–
Morphine	Tablet, 10 mg	56	–	–
Morphine	oral solution, 10 mg/5 ml	100 ml	–	–
ORS	Sachet, 500 ml	1 sachet	4.02 (2.51–5.03)	4.53 (4.15–5.53)
Paracetamol	Tablet, 250 mg	10	–	–
Paracetamol	Suppository, 125 mg	10	1.32 (1.32–1.43)	1.32 (1.32–1.43)
Paracetamol	Suppository, 250 mg	10	1.42 (1.42–1.53)	1.48 (1.42–1.53)
Paracetamol	Suspension, 125 mg/5 ml	100 ml	3.17 (3.07–6.40)	7.92 (3.26–7.92)
Phenobarbital	Tablet, 30 mg		–	–
Phenobarbital	Injection, 100 mg/ml	1 vial	–	–
Phenytoin	Tablet, 50 mg	90	–	–
Phenytoin	Suspension, 25 mg,30 mg/5 ml	500 ml	–	–
Procain penicillin	Injection, 1 g, vial	1 vial	0.06 (0.06–0.07)	0.08 (0.06–0.11)
Salbutamol	Inhaler, 100mcg	1 inhaler (200 doses)	2.26 (1.45–2.51)	2.51 (2.49–2.58)
Vitamin A	Capsule, 100.000 IU	50	1.60 (1.60–2.26)	2.45 (1.60–2.52)
Vitamin B6	Injection, 50 mg/ml	1 vial	0.14 (0.14–0.17)	0.17 (0.17–0.23)
Zinc	Tablet, 20 mg	14	1.95 (1.67–2.23)	2.08 (1.67–2.23)

Table 3 Affordability: Number of days' wages of the lowest paid government worker needed to purchase standard medications

Disease condition and 'standard' treatment			Day's wages to pay for treatment	
Condition	Drug name, strength, dosage form	Treatment schedule	LPM-Public sector	LPM-Private sector
Respiratory Tract Infections, UTIs	Amoxicllin Suspension 125 mg/5 ml	Child up to 10 years: 125 mg(=5 ml)x3x7 days = 105 ml	0.38	0.65
Respiratory Tract Infections, Otitis Media	Amoxicillin Clavulanic Acid Suspension 125–31.25 mg/5 ml	Child 1–6 years: 125 mg(=5 ml)x3x7 days = 105 ml	0.46	1.03
Respiratory Tract Infections, Otitis Media	Amoxicillin Clavulanic Acid Suspension 250–62.5 mg/5 ml	Child over 10 years: 250 mg(=5 ml)x3x7 days = 105 ml	0.85	1.00
Seizure Disorder	Carbamazepine tablet, 100 mg	Maintenance treatment: 5 mg/kg*18 kg*3*30 days = 8100 mg or 40.5 tablets for 1 month	0.34	0.54
Infections due to Susceptible Organisms	Ceftriaxone 500 mg vial	Child under 50 kg: Maximum 1 g dailyx7 days = 7 g or 14 vials	0.11	0.15
Infections due to Susceptible Organisms	Sulfamethoxazole+Trimethoprim (400 mg + 80 mg)	18kgx4 mg/kg = 72 mg TMPx2x7days = 1008 mg.126 ml or 12.6 tablets total for 7 days	0.09	0.30
Dehydration	Oral Rehydration Solution, powder to make 500 ml	Moderate Dehydration; 75 ml/kgx18kg = 1350 ml	0.06	0.12
Pneumonia	Amoxicllin Suspension 125 mg/5 ml	Child up to 10 years: 125 mg(=5 ml)x3x7 days = 105 ml	0.38	0.65
Pain/inflammation	Paracetamol Suspension 24 mg/ml	5 year old child: 15 mg/kgx18kgx4x3 = 3240 mg = (130 mL)	0.28	0.28
Pain/inflammation	Ibuprofen suspension	5 year old child: 15 mg/kgx18kgx4x3 = 3240 mg = (130 mL)	0.67	0.79
Asthma	Salbutamol inhaler 100 mcg/dose	1 inhaler 200 doses	0.38	0.65
Xerophthalmia	Vitamin A 50,000 units	Child 1–12 years: 200,000 units × 3 doses	0.12	0.18

*LPM- Lowest Price Medicine

injection [1], isoniazid- scored tablet [1], morphine-oral solution [1], phenobarbital -injection [1], phenytoin- chewable tablet [1] spacer- device [1] were not assessable, because they are not registered and unavailable in Mongolia. Similarly, lack of appropriate dosage formulations for phenobarbital, phenytoin, carbamazepine, diazepam (rectal solution) were reported in a study at a tertiary care hospital with 2000 beds, in Western India [22].

This identifies a lack of some child friendly formulations available which could be related to the difficulty of obtaining the product if it was not locally manufactured. A study has assessed the availability of essential pediatric medicines in China and reported that a dearth of registered pediatric medicines may be attributed to multiple factors including the manufacturers' lack of motivation to produce because of low demand or small profit, less effective bidding and procurement systems for pediatric medicines, hospitals' preferences for higher-priced medicines, inappropriate drug selection and weak health and supply systems [15, 23]. Additionally, insufficient knowledge or application of clinical standards and protocols [24], and exclusion from central procurement lists due to high cost may be other reasons for unavailability [25].

Amongst the surveyed medicines, originator brands were rarely available in both sectors, mainly due to high cost and the Government's effort to improve and promote the use of generic medicines in Mongolia [5]. The study results were consistent with previous studies assessing availability and affordability of essential medicines for adults [13, 16, 26–28]. These studies have shown that availability was lower in the public sector when compared to the private pharmacies.

Lack of child friendly formulations was observed in this study. Chloramphenicol injection, morphine, beclomethasone were not available in two sectors. According to other studies, similar findings have been reported [23, 29]. Medicines to treat seizure disorders (phenobarbital, phenytoin) and pain (morphine) were not found in any of the surveyed pharmacy outlets. This is due to the legislation restricting the use of narcotic and psychotropic drugs [4], only a few pharmacy outlets with special permission are eligible to stock them.

Diseases of the digestive system, including diarrhea was one of the main reasons for pediatric mortality and morbidity in Mongolia. Oral rehydration powders were available in most of pharmacy outlets in both sectors. However, dispersible tablets of Zinc as recommended in the EMLc, were available in only half of the surveyed sites (50.6%). Evidence based data suggest that zinc is beneficial for treatment of pediatric diarrhea for children aged 6 months or older [30].

Paracetamol (acetaminophen) has a unique role in children because it is the first-line choice for the treatment of both fever and pain. When used in the recommended doses, it has few side effects and is remarkably well tolerated [31]. However, the recommended pediatric dose tablet was not available in any of the surveyed pharmacies. Instead, dispensers (pharmacist or pharmacy technician) would dispense adult dose tablet (500 mg) and advise to cut the tablet into half when a pediatric dose was prescribed. Clinical data proves that in overdose, paracetamol is hepatotoxic [31].

The affordability of lowest cost medicines was compared across the country. The pediatric essential medicines were generally less affordable in the private sector and costed more than the recommended international reference prices.

Mongolia is country with seasonal variations, with winter being very long and harsh. During this time, most pediatric conditions are associated with respiratory infections. Pneumonia and other respiratory infections are reported to be the main reason for children's hospitalization in Mongolia [3]. Empiric treatment with appropriate antibiotics for respiratory infections, including pneumonia is crucial in the reduction of mortality from pneumonia [32]. Treatment of pneumonia with amoxicillin suspension would cost more than a half day's wage, whereas for other respiratory infections (otitis media), the cost of treatment would be 1 day's wage.

When compared to other countries, this result is comparably low [29]. Considering the fact that 14% of Mongolians live on less than USD 1 per day [2], treatments seem to be too expensive. On the other hand, treatment cost reflects medicines cost only, excluding any additional consultation or diagnostic costs. Additionally, treatment was estimated only for one child, indicating that families with more children and their treatment would endure an overwhelming cost. Similar to previous findings, essential medicines are often not affordable for many populations [13, 16, 27, 33].

Limitations

The study has several limitations that are consistent with previous surveys. The WHO/HAI methodology did not assess the therapeutic alternatives or alternative dosage forms. The study results reflect the status of availability and cost based on the day of data collection. They do not necessarily reflect the monthly or yearly availability of essential pediatric medicines at the national level or individual pharmacy outlets. In addition, the median cost ratio was estimated using the supplier cost. Although, when the supplier cost was not available, buyer costs were used to calculate the median international reference cost. Substituting the supplier with buyer cost could result in inaccurate prices and therefore influence the true median price [15].

On the other hand, the study has utilized a previously validated methodology using a standardized way to evaluate the availability and costs of essential pediatric medicines in the country [34]. Furthermore, training and using multiple checkpoints have improved the quality of data collection, data entry and interpretation.

Conclusion

The findings of this study can serve as basic data to develop and revise the National Policy in order to improve the accessibility and availability of essential pediatric medicines in Mongolia. Furthermore, control, monitoring and comparing pediatric medicines costs not just across the country but also at the international level would help to increase transparency of different tasks including registration, procurement and reimbursement decision making procedures. A detailed investigation regarding the prescribing of pediatric medicines should be completed to identify the challenges and barriers. Finally, the procurement, supply and distribution of essential pediatric medicines needs to be examined in order to identify the lack of availability and higher costs of some essential pediatric medicines in Mongolia.

Abbreviations

DRF: Drug Revolving Fund; EMLc: The Essential Medicines List for Children; GDP: Gross Domestic Product; HAI: Health Action International; IRP: International Reference Price; MDG: Millennium Development Goals; NDPM: National Drug Policy of Mongolia; NEDL: National Essential Drug List; NSAID: Non steroidal anti-inflammatory drugs; WHO: World Health Organization

Acknowledgements

Authors would like to acknowledge all pharmacists consenting to participate as well as Dr. Marg Ewen, Health Action International, who provided necessary materials for data collection and analysis.

Authors' contributions

GD, BS, TS, BG - conceived of the study, and participated in its design and coordination and helped to draft the manuscript. All authors have read and approved the manuscript.

Competing interests

We declare that there was no funding for publication of this manuscript and we have no financial or non-financial competing interests.

Author details

[1]School of Pharmacy and Biomedicine, Mongolian National University of Medical Sciences, S.Zorig Street, Ulaanbaatar 14210, Mongolia. [2]School of Pharmacy, Bentley, Curtin University, GPO Box U1987, Bentley, WA 6845, Australia. [3]School of Public Health, Mongolian National University of Medical Sciences, S. Zorig Street, Ulaanbaatar 14210, Mongolia.

References

1. National Statistics Office of Mongolia. National Statistics Office of Mongolia.,, 2016.
2. World Bank. Poverty Rate in Mongolia Estimated at 29.6 Percent. 2016. Available from http://www.worldbank.org/en/news/press-release/2017/10/17/2016-poverty-rate-in-mongolia-estimated-at-296-percent.
3. Health Development Centre of Mongolia. Health indicators of Mongolia 2014.
4. Ministry of Health Mongolia. The drugs act of Mongolia 1998.
5. Ministry of Health Mongolia. National Drug Policy of Mongolia, 2014.
6. Ariuntuya S, Narantuya Kh, Davaajargal S, Enkhjargal TS, Unurtsetseg T. Health Indicators of Mongolia 2014. Ulaanbaatar Mongolia Health Department of Mongolia.
7. World Health Organization. Priority life-saving medicines for women and children. Geneva: WHO; 2012. Available.

8. Murray CJ, Laakso T, Shibuya K, Hill K, Lopez AD. Can we achieve millennium development goal 4? New analysis of country trends and forecasts of under-5 mortality to 2015. Lancet. 2007;370(9592): 1040–54. Available.
9. World Health Organization. Make medicines child size, 2010.
10. World Health Organization. Promoting rational use of medicines: Core components, 1977.
11. Ministry of Health Mongolia. The National Essential Drug List of Mongolia (7th revision) 2014.
12. Ministry of Health and Sports Mongolia. Pharmaceutical sector indicators of Mongolia, 2014.
13. Munkhdelger Ch. Medicine Prices, Availability, Affordability and Price Components in Mongolia. 2013 [cited 1st of April]. Available from: http://haiweb.org/wp-content/uploads/2015/07/Mongolia-Report-Pricing-Surveys.pdf.
14. World Health Organization. Health Action International. Medicine prices: a new approach to measurement. Working draft for field testing and revision. WHO/EDM/PAR/2003.2), 2003. Available from: http://www.haiweb.org/medicineprices/manual/manuals/MedicinePrices.pdf; 2003.
15. Cameron A, Ewen M, Ross-Degnan D, Ball D, Laing R. Medicine prices, availability, and affordability in 36 developing and middle-income countries: a secondary analysis. Lancet. 2009;373(9659):240–9. Available.
16. Cameron A, Roubos I, Ewen M, Mantel-Teeuwisse AK, Leufkens HG, Laing RO. Differences in the availability of medicines for chronic and acute conditions in the public and private sectors of developing countries. Bull World Health Organ. 2011;89:412–21. Available.
17. Ministry of Health Mongolia. Health indicators of Mongolia 2015.
18. World Health Organization. Overview of methods for medicines availability and pricing surveys: better medicines for children project., 2009.
19. Management Sciences for Health. International drug price Indicator 2003.
20. State Bank of Mongolia. Currency exchange rate 2016.
21. Health Action International: World Health Organization. Meassuring medicine prices, availability, affordability and price components., 2002.
22. Desai M, Jain K, Shah S, Dikshit R. Availability of pediatric medicines and their perception among prescribers at a tertiary care teaching hospital. Available; 2012.
23. Chen W, Tang S, Sun J, Ross-Degnan D, Wagner AK. Availability and use of essential medicines in China: manufacturing, supply, and prescribing in Shandong and Gansu provinces. BMC Health Serv Res. 2010;10(1):1. Available.
24. Chisholm D, David B. Evans. Improving health system e ciency as a means of moving towards universal coverage, 2010.
25. Robertson J, Forte G, Trapsida J-M, Hill S. What essential medicines for children are on the shelf? Bull World Health Organ. 2009;87(3):231–7. Available.
26. Anson A, Ramay B, de Esparza AR, Bero L. Availability, prices and affordability of the World Health Organization's essential medicines for children in Guatemala. Glob Health. 2012;8(1):22. Available.
27. Mendis S, Fukino K, Cameron A, Laing R, Filipe Jr A, Khatib O, et al. The availability and affordability of selected essential medicines for chronic diseases in six low-and middle-income countries. Bull World Health Organ. 2007;85(4):279–88. Available.
28. van Mourik MS, Cameron A, Ewen M, Laing RO. Availability, price and affordability of cardiovascular medicines: a comparison across 36 countries using WHO/HAI data. BMC Cardiovasc Disord. 2010;10(1):25. Available.
29. Anson A, Ramay B, de Esparza AR, Bero L. Availability, prices and affordability of the World Health Organization's essential medicines for children in Guatemala. Glob Health. 2012;8(1):1. Available.
30. Lazzerini M, Ronfani L. Oral zinc for treating diarrhoea in children. The Cochrane Library. 2008; Available.
31. Cranswick N, Coghlan D. Paracetamol efficacy and safety in children: the first 40 years. Am J Ther. 2000;7(2):135–42. Available.
32. World Health Organization. Technical bases for the WHO recommendations on the management of pneumonia in children at first-level health facilities. 1991; Available.
33. Niëns LM, Cameron A, Van de Poel E, Ewen M, Brouwer WB, Laing R. Quantifying the impoverishing effects of purchasing medicines: a cross-country comparison of the affordability of medicines in the developing world. PLoS Med. 2010;7(8):e1000333. Available.
34. Madden JM, Meza E, Ewen M, Laing RO, Stephens P, Ross-Degnan D. Measuring medicine prices in Peru: validation of key aspects of WHO/HAI survey methodology. Rev Panam Salud Publica. 2010;27(4):291–9. Available.

24

A case report of parapneumonic pleural effusion caused by *Streptococcus pneumoniae* serotype 19A in a child immunized with 13-valent conjugate pneumococcal vaccine

Idrissa Diawara[1,2*], Khalid Zerouali[1,2], Naima Elmdaghri[1,2,3] and Abderrahman Abid[4]

Abstract

Background: Simple parapneumonic effusion is a pleural effusion associated with lung infection (i.e., pneumonia). *Streptococcus pneumoniae* remains the most common pathogen causing parapneumonic effusions. In Morocco, the pneumococcal conjugate vaccine 13-valent (PCV13) was introduced in the national immunization program in October 2010 in 2 + 1 schedule for prevention of pneumococcal disease, and replaced by the PCV10 in July 2012 in the same schedule. We report a case of parapneumonic pleural effusions caused by *S. pneumoniae* serotype 19A in a child immunized with 3 doses of PCV13.

Case presentation: This is a 2.5 years old previously healthy Moroccan female, fully vaccinated by PCV13 and immunocompetent, admitted to a private medical clinic with a six months history of persistent asthma. On arrival (7 February 2015), she was febrile to 40.3 °C with a brutal flu syndrome, chills, dry cough and serous rhinitis, for which she received symptomatic treatment. A biological assessment was done that confirmed the clinical diagnosis of flu. Seven days after, she presented a progressive deterioration of its general condition and the onset of severe abdominal pain. She was hospitalized and a second biological assessment, computed tomography scans and chest radiography were done that confirmed a diagnosis of a pneumococcal parapneumonia with abscess of the left lower lobe with encysted empyema. Microbiological analysis of the pleural fluid showed a *S. pneumoniae* serotype 19A with susceptibility intermediate to penicillin. The patient was treated by antibiotics including amoxicillin, cefixime ceftriaxone and vancomycin.

Conclusions: We reported a case of parapneumonic pleural effusions caused by a vaccine serotype pneumococcal 19A occurring in an immunocompetent child immunized with 3 doses of PCV13.

Keywords: *Streptococcus pneumoniae*, Serotype 19A, Parapneumonic effusion, Pneumococcal conjugate vaccine 13-valent

* Correspondence: diawaraidris@gmail.com
[1]Laboratoire de Microbiologie, Faculté de Médecine et de Pharmacie, Hassan II University of Casablanca, B.P 5696 Casablanca, Morocco
[2]Service de Microbiologie, CHU Ibn Rochd, B.P 2698 Casablanca, Morocco

Background

Simple parapneumonic effusion is defined as pleural effusion associated with lung infection (i.e., pneumonia). Indeed, parapneumonic pleural effusion is a complicated state that occurs subsequently in community-acquired pneumonia. This Complication often necessitates drainage and is associated with prolonged hospitalization [1]. *Streptococcus pneumoniae* remains the most common pathogen causing parapneumonic effusions [2]. In Morocco, the PCV13 was introduced in the national immunization program in October 2010 in 2 + 1 schedule for prevention of pneumococcal disease caused by vaccine serotypes, such as 4, 6B, 9 V, 14, 18C, 19F, 23F (included in PCV7) plus 1, 3, 5, 6A, 7F and 19A. The PCV13 was replaced by the PCV10 in July 2012. Before the PCV introduction, serotypes included in PCV10 and PCV13 covered 71.6 and 82.4% of serotypes associated with IPD among children under five years of age in Casablanca, respectively [3]. However, pneumococcal pneumonia in children or adult is not documented in Morocco. Reports of vaccine failure from PCV13 have been documented most frequently for serotype 3 causing parapneumonic effusion. We reported a case of parapneumonic pleural effusion caused by *S. pneumoniae* serotype 19A in a child immunized with 3 doses of PCV13.

Case presentation

A 2.5 years old previously healthy Moroccan female was admitted to a private medical clinic with an antecedent of six months of persistent asthma that was controlled by inhaled corticosteroid therapy. On admission at the private medical clinic (7 February 2015), she was febrile to 40.3 °C with a brutal flu syndromes: chills, dry cough and serous rhinitis, for which she received symptomatic treatment, comprising bed rest and paracetamol. Moreover, she had no dyspnoea, wheezing or crackles on auscultation. After four days, she presented the same symptoms, and a biological assessment was done that confirmed the clinical diagnosis of flu: her white blood cell count was 9540 cells/mm^3 with 69.7% neutrophils, hemoglobin at 11 g/dL, platelet count at 288,000/mm^3, C-reactive protein (CRP) was 2.3 mg/L. After seven days, she presented a progressive deterioration of her general conditions and the onset of severe abdominal pain that led to the hospitalization and a second biological assessment was done. According to this biological assessment, her white blood cell count was 17,090 cells/mm^3 with 85% neutrophils, hemoglobin at 11.1 g/dL, platelet count at 338,000/mm^3 and the CRP was elevated at 319.28 mg/L. The abdominal-pelvic ultrasound performed in a context of abdominal pain showed no abnormality. A specialized Otorhinolaryngologic examination established the diagnosis of bilateral acute otitis media (AOM), but the child did not complain of earaches and showed no ear discharge. A Treatment with ceftriaxone at 100 mg/kg/day for 3 days was started. On the third day of this treatment, she became afebrile and she left the clinic with the diagnosis of AOM and the treatment of ceftriaxone was replaced by cefixime per os at 8 mg/kg/day every 12 h for four days. At home, because she developed once again a rapid fever, cefixime was replaced by amoxicillin/clavulanate at 80 mg/kg/day every 8 h for seven days, but this changing did not provide any favourable clinical result. However, chest radiography of front that was made in these hospital records was initially misinterpreted and was wrongly considered as normal. Thereafter, an extensive analysis of this first chest radiograph showed an opacity of the left thoracic base, erasing the totality of diaphragmatic cupola and filling the pleural cul-de-sac with a pleural band of 1 cm thick (Fig. 1). Moreover, the child has begun having evident difficulties to breath with a chest pain, dyspnoea and expiratory moaning. A second chest radiography was performed after thirteenth day of disease. The result of this radiography rectified the diagnosis and showed an excavated pneumonia in the lower left lobe with a pleural effusion of 3 cm thick (Fig. 2). Finally, a chest computed tomography scan confirmed the diagnosis of abscess pneumonia with empyema (Fig. 3).

After 23rd day of the disease, the absence of apyrexia despite amoxicillin/clavulanate treatment and the need to identify the etiologic agent, the child was re-hospitalized and a pleural puncture under general anaesthesia was performed at two intercostal spaces (5th axillary and 6th posterior). The 5th pleural space allowed to withdraw more than 6 mL of pus and sent to the laboratory for analysis.

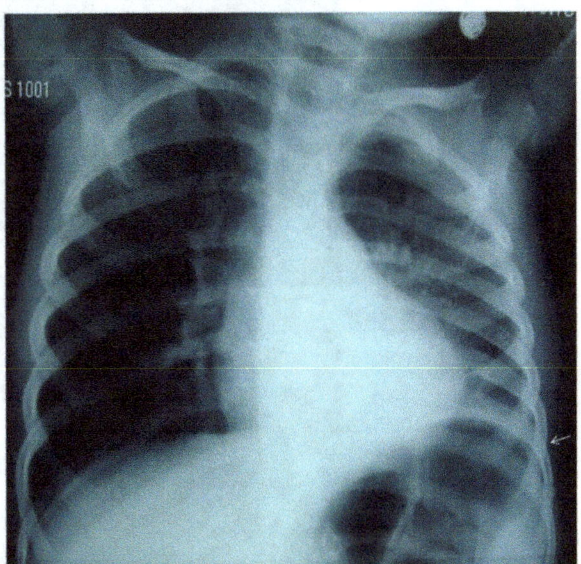

Fig. 1 Chest radiograph showed opacity of the left rib base (see *arrow*), erasing the totality of the diaphragmatic cupola filling the pleural cul-de-sac with a pleural band

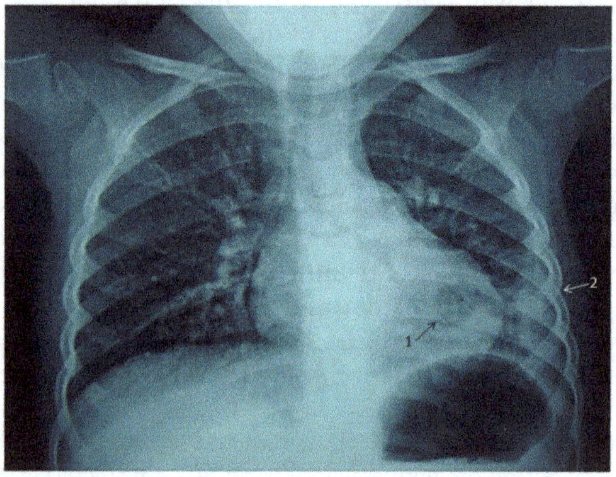

Fig. 2 Excavated pneumonia in the lower left lobe (*arrow 1*) with a pleural effusion of 3 cm thick (*arrow 2*)

Laboratory analysis was performed at the Microbiology Laboratory of Ibn Rochd University Hospital Centre of Casablanca. This analysis showed a diplococci positive Gram in direct examination and bacterial culture revealed the presence of *S. pneumoniae*. Serogrouping was done by the checkerboard method with Pneumotest-latex (Statens Serum Institute antisera, Copenhague, Denmark) and serotyping was performed by Quellung capsule swelling using Statens Serum Institute antisera (Copenhague, Denmark). These methods of serogrouping/serotyping classified the serotype as 19A. Antibiotic susceptibility testing was done following the Clinical Laboratory Standard Institute guidelines (CLSI, 2015). Erythromycin, tetracycline, choramphenicol, vancomycin, levofloxacin, rifampicin and cotrimoxazole were tested by disk diffusion; penicillin and ceftriaxone by E-test on Mueller Hinton Agar supplemented with 5% sheep blood. The strain was susceptible to vancomycin, chloramphenicol, rifampicin and levofloxacin; intermediate susceptibility to tetracycline, ceftriaxone (MIC = 2 μg/mL) and penicillin (MIC = 4 μg/mL); and resistant to erythromycin, and cotrimoxazole. Quality control of antibiotic susceptibility testing was conducted using *S. pneumoniae* ATCC 49619.

The final diagnosis of the disease was a pneumococcal pneumonia with abscess of the left lower lobe with encysted empyema: a pneumococcal parapneumonic pleural effusion. The treatment with amoxicillin/clavulanate was stopped and replaced by ceftriaxone at 100 mg/kg/day by slow intravenous injection and vancomycin 60 mg/kg/day by continuous infusion. After 10 days of these treatments, she continued as outpatients with ceftriaxone in the same doses and teicoplanin by slow intravenous injection in a single dose by day. After eight days of these treatments, she was apyretic, her white blood cell count was 4420 cells/mm^3 with 15% neutrophils, hemoglobin at 10.7 g/dL, platelet count at 308,000/mm^3, and CRP was normal at 0.6 mg/L. The

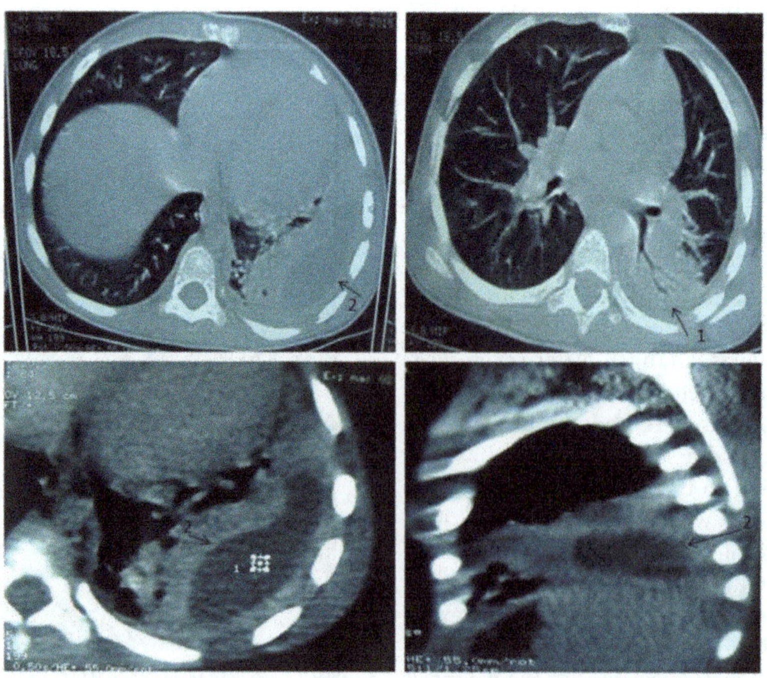

Fig. 3 Computed tomography scans of the chest showing a significant parenchymal condensation and shrinking of the left basal pyramid (*narrow 1*) with fluid collection of the convex, suggesting a pleural empyema on the left (*narrow 2*)

pneumonia was completely treated as showed on chest radiography (Fig. 4). After two weeks (24 march 2015), antibiotic treatments were stopped.

The examination of her vaccine status showed that she received PCV13 vaccine at 2 months of age, 4 months of age and the third dose at 12 months of age (2 + 1 doses). The development of IPD despite the complete vaccination, led us to undertake an immune deficiency evaluation three months after the disease (on June). This assessment revealed that the total classic complement pathway screen was within normal range and Immunoglobulin (Ig) Gamma and its subclasse, IgA and IgM levels were normal. Furthermore, she has not presented any high risk for invasive *S. pneumoniae* disease in children included chronic heart disease (particularly cyanotic congenital heart disease and cardiac failure); diabetes mellitus; cerebrospinal fluid leak; cochlear implant; sickle cell disease and other hemoglobinopathies; anatomic or functional asplenia; HIV infection; chronic renal failure and nephrotic syndrome.

Discussion

In a previous study, we reported data about IPD from children less than five years of age in Casablanca [4]. We showed that after vaccine implementation, the main IPD that affected children were meningitis, bacteremia and some rare cases of pleural infections. The examination of vaccine status showed that 40% of vaccine serotypes were isolated from children who received at least one dose of PCV10 or PCV13 in Casablanca. Vaccination schedule was incomplete for all vaccine failures described in this last study [4]. Furthermore, the replacement of PCV13 by PCV10 vaccine in the Moroccan NIP could affect serotype distribution at national scale, because PCV10 does not contain serotypes 3, 6A and 19A. Elsewhere, Vaccine coverage of PCVs vaccines in children aged to 2 years of age was estimated to 88% at the Grand Casablanca in 2014 as declared by the observatory regional of epidemiology service of health of Casablanca. In the present case report, we reported a pneumococcal parapneumonia in a child that previously presented a flu infection associated with an AOM. Influenza infections can make some people more susceptible to develop bacterial pneumonia. *S. pneumoniae* is the most common cause of this bacterial pneumonia among children. Pneumococcal infections can be a serious complication of seasonal influenza infections [5].

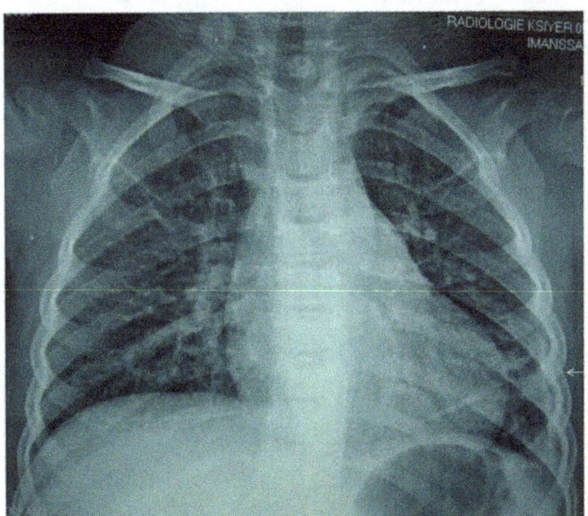

Fig. 4 Chest radiograph showing the cleaning of pneumonia and empyema (see *arrow*)

Pneumococcal infections are mainly caused by the colonizing serotypes and are therefore more susceptible to develop antibiotic resistance [6]. Moreover, antibiotic pressure has a continuing role in increasing pneumococcal resistant strains in respiratory infections. Pneumococcal serotype 19A remains a redoubtable serotype because of its clinical implication of pneumococcal disease and its ability to develop higher level of antibiotics resistance [7].

As for the diagnosis of flu, it was based mainly on clinical diagnosis because the child presented the majors clinical symptoms of flu and the first biological assessment showed no sign of inflammation in favour of bacterial infection.

Concerning the management of empyema, in most cases, it is managed by drainage [8]. For the case presented here, due to the low abundance of pus in the empyema, we did not practice the pleural drainage. We adopted the strategy of the use of antibiotic therapy alone without drainage, nor early decortications. The persistence of fever for more than 10 days remains for us a classical data in a context of empyema of the child.

Parapneumonic effusion and empyema are disease processes that evolve over time and involve different management strategies [8]. To prevent pneumococcal diseases, WHO recommended the inclusion of PCVs in childhood immunization programmes worldwide [9]. Surveillance after the introduction of a PCV to the standard childhood immunization schedule demonstrated that the vaccines were effective in preventing IPD and providing herd immunity [10]. In the United States after the introduction of PCV to the standard childhood immunization schedule, the overall rate of pneumococcal pneumonia has declined but the absolute number of cases of complicated pneumococcal pneumonia and the proportion of invasive pneumococcal disease caused by pneumonia had increased [11].

Pneumococcal antibody titers vary over time, even in healthy subjects. With the change of vaccine strategy, waning coverage can occur for serotypes that not include in the new vaccine. Vaccine failure has been reported in fully immunized children, due to serotype 3 in the parapneumonic pleural effusion context after 3 + 1 doses of PCV13 [12], but also serotype 19A in bacteremic pneumococcal pneumonia after 3 + 1 doses PCV13 [13]. There are currently no reports of PCV13 failure in preventing complicated pneumonia caused by serotype 19A among children vaccinated with the full 2 + 1 schedule. These reported cases highlighted that pneumococcal serotypes can differ in their abilities to colonize the nasopharynx, and in whether they are likely to cause invasive disease once they do colonization. The serotypes can differ also in what disease manifestations (e.g., conjunctivitis, otitis media, pneumonia, bacteremia, or meningitis) they are more likely to cause and with what complication, whether they are likely to be resistant to antimicrobial agents or to escape vaccination, where they are most predominant geographically [7].

It is typical when describing vaccine failures, to verify whether or not the PCV13 was administered correctly with the correct formulation, no storage issues with the doses, on the correct dates according to the child's age. According to the information provided by the paediatrician who vaccinated the child, the three doses of PCV13 have been correctly administered in the antero-external face of the thigh. Moreover, the vaccine complied with the recommended cold chain.

A potential limitation of this case report is that we were not able to determine the pneumococcal serotype 19A IgG level for the patient during her illness and after disease.

Conclusions

This is the first documented case of parapneumonic pleural effusions caused by vaccine serotype 19A occurring in an immunocompetent child immunized with 3 doses of PCV13. Further surveillance is necessary to see how the effectiveness of PCV10 vaccine will reduce IPD caused by non-PCV10 vaccine serotypes.

Abbreviations

AOM: Acute otitis media; CRP: C-reactive protein; IPD: Invasive pneumococcal disease; MIC: Minimum inhibitory concentration; PCV10: Pneumococcal conjugate vaccine 10-valent; PCV13: Pneumococcal conjugate vaccine 13-valent; PCV7: Pneumococcal conjugate vaccine 7-valent

Acknowledgements

The authors thank Prof. Houria Belabbes, Department of Microbiology, Faculty of Medicine and Pharmacy, Casablanca, Morocco and Dr. Katfy Khalid, Bacteriology-Virology and Hospital Hygiene Laboratory, University Hospital Centre Ibn Rochd of Casablanca, Morocco for their assistance.

Funding

No funding was obtained for this study.

Authors' contributions

NE and AA are responsible for general conception and design, coordinated and helped to draft the manuscript. AA and ID carried out the analysis are responsible for data collection. They performed interpretation of clinical data and drafted the manuscript. KZ and AA are responsible for the final approval of the article. All authors read and approved the final manuscript.

Competing interests

The authors declare that they have no competing interests.

Author details

[1]Laboratoire de Microbiologie, Faculté de Médecine et de Pharmacie, Hassan II University of Casablanca, B.P 5696 Casablanca, Morocco. [2]Service de Microbiologie, CHU Ibn Rochd, B.P 2698 Casablanca, Morocco. [3]Institut Pasteur du Maroc, 1 Louis Pasteur place, Casablanca, Morocco. [4]Service des Maladies Infectieuses Pédiatriques, Hôpital d'Enfants Abderrahim Harouchi, CHU Ibn Rochd, Casablanca, Morocco.

References

1. Resti M, Moriondo M, Cortimiglia M, et al. Italian Group for the Study of Invasive Pneumococcal Disease. Community-acquired bacteremic pneumococcal pneumonia in children: diagnosis and serotyping by real-time polymerase chain reaction using blood samples. Clin Infect Dis. 2010;51:1042–9.
2. Li ST, Tancredi DJ. Empyema hospitalizations increased in US children despite pneumococcal conjugate vaccine. Pediatrics. 2010;125:26.
3. Elmdaghri N, Benbachir M, Belabbes H, Zaki B, Benzaid H. Changing epidemiology of pediatric *Streptococcus pneumoniae* isolates before vaccine introduction in Casablanca (Morocco). Vaccine. 2012;30(Suppl 6):G46–50.
4. Diawara I, Zerouali K, Katfy K, Zaki B, Belabbes H, Najib J, Elmdaghri N. Invasive pneumococcal disease among children younger than 5 years of age before and after introduction of pneumococcal conjugate vaccine in Casablanca, Morocco. Int J Infect Dis. 2015;40:95–101.
5. Dawood FS, Fiore A, Kamimoto L, Nowell M, Reingold A, Gershman K, Meek J, Hadler J, Arnold KE, Ryan P, Lynfield R, Morin C, Baumbach J, Zansky S, Bennett NM, Thomas A, Schaffner W, Kirschke D, Finelli L. Emerging Infections Program (EIP) Network. Influenza-associated pneumonia in children hospitalized with laboratory-confirmed influenza, 2003-2008. Pediatr Infect Dis J. 2010;29(7):585–90.
6. Simell B, Auranen K, Kayhty H, Goldblatt D, Dagan R, O'Brien KL. The fundamental link between pneumococcal carriage and disease. Expert Rev Vaccines. 2012;11:841–55.
7. Hausdorff WP, Brueggemann AB, Hackell JG, Scott JAG. Pneumococcal Serotype Epidemiology. In: Siber GR, Klugman KP, Mäkelä PH, editors. Pneumococal Vaccines. Washington DC: ASM press; 2008. p. 139–60.
8. Jaffé A, Balfour-Lynn IM. Management of empyema in children. Pediatr Pulmonol. 2005;40:148.
9. World Health Organization (b). Pneumococcal conjugate vaccine for childhood immunization-WHO position paper. Wkly Epidemiol Rec. 2012;87:129–44.
10. Harboe ZB, Dalby T, Weinberger DM, et al. Impact of 13-valent pneumococcal conjugate vaccination in invasive pneumococcal disease incidence and mortality. Clin Infect Dis. 2014;59:1066.
11. Grijalva CG, Nuorti JP, Zhu Y, Griffin MR. Increasing incidence of empyema complicating childhood community-acquired pneumonia in the United States. Clin Infect Dis. 2010;50:805.
12. Antachopoulos C, Tsolia MN, Tzanakaki G, Xirogianni A, Dedousi O, Markou G, Zografou SM, Eliades A, Kirvassilis F, Kesanopoulos K, Roilides E. Parapneumonic pleural effusions caused by Streptococcus pneumoniae serotype 3 in children immunized with 13-valent conjugated pneumococcal vaccine. Pediatr Infect Dis J. 2014;33(1):81–3.
13. Iroh Tam PY, Hanisch BR, Forward B. Serotype 19A Bacteremic Pneumococcal Pneumonia After 4 Doses of 13-Valent Conjugate Vaccine: A Review of Pneumococcal Conjugate Vaccine Effectiveness. Clin Pediatr (Phila). 2014; doi:10.1177/0009922814562550.

25

Addressing asthma and obesity in children with community health workers: proof-of-concept intervention development

Molly A Martin[1*], Steven K. Rothschild[2], Elizabeth Lynch[2], Katherine Kaufer Christoffel[3], Militza M. Pagán[4], Jose Luis Rodriguez[5], Anna Barnes[3], Kelly Karavolos[2], Antonieta Diaz[6], Lucretia M. Hoffman[7], Diana Plata[8] and Sandra Villalpando[9]

Abstract

Background: The objective of this study was to design and test the feasibility and impact of a community health worker (CHW) intervention for comorbid asthma and obesity.

Methods: Using a proof of concept study design, we collected pre/post outcomes from a single intervention cohort of urban low-income in a single community area. A community-based participatory research approach was employed. Forty-six children and their caregivers were recruited. Children were 5–12 years old with physician-diagnosed asthma and body mass index (BMI) > 85%. Families were offered 12 home visits from CHWs that integrated asthma and obesity core curriculums. The primary asthma outcome was asthma control, measured via the Childhood Asthma Control Test (cACT). The primary obesity outcome was child body mass index (BMI).

Results: Families received a median of 10 out of the 12 home visits over 1 year. At 1 year, there was a significant improvement in the number of children with controlled asthma as measured via cACT (85.7% at 1 year compared to 61.9% at baseline, $p = 0.01$). Activity limitations and emergency utilization were reduced while inhaler technique improved ($p < 0.01$ for all). Child BMI z-score was reduced: mean = 1.97 (SD 0.79) at 1 year compared to mean = 2.13 (SD 0.40) at baseline, $p < 0.01$. No association was seen between change in child BMI and change in asthma control. Worse baseline child depression scores were associated with less improvement in asthma control ($p = 0.003$) and higher baseline caregiver post-traumatic stress disorder scores were associated with increased child BMI ($p = 0.012$).

Conclusions: The CHW intervention has promise for improving asthma and weight outcomes in high-risk children with comorbid asthma and obesity; this model warrants further development and investigation.

Keywords: Asthma, Obesity, Pediatrics, Community health worker

Background

Obesity constitutes an important risk factor for asthma. Asthma prevalence is higher in overweight and obese children [1, 2] and obesity frequently precedes asthma development, suggesting a causal role [3, 4]. Obese children with asthma use more medicine, wheeze more, and have more unscheduled emergency department visits than non-obese children with asthma [4].

Despite these strong associations, interventions targeting children with both asthma and obesity are limited [5–9]. This gap in the field prompted the formation of the Community United to Raise Awareness: Asthma and Active Living study (CURA 2) with the goal of developing a behavioral intervention for children with both asthma and obesity. The home-based intervention used a community health worker (CHW) asthma model that had previously been tested in the target community [10]. The intervention was strengthened by increasing the dose and duration, and by adding pediatric obesity modules. The CURA 2 intervention was then tested in a proof of concept study to assess if these changes resulted in a feasible

* Correspondence: mollyma@uic.edu
[1]University of Illinois at Chicago, 840 South Wood Street, M/C 856, Chicago, IL 60612, USA

intervention that could improve asthma control and reduced body mass index (BMI).

Methods

Theoretical model

This study is part of the Rush Center for Urban Health Equity which adapts the Warnecke model for population health disparities [11]. Proximal, intermediate, and distal factors and their contributions to disparities are considered. The portion of the CURA 2 study described in this manuscript focused on the home and aimed to address family social relationships, risk behaviors, psychosocial factors, and the physical environment. Other study phases not described here targeted schools. Social Cognitive Theory guides the CHW intervention [12]. Behavior is shaped and maintained by consequences, particularly by immediate feedback from both objective sources (such as observation of inhaler technique or home triggers) and an individual's social network (beliefs and traditions of family and friends). The asthma CHW home intervention measures and supports these behaviors and social networks using self-management skills (self-monitoring, social support, environmental rearrangement, problem solving, and behavior change plans).

Study design

This proof of concept study was uncontrolled with data collection at baseline (pre) and 12-months (post) in the homes by research assistants (RAs), and 12 CHW home visits offered over the 12-month intervention period. A community-based participatory research approach was employed to design and oversee the study. The study built off of partnerships developed in previous research in a low income community area in Chicago with high documented asthma prevalence and morbidity [10, 13]. The study team included clinician researchers with expertise in behavioral interventions, asthma, obesity, and child development. Community partners on the study team included a local health coalition (Greater Humboldt Park Community of Wellness), a social service organization (Puerto Rican Cultural Center), a parent-led service organization (Women Living with Hope), and an obesity advocacy organization (Consortium to Lower Obesity in Chicago Children).

The recruitment goal for this uncontrolled cohort was 30–50 children that met the following inclusion criteria: 5–12 years old, residence within defined geographic boundaries, physician-diagnosed asthma (per caregiver report), overweight or obese (BMI > 85%), and not attending a school with a planned subsequent school-level intervention. Participants were recruited via community events, schools, and local clinics. Written informed consent from caregivers and child assent were obtained in the home by research assistants in the family's preferred language (English or Spanish). The study was approved by the Rush University Medical Center Institutional Review Board and Chicago Public Schools Research Review Board.

Outcomes

Outcomes were assessed by bilingual RAs in the home at baseline and 12-months. Survey questions were asked verbally to the caregiver/child with the exception of the mental health instruments which were self-administered. Families received \$50 both at the baseline and 12-month data collections for a total of \$100 by the end of the study.

Asthma control

Asthma control was determined using the Childhood Asthma Control Test (cACT) [14]. A score of >19 is considered uncontrolled [14]. The Expert Panel Report 3 guidelines to assess control using questions on symptoms, medication usage, missed activities, and prednisone use were also used [15]. Families self-reported emergency department visits and hospitalizations.

Asthma medications

RAs asked to see all of the children's asthma medications. For children with an inhaled corticosteroid (ICS), adherence was determined using a medication dose counter placed on the inhaler that documented the number of times the inhaler was actuated daily (Doser CT, MediTrack, Inc., South Easton, MA) or using the ICS canister's integrated dose counter [10, 16]. Children were asked to demonstrate their medication technique [17].

Home triggers

Home asthma trigger data were obtained by caregiver report, a visual home assessment, and objective measurement [18]. Families were asked about behaviors related to allergens such as dust mites, pets, roaches and rodents, and exposures to irritants such as cigarette smoke. The visual home assessment included visual and olfactory examination of the child's bedroom, main living area, kitchen, bathroom, and heating source. Saliva was taken from children and tested for cotinine with an ELISA using a high sensitivity quantitative immunoassay (Salimetrics, Inc, State College, PA), with calibrator range 0.8–200 ng/mL, sensitivity 0.05 ng/mL. Salivary cotinine levels ranging from 1–7 ng/ml were coded as environmental tobacco smoke (ETS) exposure [19]. A positive report of a trigger from any one of the three data sources resulted in a positive score for that trigger.

Allergen sensitivity

Aeroallergen sensitivity of children was assessed in the home at baseline using the ImmunoCAP® Rapid Inhalant Profile 1, an in vitro semi-quantitative assay for measurement of allergen specific IgE in whole blood (http://www.phadia.com/en/Products/Allergy-testing-products/ImmunoCAP-Rapid/).

Child and caregiver anthropometrics

Height was measured using a tape measure and straight edge. Weight was measured using a calibrated portable digital scale. BMI was calculated as kilograms/meters squared using CDC age/sex specific growth charts formulas.

Child and caregiver hemoglobin A1c and lipid profiles

One caregiver per family and the child were asked to fast before the data collection visit, and blood was collected using dried blood kits. Hemoglobin A1c assays were performed using a standard procedure developed by ZRT laboratory [20]. Lipid profiles were measured using commercial kits (Randox Laboratory, UK) and reagents (e.g., enzymatic reagents, standards and control sera) [21].

Child physical activity

Children wore ActiGraph Accelerometers (GT1M and GT3X units) around their waists. Accelerometers were set for 15 s epochs and were worn for a minimum of 10 h/day for 4 days (including 1 weekend day). Physical activity levels were set using the Evenson cut points [22]. Children (or caregivers for children under 8) also completed a 7 day physical activity recall [23].

Home food environment

Visual inspection of the home food environment for obesogenic foods was conducted using the Home Food Inventory [24]. Caregivers were asked nutrition behavior questions from the Family Nutrition and Physical Activity screening tool [25]. Food security was assessed using the USDA Food Security Survey [26].

Other

Sleep disordered breathing was assessed using the snoring portion of the Pediatric Sleep Questionnaire [27]. Caregivers were asked about self-efficacy for asthma management using the Parent Asthma Self-Efficacy Scale [28]. A similar 10-item scale about self-efficacy nutrition and physical activity was created. Caregivers were screened for depression symptoms using the PHQ-9 [29] and for trauma using the Short Form of the PTSD Checklist - Civilian Version [30]. Children were screened for depression using the Child Depression Inventory 2 Short Form [31].

Intervention

CHWs were trained by investigators using a 40 h curriculum that contained established asthma training [10] and newly created pediatric obesity modules (http://cuhe.rush.edu/Cura%202/Pages/CommunityHealthWorkerTraining.aspx.) Families were offered 12 home visits over 12 months from CHWs. Each home visit was expected to last about 60 min. Visits began with several minutes of social discussion for the purpose of connection. The CHWs approached each visit with the intention to teach one or two of the core curriculum topics (Table 1). The order of topics was developed based on the individual family's interest and needs. The asthma and obesity curriculum topics were interconnected to address potential conflicts in messaging. For example, when discussing steroid medications, CHWs strongly emphasized that these are not the steroids associated with weight gain. When a CHW noted a barrier in the delivery or understanding of the education, she applied self-management skills. Behavior change plans were reviewed and new plans made at the end of each visit; behavior change plans are small goals for a specific change over a 2-week period. Examples include: "getting a prescription from my doctor" or "increasing exercise by 5 min a day".

Analysis

Basic summary statistics were calculated for baseline variables. Changes in the primary outcome of asthma control (cACT) from baseline to 1 year were assessed using McNemar's exact test or paired samples *t*-test. Regression models were used to test the influence of dose, BMI, and baseline variables on primary asthma outcomes. Asthma secondary variables (Table 2) were tested for change from baseline to 1 year using McNemar's exact test or t-test. Finally, variables with statistically significant changes were included in mediation analyses to determine their influence on primary asthma outcomes. These same series of analyses were repeated with the obesity primary outcome (child BMI z-score) and obesity secondary variables (Table 2).

Table 1 Community health worker home visit topics

Asthma Core Curriculum	Obesity Core Curriculum	Self-Management Skills
General asthma facts	General obesity facts	Problem solving
Controller medications	Healthy foods	Social support
Inhalers and spacers	Beverages	Environmental rearrangement
Symptom recognition	Portions and labels	Self-monitoring
Asthma triggers	Physical activity	
Communicating with providers	Screen time	
Asthma and schools	Communicating with providers	
Asthma and obesity	Obesity and schools	

Table 2 Clinical characteristics ($N = 46$)

Asthma control	
cACT, mean (SD)	20.9 (3.6)
cACT <20 (uncontrolled), N (%)	18 (40.0)
Uncontrolled in last 30 days, N (%)	
Day symptoms	17 (37.0)
Night symptoms	23 (50.0)
Excess quick reliever use	16 (34.8)
Activity limitations	16 (34.8)
Healthcare utilization for asthma over last 12 months, N (%)	
Emergency room	15 (32.6)
Hospitalization	6 (13.0)
Prednisone/prednisolone use	12 (26.1)
Medications	
Have a quick relief medication, N (%)	29 (63.0)
Have an inhaled corticosteroid, N (%)	20 (43.0)
Puffs/day inhaled corticosteroid, median (25th, 75th percentile)	0.6 (0.2, 1.4)
Have a spacer, N (%)	16 (34.8)
Percent correct technique, mean (SD)	58 (18.3)
Tobacco exposure, N (%)	
Self-reported smoker in the home	21 (45.7)
Cotinine level >1.0	11 (23.9)
Home triggers, N (%)	
Working vacuum	23 (50.0)
Dogs	17 (37.0)
Cats	4 (8.7)
Problem with roaches	18 (39.1)
Problem with rats/mice	14 (30.4)
Problem with mold	22 (47.8)
Allergen sensitivity, N (%)	
Dog	6 (18.0)
Cat	8 (24.0)
Dust mite 1 (*D. pteronyssinus*)	14 (42.0)
Dust mite 2 (*D. farina*)	13 (39.0)
Child anthropometrics	
Overweight (BMI 85–95%), N (%)	7 (15)
Obese (BMI ≥95%), N (%)	39 (84)
Child,[a] N (%)	
Hemoglobin A1c borderline high (5.7–6.4)	16 (36)
Hemoglobin A1c elevated (≥6.5)	1 (2)
LDL cholesterol borderline high (110–129)	4 (9)
LDL cholesterol elevated (≥130)	6 (13)
HDL cholesterol borderline low (40–45)	8 (18)
HDL cholesterol low (<40)	18 (40)
Triglycerides borderline high[b]	6 (13)
Triglycerides elevated[b]	29 (64)
Child physical activity	
Minutes of moderate/vigorous physical activity, median (25th, 75th percentile)	39 (29,59)
Physical activity 60 min/day, N (%)	10 (21.7)
Self-reported physical activity,[c] mean (SD)	2.8 (0.7)
Caregiver obese (BMI ≥30), N (%)	28 (60.9)
Caregiver,[d] N (%)	
Hemoglobin A1c elevated (≥6.5)	10 (31)
LDL cholesterol elevated (≥160)	2 (5)
HDL cholesterol low (<40)	10 (23)
Triglycerides elevated (≥200)	17 (39)
Child screen time >2 hrs/day, N (%)	43 (93.5)
Child seems to stop breathing at night (obstructive sleep apnea), N (%)	10 (21.7)
Food security, N (%)	
Marginal	10 (23.0)
Low/very low	23 (50.0)
Percent of home food obesogenic, mean (SD)	35 (14)
Self-reported family nutrition in high risk category, N (%)	14 (30.4)

[a] $N = 45$
[b] Age 0–9: 75–99 = borderline high, ≥100 = elevated. Age 10–19: 90–129 = borderline high, ≥130 = elevated
[c] A score of 1 indicates low physical activity, whereas a score of 5 indicates high physical activity
[d] $N = 44$

Results

The participating families ($N = 46$) were primarily low income and Hispanic which reflects the demographics of the target community (Table 3). Their clinical data are shown in Table 2. While only 40% of children had cACT scores indicating poor asthma control over the past 30 days, 74% were uncontrolled over the past year based on the EPR3 guidelines for control that include emergency room or hospitalization. Inhaled corticosteroid presence was low (43%) but only persistent asthma requires these medications. Quick relief medicines are essential for all children with asthma; however, 37% of children did not have a quick relief medication and 65% did not have a spacer. Technique with their devices was suboptimal. Across all devices, the mean number of demonstrated correct steps for usage was 58% (SD 18.3). Triggers in the home were common, as were allergies to common triggers. Almost a quarter of children had cotinine levels suggesting recent ETS exposure. The majority of children were obese (84%) and the rest overweight. Screen time exceeded recommendations (93.5% reported more than two hours per day) and few children (22%) met the requirements for 60 min/day of moderate/vigorous physical activity.

Many psychosocial stressors were identified. Among caregivers, 28.9% had symptoms of moderate-to-severe

Table 3 Baseline demographics ($N = 46$)

Caregiver	
Female, N (%)	44 (95.7)
Age, mean (SD)	37.9 (7.6)
Years of school completed, median (Q1, Q3)	12 (9,13)
Hispanic, N[a] (%)	39 (84.8)
Mexican	19 (48.7)
Puerto Rican	16 (41.0)
Other Hispanic	3 (7.7)
Refuse	1 (2.2)
Race, N[a] (%)	
Black/non-Hispanic	7 (15.2)
White/non-Hispanic	3 (6.5)
Other	37 (80.4)
Place of birth, N (%)	
United States	18 (39.1)
Mexico	15 (32.6)
Puerto Rico	10 (21.7)
Other	3 (6.5)
If not born in US, years on mainland US, median (Q1, Q3)	15.5 (12, 24)
Income, N (%)	
< $5,000	9 (19.6)
$5,000–$14,999	12 (26.0)
$15,000–$19,999	14 (30.4)
$20,000–$59,999	11 (23.9)
Home ownership, N(%)	
Own outright/mortgage	5 (10.9)
Rent	36 (78.3)
Live with others rent free	4 (8.7)
Other	1 (2.2)
Marital Status, N(%)	
Married/live with partner	25 (54.3)
Single	18 (39.1)
Separate/Divorced/Widowed	3 (7.7)
Child	
Age, mean (SD)	9.7 (2.2)
Female, N (%)	31 (67.4)
Grade, median (Q1, Q3)	4 (2,5)
Place of birth, N (%)	
United States	42 (91.3)
Mexico	1 (2.2)
Puerto Rico	3 (6.5)
Child health insurance Medicaid, N (%)	44 (95.7)

[a]For race and ethnicity, participants were allowed to endorse multiple categories if they applied

depression, 66% had experienced at least one traumatic life event, and 33.8% screened positive for probable PTSD. In children, 5.3% had depression scores in the "high average" range while 13.2% in the "elevated" range.

Families received a median of 10 out of the 12 home visits over 1 year (Fig. 1). Three families refused all home visits; one of these refused the 1 year data collection as well. Two other families accepted CHW visits but refused the 1 year data collection. As shown in Table 4, there was a significant improvement in children with controlled asthma as measured via cACT (85.7% at 1 year compared to 61.9% at baseline, $p = 0.01$) but this represented only a mean change in cACT score of 1.9 (SD 4.4). The minimally important difference for the cACT is 2 [32]. Activity limitations were reduced (7% at 1 year compared to 32.6% at baseline, $p = 0.002$) and emergency department/hospital use decreased (27.9% at 1 year compared to 53.5% at baseline, $p = 0.003$). Inhaler technique improved (90% correct at 1 year compared to 60% at baseline, $p < 0.01$). Child BMI z-score was reduced at 1 year: mean = 1.97 (SD 0.79) at 1 year compared to mean = 2.13 (SD 0.40) at baseline, $p < 0.01$. The number of CHW home visits received was weakly associated with healthcare utilization at 1 year ($p = 0.049$) but no other asthma outcomes were associated with number of visits received. Also, no association was seen between change in child BMI and change in asthma control ($p = 0.188$).

Secondary analyses were conducted to better understand the primary outcomes. None of the baseline asthma and obesity supporting variables predicted change in asthma control or child BMI. However, worse baseline child depression scores were associated with less improvement in asthma control ($p = 0.003$) and higher baseline caregiver PTSD scores were associated with more child BMI change in the direction of weight gain ($p = 0.012$). Many of the supporting variables did improve over the year, including nighttime asthma symptoms ($p = 0.041$), activity limitation ($p = 0.002$), ED/hospitalizations ($p = 0.003$), inhaler technique ($p < 0.001$), child hemoglobin A1c ($p = 0.027$), child HDL cholesterol ($p = 0.013$), and sleep disordered breathing ($p = 0.027$). Although caregivers were not the focus of the intervention, they gained weight (baseline BMI mean = 34.8, SD 9.6; 1 year BMI mean = 36.2, SD 10.1; $p = 0.008$) while showing improvements in hemoglobin A1c ($p = 0.012$) and HDL cholesterol ($p = 0.036$). However, none of the supporting variables that showed positive changes over the year mediated child asthma control or BMI. Caregiver depression decreased from baseline to 1 year (PHQ9 baseline mean = 7.5, SD 7.1; 1 year mean = 5.6, SD 6; $p = 0.039$). Change in caregiver depression score was weakly associated with change in child BMI z-score ($p = 0.079$) but not asthma control.

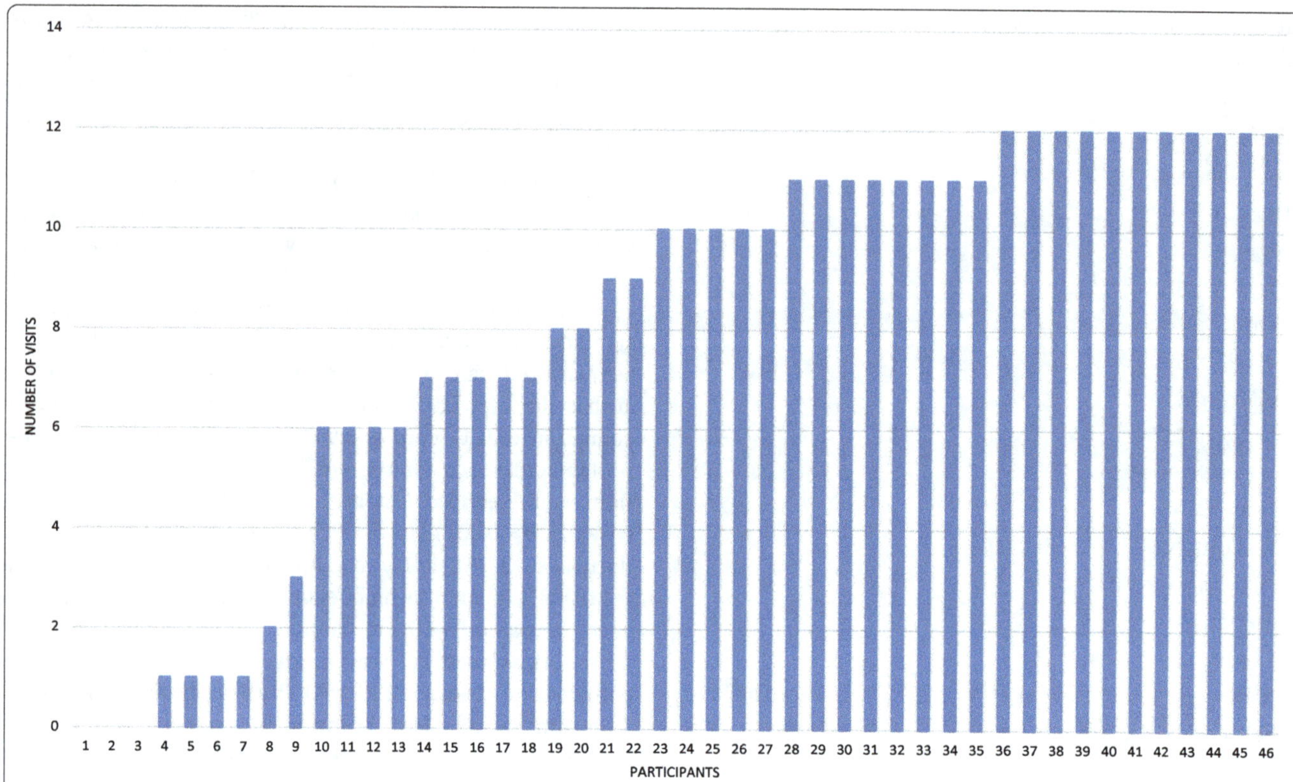

Fig. 1 Completed CHW Visits in One Year

Discussion

CURA 2 sought to test the feasibility of a home CHW intervention targeting both asthma and obesity, and to generate estimates for the potential of this intervention to improve child asthma control and BMI. The CHW intervention was well received. Only three families refused the CHW home visits. We strove to deliver 12 home visits but only 30% were able to complete all 12, and that was with difficulty. The primary content was intended to be delivered in visits one through ten, with visits 11–12 used for review and reinforcement. For asthma CHW intervention alone, Postma et al found that six visits were acceptable [33]. Campbell et al. showed that four home visits were associated with improved outcomes and a significant return on investment [34]. Because CURA 2 combined both asthma and obesity content, we suggest 10 home visits in a year would have been a more feasible goal.

While efficacy of the intervention cannot be definitively determined due to limited power and a lack of a control group, comparison of pre/post data suggest a possible benefit for asthma. The asthma control score, nighttime symptoms, activity limitations, ED/hospitalizations, and medication technique all improved at 1 year. However, the change in asthma control was modest and some of the children seemed to have mild intermittent controlled asthma from the start. Medication use and triggers in the home did not change, making it difficult to understand how changes in asthma occurred and whether they can be attributed to the intervention. Observed changes may simply be a result of natural improvements in asthma control as children grow. Future studies should consider restricting their sample to children with uncontrolled persistent asthma to reduce these limitations.

The outcomes for obesity were more robust. As children approach adolescence, it is typical for BMI to increase [35]. However, CURA 2 study participants had an overall decrease in BMI. A 0.25 BMI Z-score reduction is associated with reduced inflammation and improved insulin sensitivity in children; [36] the mean reduction in this study was 0.16. We saw some improvements at 1 year in markers of diabetes and lipids (for children and their caregivers) as well as obstructive sleep apnea, but we did not see anticipated changes in food environment, screen time, or activity level. The CHW intervention targeted healthy foods, screen time and physical activity as steps toward weight management which makes the mechanism for BMI reduction more difficult to understand and limits our ability to attribute it to the intervention.

Several key barriers to implementing the asthma control and obesity reduction strategies were identified. The first was lack of communication between the CHWs and clinical providers. CHWs (and potentially providers) could have

Table 4 Primary and secondary outcomes

	Baseline	One Year	*P* value
Asthma			
Asthma Control			
cACT[a] <20	16 (38.1%)	6 (14.3%)	0.013
Uncontrolled day symptoms	16 (37.2%)	10 (23.3%)	0.109
Uncontrolled night symptoms	21 (48.8%)	11 (25.6%)	0.041
Excess quick reliever use	14 (32.6%)	13 (30.2%)	0.819
Activity limitations	14 (32.6%)	3 (7.0%)	0.002
ED/hospitalization in past year	23 (53.5%)	12 (27.9%)	0.003
Asthma self-efficacy, mean (SD)	4.1 (0.8)	4.4 (0.5)	0.006
Inhaler technique (% of steps correct), mean (SD)	60% (20)	90% (10)	<0.001
Obesity			
Weight control			
BMI z-score,[a] mean (SD)	2.13 (0.40)	1.97 (0.70)	0.002
BMI percentile, mean (SD)	97.6 (2.2)	96.1 (4.4)	0.011
Obese (BMI ≥ 95%)	84%	74%	
Nutrition self-efficacy, mean (SD)	3.6 (0.8)	3.9 (0.7)	0.007
Child hemoglobin A1c, mean (SD)	5.6 (1)	5.3 (1.2)	0.027
Child HDL cholesterol, mean (SD)	44.9 (12.3)	52.3 (12.7)	0.013
Child sleep disordered breathing, mean (SD)	2 (2)	1.5 (1.8)	0.027
Caregiver BMI, mean (SD)	34.8 (9.6)	36.2 (10.1)	0.008
Caregiver hemoglobin A1c, mean (SD)	6 (1.3)	5.6 (1.8)	0.012
Caregiver HDL cholesterol, mean (SD)	50.2 (11.4)	54.7 (9.4)	0.036

[a]Primary outcomes

No significant changes from baseline to one year for presence of a quick relief or controller medication, controller medication adherence, prednisone use, cotinine level, observed triggers in the home, self-reported physical activity, screen time, accelerometry, food security, self-reported food in the home, observed obesogenic food in the home, child triglyceride, child LDL cholesterol, caregiver triglycerides, and caregiver LDL cholesterol

benefitted from the ability to discuss care plans with providers. Second, mental health issues were prevalent; caregivers endorsed high levels of trauma and depression, and these variables appeared to have mediating effects on child BMI. Poorer psychological functioning has been associated with increased asthma morbidity [37] and similar associations are also seen in obesity [38, 39]. The impact of the CHW intervention on psychological functioning remains unclear [40] and requires further investigation.

Conclusions

While the small sample size and lack of a control group limits our interpretation of intervention effects, we demonstrated feasibility and potential effects of a CHW intervention for children with both asthma and obesity. CHW asthma interventions have already shown benefits in asthma symptom control and healthcare utilization [41]. Our study is novel in that the intervention targets a subpopulation of children with both asthma and obesity. These children typically suffer worse asthma morbidity and their asthma is more challenging to control, [1, 2] yet few studies have published interventions specifically targeting these children [5–9]. None of these used CHWs and no pediatric obesity CHW training curriculum had been published to date. Therefore we created a curriculum, merged it with asthma training, and then delivered the combined asthma/obesity intervention to a high risk cohort of urban children and their families. For asthma medication adherence, medication technique, and triggers, outcomes were measured objectively; this limits the sometimes inaccurate results generated from self-reported data. The measured changes in asthma control and child BMI, while not large, warrant further study. Our small study could not address the full spectrum of social, behavioral, and environmental contributors to asthma and obesity [11, 41]. However our findings suggest that the CURA 2 CHW intervention, which could be expanded to include clinical and community partners and mental health resources, has promise for improving asthma and weight outcomes in the high-risk population of children with comorbid asthma and obesity.

Abbreviations

CURA 2: Community united to raise awareness: asthma and active living; BMI: Body mass index; cACT: Childhood asthma control test; CHW: Community health worker; ETS: Environmental tobacco smoke; ICS: Inhaled corticosteroid; PTSD: Post-traumatic stress disorder; RAs: Research assistants

Acknowledgements

This study is part of the Rush Center for Urban Health Equity which is funded by the National Institutes of Health (NIH) through the National Institute for Heart Lung and Blood (NHLBI), grant number 1P50HL105189-01. The content of this manuscript is solely the responsibility of the authors and does not necessarily represent the official views of the NIH or NHLBI. The authors would like to thank the rest of the co-investigators and staff: Gilma Arguello, Jaime Arteaga, Rosalinda Campos, Rose de Jesus, Sheila Dugan, Dora Flores-Albert, Eleanor Floyd, Matt Greve, Hong Li, Lolita Lopez, Dorian Ortega, Sara Nixon, Janet Rocha, Madeleine Shalowitz, Serina Silvestry, Julio Urrutia, Sandra Villalpando, and Grant Vitale. We would like to thank the Rush Center for Urban Health Equity Principal Investigator Lynda H Powell, and Director of the Data Core DeJuran Richardson. We also want to thank our fantastic Community Advisory Board and our partners: The Puerto Rican Cultural Center, Women Living with Hope, the Greater Humboldt Park Community of Wellness, and the Consortium to Lower Obesity in Chicago Children. Finally, thanks to the many other organizations, schools, and families who made this study possible.

Funding

This study is part of the Rush Center for Urban Health Equity which is funded by the National Institutes of Health (NIH) through the National Institute for Heart Lung and Blood (NHLBI), grant number 1P50HL105189-01. The content of this manuscript is solely the responsibility of the authors and does not necessarily represent the official views of the NIH or NHLBI.

Authors' contributions

All authors contributed to the preparation of this manuscript and have approved it. The following authors participated in study design, implementation, and analysis: MAM, SKR, EL, KKC, MLP, JLR, AB. The following authors participated in data analysis: KK, DP. AD contributed to study implementation and analysis. LH and SV contributed to parts of study design and implementation.

Competing interests

The authors declare that they have no competing interests.

Author details

[1]University of Illinois at Chicago, 840 South Wood Street, M/C 856, Chicago, IL 60612, USA. [2]Rush University Medical Center, 1700 W Van Buren, Suite 470, Chicago, IL 60612, USA. [3]Lurie Children's Hospital, 225 E Chicago Ave, Chicago, IL 60611, USA. [4]Puerto Rican Cultural Center, 2700 W Haddon Ave, Chicago, IL 60622, USA. [5]Greater Humboldt Park Community of Wellness, 1116 N. Kedzie, Chicago, IL 60651, USA. [6]University of Illinois at Chicago, Jane Addams College of Social Work, 1040 West Harrison Street, Chicago, IL 60607, USA. [7]Forsyth County Department of Public Health, 201 N Chestnut St, Winston-Salem, NC, USA. [8]Rush University Medical Center, College of Medicine, 600 S Paulina St, Chicago, IL 60612, USA. [9]University of Illinois at Chicago, College of Medicine, 808 S Wood St, Chicago, IL 60612, USA.

References

1. Belamarich PF, Luder E, Kattan M, et al. Do obese inner-city children with asthma have more symptoms than nonobese children with asthma? Pediatrics. 2000;106(6):1436–41.
2. Halfon N, Larson K, Slusser W. Associations between obesity and comorbid mental health, developmental, and physical health conditions in a nationally representative sample of US children aged 10 to 17. Acad Pediatr. 2013;13(1):6–13.
3. Chen YC, Dong GH, Lin KC, et al. Gender difference of childhood overweight and obesity in predicting the risk of incident asthma: a systematic review and meta-analysis. Obes Rev. 2012;13 Suppl 3:222–31.
4. Shore SA. Obesity and asthma: possible mechanisms. J Allergy Clin Immunol. 2008;121(5):1087–93.
5. Adeniyi FB, Young T. Weight loss interventions for chronic asthma. Cochrane Database Syst Rev. 2012;7:CD009339.
6. Lang JE. Obesity and asthma in children: current and future therapeutic options. Paediatr Drugs. 2014;16(3):179–88.
7. da Silva PL, de Mello MT, Cheik NC, et al. Interdisciplinary therapy improves biomarkers profile and lung function in asthmatic obese adolescents. Pediatr Pulm. 2012;47(1):8–17.
8. Lin JH. Normocaloric diet improves asthma-related quality of life in obese pubertal adolescents. Pediatrics. 2014;134 Suppl 3:S170–1.
9. Spriet SW, Davis KL. Diet-induced weight loss in obese children with asthma: a randomized controlled trial. Pediatrics. 2014;134 Suppl 3:S170.
10. Martin MA, Mosnaim GS, Olson D, et al. Results from a community-based trial testing a community health worker asthma intervention in Puerto Rican youth in Chicago. J Asthma. 2014;27:1–12.
11. Warnecke RB, Oh A, Breen N, Gehlert S, Paskett E, Tucker KL, Lurie N, Rebbeck T, Goodwin J, Flack J, Srinivasan S, Kerner J, Heurtin-Roberts S, Abeles R, Tyson FL, Patmios G, Hiatt RA. Approaching health disparities from a population perspective: the National Institutes of Health Centers for Population Health and Health Disparities. Am J Public Health. 2008;98(9):1608–15.
12. Bandura A. Self-efficacy: toward a unifying theory of behavioral change. Psychol Rev. 1977;84:191–215.
13. Martin MA, Olson D, Mosnaim GS, et al. Recruitment, asthma characteristics, and medication behaviors in Midwest Puerto Rican Youth: data from project CURA. Ann Allerg Asthma Im. 2012;109:121–7.
14. Liu AH, Zeiger R, Sorkness C, et al. Development and cross-sectional validation of the childhood asthma control test. J Allergy Clin Immunol. 2007;119(4):817–25.
15. Expert Panel Report 3. Guidelines for Diagnosis and Management of Asthma. National Asthma Education and Prevention Program, 2007. Available at https://www.ncbi.nlm.nih.gov/books/NBK7232/. Accessed 21 Oct 2013.
16. Bender BG, Wamboldt FS, O'Connor SL, et al. Measurement of children's asthma medication adherence by self-report, mother report, canister weight, and Doser CT. Ann Allerg Asthma Im. 2000;85:416–21.
17. American College of Chest Physicians. The American College of Chest Physicians Patient Education Guide: using your MDI with a spacer. 2006. Web site. Available at http://www.chestnet.org/Publications/Other-Publications/Patient-Education-Guides. Accessed 18 Oct 2013.
18. Martin MA, Thomas AM, Mosnaim GS, et al. Home asthma triggers: barriers to asthma control in Chicago Puerto Rican children. J Health Care Poor U. 2013;24(2):813–27.
19. Kumar R, Curtis LM, Khiani S, et al. A community-based study of tobacco smoke exposure among inner-city children with asthma in Chicago. J Allergy Clin Immunol. 2008;122(4):754–9.
20. Lakshmy R, Gupta R. Measurement of glycated hemoglobin A1c from dried blood by turbidimetric immunoassay. J Diabetes Sci Technol. 2009;3(5): 1203–6.
21. Kapur S, Kapur S, Zava D. Cardiometabolic risk factors assessed by a finger stick dried blood spot method. J Diabetes Sci Technol. 2008;2(2):236–41.
22. Evenson KR, Catellier DJ, Gill K, et al. Calibration of two objective measures of physical activity for children. J Sports Sci. 2008;26(14):1557–65.
23. Janz KF, Lutuchy EM, Wenthe P, et al. Measuring activity in children and adolescents using self-report: PAQ-C and PAQ-A. Med Sci Sports Exerc. 2008;40(4):767–72.
24. Fulkerson JA, Nelson MC, Lytle LA, et al. The validation of a home food inventory. Int J Behav Nutr Phys Act. 2008;5:55.
25. Ihmels MA, Welk GJ, Eisenmann JC, et al. Development and preliminary validation of a Family Nutrition and Physical Activity (FNPA) screening tool. Int J Behav Nutr Phys Act. 2009;6:14.

26. U.S. Household Food Security Survey Module: Three-Stage Design, with Screeners. Economic Research Service, USDA. July 2008. Available at https://www.ers.usda.gov/topics/food-nutrition-assistance/food-security-in-the-us/surveytools/. Accessed 29 Nov 2016.
27. Chervin RD, Hedger K, Dillon JE, et al. Pediatric Sleep Questionnaire (PSQ): validity and reliability of scales for sleep-disordered breathing, snoring, sleepiness, and behavior problems. Sleep Med. 2000;1:21–32.
28. Bursch B, Schwankovsky L, Gilbert J, et al. Construction and validation of four childhood asthma self-management scales: parent barriers, child and parent self-efficacy, and parent belief in treatment efficacy. J Asthma. 1999;36:115–28.
29. Kroenke K, Spitzer RL, Williams JB. The PHQ-9: validity of a brief depression severity measure. J Gen Intern Med. 2001;16(9):606–13.
30. Lang AJ, Stein MB. An abbreviated PTSD checklist for use as a screening instrument in primary care. Behav Res Ther. 2005;43(5):585–94.
31. Child Depression Inventory 2 Short Form. Available at http://www.mhs.com/product.aspx?gr=edu&prod=cdi2&id=overview. Accessed 15 May 2015.
32. Voorend-van Bergen S, Vaessen-Verberne AA, Landstra AM, Brackel HJ, van den Berg NJ, Caudri D, de Jongste JC, Merkus PJ, Pijnenburg MW. Monitoring childhood asthma: web-based diaries and the asthma control test. J Allergy Clin Immunol. 2013;133:1599–605. e2.
33. Postma J, Smalley K, Ybarra V, Kieckhefer G. The feasibility and acceptability of a home visitation, asthma education program in a rural, Latino/a population. J Asthma. 2001;48(2):139–46.
34. Campbell JD, Brooks M, Hosokawa P, Robinson J, Song L, Krieger J. Community health worker home visits for Medicaid-enrolled children with asthma: effects on asthma outcomes and costs. Am J Public Health. 2015;105(11):2366–72.
35. Ogden CL, Carroll MD, Kit BK, et al. Prevalence of childhood and adult obesity in the United States, 2011–2012. JAMA. 2014;311(8):806–14.
36. Ford AL, Hunt LP, Cooper A, et al. What reduction in BMI SDS is required in obese adolescents to improve body composition and cardiometabolic health? Arch Dis Child. 2010;95(4):256–61.
37. Goodwin RD, Bandiera FC, Steinberg D, et al. Asthma and mental health among youth: etiology, current knowledge and future directions. Expert Rev Respir Med. 2012;6(4):397–406.
38. Gundersen C, Lohman BJ, Garasky S, et al. Food security, maternal stressors, and overweight among low-income US children: results from the National Health and Nutrition Examination Survey (1999–2002). Pediatrics. 2008;122(3):e529–40.
39. Farr OM, Sloan DM, Keane TM, et al. Stress- and PTSD-associated obesity and metabolic dysfunction: a growing problem requiring further research and novel treatments. Metabolism. 2014;63(12):1463–8.
40. Stacciarini JM, Rosa A, Ortiz M, et al. Promotoras in mental health: a review of English, Spanish, and Portuguese literature. Fam Community Health. 2012;35(2):92–102.
41. Postma J, Karr C, Kieckhefer G. Community health workers and environmental interventions for children with asthma: a systematic review. J Asthma. 2009;46(6):564–76.

26

Using a practical molecular capsular serotype prediction strategy to investigate *Streptococcus pneumoniae* serotype distribution and antimicrobial resistance in Chinese local hospitalized children

Ping Jin[1,2†], Lijuan Wu[3†], Shahin Oftadeh[4], Timothy Kudinha[4,5], Fanrong Kong[4] and Qiyi Zeng[1*]

Abstract

Background: China is one of ten countries with the highest prevalence rate of pneumococcal infections. However, there is limited serotype surveillance data for *Streptococcus pneumoniae*, especially from the community or rural regions, partly due to limited serotyping capacity because Quellung serotyping is only available in few centers in China. The aim of this study was to develop a simple, practical and economic pneumococcal serotype prediction strategy suitable for future serotype surveillance in China.

Methods: In this study, 193 *S. pneumoniae* isolates were collected from hospitalized children, 96.9 % of whom were < 5 years old. The *cpsB* sequetyping, complemented by selective and modified USA CDC sequential multiplex-PCR, was performed on all the isolates, and serotypes 6A-6D specific PCRs were done on all serogroup 6 isolates. Based on systematic analysis of available GenBank *cpsB* sequences, we established a more comprehensive *cpsB* sequence database than originally published for *cpsB* sequetyping. Antibiotic susceptibility of all isolates was determined using the disk diffusion or E-test assays.

Results: We built up a comprehensive *S. pneumoniae* serotype *cpsB* sequetyping database for all the 95 described serotypes first, and then developed a simple strategy for serotype prediction based on the improved *cpsB* sequetyping and selective multiplex-PCR. Using the developed serotype prediction strategy, 191 of 193 isolates were successfully "serotyped", and only two isolates were "non-serotypeable". Sixteen serotypes were identified among the 191 "serotypeable" isolates. The serotype distribution of the isolates from high to low was: 19 F (34.7 %), 23 F (17.1 %), 19A (11.9 %), 14 (7.3 %), 15B/15C (6.7 %), 6B (6.7 %), 6A (6.2 %), 9 V/9A (1.6 %); serotypes 6C, 3, 15 F/15A, 23A and 20 (each 1.1 %); serotypes 10B, 28 F/28A and 34 (each 0.5 %). The prevalence of parenteral penicillin resistance was 1.0 % in the non-meningitis isolates and 88.6 % in meningitis isolates. The total rate of multidrug resistance was 86.8 %.

(Continued on next page)

* Correspondence: qiyizengshenzhen@163.com
†Equal contributors
[1]Pediatric Center, Zhujiang Hospital, Southern Medical University, Guangzhou 510282, P. R. China

(Continued from previous page)

Conclusions: The integrated *cpsB* sequetyping supplemented with selective mPCR and serotypes 6A-6D specific PCRs "cocktail" strategy is practical, simple and cost-effective for use in pneumococcal infection serotype surveillance in China. For hospitalized children with non-meningitis penicillin-susceptible pneumococcal infections, clinicians still can use narrow-spectrum and cheaper penicillin, using the parenteral route, rather than using broader-spectrum and more expensive antimicrobials.

Keywords: *Streptococcus pneumoniae*, serotype prediction, *cpsB* sequetyping, Sequential multiplex PCR, Antibiotic multidrug resistance

Background

Streptococcus pneumoniae is a leading cause of bacterial pneumonia, meningitis, and sepsis in children worldwide. Although China is among the ten countries with the highest prevalence of pneumococcal cases [1], there is limited epidemiological data on invasive pneumococcal disease in mainland China. Vaccination, targeting the pneumococcal polysaccharide capsule, is the best way to prevent pneumococcal disease, especially in children. The 7-valent pneumococcal conjugate vaccine (PCV7), which is no longer available, became accessible for the private sector in China in September 2008 [2], but was never part of the universal immunization program in this country. Even in Shenzhen (one of the biggest cities in China which borders Hong Kong), the PCV7 immunization rate is still less than 1 % [3].

The capsular polysaccharide is the main virulence determinant of *S. pneumoniae*, and structural differences of this polysaccharide, can divide *S. pneumoniae* into many serotypes. After including the newly identified serotypes 6D, 6E and 11E, there are 46 different serogroups and 95 serotypes of *S. pneumoniae* that have been described to date [4–6]. Conventional serotyping by the Quellung reaction is complex, costly, and requires highly skilled personnel. On the other hand, latex agglutination is a simple and efficient alternative method to Quellung reaction serotyping, but still needs further work to improve its capacity to detect colonizing pneumococcal strains at low density [7]. In recent years, a variety of DNA-based methods that rely on the capsular polysaccharide synthesis locus for the detection of pneumococcal serotypes, have been described, including approaches based on sequencing, restriction fragment length polymorphisms, hybridization assays, microarrays, and different PCR strategies [8–15]. For many developing countries including China, it is crucial to find a practical, simple and cost-effective strategy for routine serotype prediction and pneumococcal serogroup/serotype surveillance.

In a previous study, Leung and collaborators used a single PCR sequencing method targeting *cpsB* gene (sequetyping) to identify *S. pneumoniae* serotypes [13]. The USA Centers for Disease Control and Prevention (CDC) has published a sequential multiplex PCR (mPCR) protocol, which, although is the most commonly used molecular assay for identification of *S. pneumoniae* serotypes, is complicated by the need to perform eight sets of multiplex PCRs. Here, we employed *cpsB* sequetyping coupled with local based selective and modified sequential multiplex PCR, and serotypes 6A-6D specific PCRs, to predict the serotypes of 193 *S. pneumoniae* isolates from hospitalized children with pneumococcal infection in our district hospital.

The aim of this study was, as a showcase, to investigate the best combination of the aforementioned methods for use as an initial serotype screening method especially for developing countries. Furthermore, in order to provide some local epidemiological data for current and future planning purposes, we studied the serotype distribution, antibiotic susceptibility and clinical presentation, amongst the 193 *S. pneumoniae* isolates.

Methods

S. pneumoniae isolates

S. pneumoniae isolates (n =193) from children, were provided by Shenzhen Bao'an Maternity & Child Health Hospital, during the period January 2009 to December 2013. The identity of the isolates was confirmed using standard microbiological tests, including colony morphology, optochin susceptibility and bile solubility.

Among the 193 isolates, 169 (87.6 %) isolates were from sputum, 17 (8.8 %) from blood, 3 (1.6 %) from pleural fluid, 2 (1.0 %) from cerebrospinal fluid and 2 (1.0 %) from other normally sterile body sites (Additional file 1: Table S1). All the children with pneumonia imply satisfied the World Health Organization standard definition for pneumonia, including classification as non-severe, severe and very severe pneumonia [16]. The serotypes of all the isolates were unknown at the time of receipt and testing. When two isolates from the same subject had an identical serotype, only one isolate was included in the study.

In children with pneumonia (severe or non-severe), sputum was collected with a small suction catheter, which was passed through the nose into the laryngopharynx. The length of the catheter into the respiratory tract was equal to the distance from the apex of the nose to the earlobe, and then to the thyroid cartilage. Upon eliciting a cough reflex, respiratory tract secretions were aspirated. In patients with very severe pneumonia who were under mechanical ventilation, sputum was collected from an endotracheal tube. The squamous epithelial cell numbers of <10 per 10 x objective microscopic field was used as an indicator of good quality sputum for culture [17], and only samples that met this quality criteria were cultured.

The study was approved by the Medical Ethics Committee of Shenzhen Bao'an Maternity & Child Health Hospital affiliated with Jinan University (No. S-2013002); and signed informed consents were obtained from patient's parents or guardians.

DNA extraction from bacterial isolates

Pneumococcal isolates were retrieved from storage by subculture on blood agar plates (Columbia II agar base supplemented with 5 % horse blood) and incubated overnight at 37 °C in 5 % CO_2. Genomic DNA was extracted from bacteria using the AxyGenamp DNA Mini Extraction Kit (Axygen, USA) according to the manufacturer's instructions, and the purified DNA was diluted in a final volume of 100 μL Tris EDTA buffer and stored at - 20 °C until use.

Building up a comprehensive 95 serotypes *cpsB* sequetyping database based on GenBank sequences (Additional file 2: Figure S1)

The previous *cpsB* sequetyping database designed by Leung et al. [13] didn't include all the 95 serotype *cpsB* sequences. Our aim was to extend this work by including all the serotypes described to date in a new sequetyping database. All the *S. pneumoniae* sequences in the GenBank that contained the full-length of *cpsB* (as of Jan 1, 2015) were downloaded, and after sequence alignment using ClustalW and/or Blastn, each GenBank sequence was given a unique *cpsB* sequetype name (see Additional file 3: Table S2 and Additional file 2: Figure S1), ensuring that all GenBank sequences with the same *cpsB* sequence, were given the same sequetype name. The given *cpsB* sequetype name was chosen to reflect the specific serotype (if only one serotype had the sequence) or combination of serotypes (when more than one serotype have a common sequence) it represented. If multiple GenBank sequences had an identical *cpsB* sequetype, only one GenBank sequence was selected as reference to represent the sequetype (Additional file 3: Table S2). All sequences for the 90 Statens Serum Institut serotype reference strains were used as references for the relevant serotypes/sequetypes, whilst for the other sequetype references, we used those from Leung et al. [13] or other publications, and those with longer *cps* gene cluster sequences, because they were well-characterized compared with the other GenBank sequences (Additional file 2: Figure S1). As shown in Additional file 3: Table S2, if any of the reference sequences were longer than *cpsB* sequences (732-bp), the position of full length of *cpsB* (732-bp) was clearly shown on the GenBank sequences. Based on our database, all of the *S. pneumoniae* full-length *cpsB* GenBank sequences (as of Jan 1, 2015) with known serotypes and sequetypes were included (see Additional file 3: Table S2 & Additional file 2: Figure S1).

The *cpsB* sequetyping workflow for our local isolates (Fig. 1)

The *cpsB* sequetyping was performed on all 193 *S. pneumoniae* isolates as previously described [13] using our newly designed comprehensive *cpsB* sequetyping database, as shown in the workflow algorithm in Fig. 1. In brief, as described by Leung et al. [13], a region spanning the *cpsB* gene was amplified by single PCR, the amplicon purified, and the nucleotide sequence determined by double strand sequencing. The amplicon nucleotide sequences were then used to Blastn GenBank database, and if it was identical to any one or more of the GenBank sequences, the serotype (s)/*cpsB* sequetype was decided according to our *cpsB* sequetyping database (see Additional file 3: Table S2). Any mismatch between the sequences and reference sequences in GenBank were manually checked to ascertain the mismatch. Furthermore, USA CDC sequential multiplex PCRs were performed on all 193 *S. pneumoniae* isolates, and serotypes 6A-6D specific PCRs were performed on all serogroup 6 isolates. The results were checked against *cpsB* sequetyping results, before submitting the new sequences to GenBank (Additional file 4: Table S3).

Sequential multiplex PCR and local data based primer sets selection

Sequential multiplex PCR, as per CDC scheme, was employed to predict the isolate serotype(s) by targeting serotype-specific *cps* regions [11]. The primer sequences, PCR reactions and product detection are as published by the CDC and were updated in Feb 2014. (http://www.cdc.gov/streplab/pcr.html). We further designed combinations of primer sets in the first three reactions to identify the six most predominant serotypes (19 F, 19A, 14, 23 F, 15, 6) in China based on previous studies [18, 19], and three PCV7 vaccine serotypes (4, 9 V/9A, 18). In these modified reactions, reaction 1 contained primers for serotypes 4, 6 and 18; reaction 2 contained primers for serotypes 14, 9 V/9A, 15 F/15A and 19A; and reaction 3 contained primers for serotypes 15B/15C, 19 F and 23 F. If a sample was negative in the first three reactions, eight sequential multiplex PCR reactions were performed as previously described in CDC (USA) webpage (http://www.cdc.gov/streplab/pcr.html).

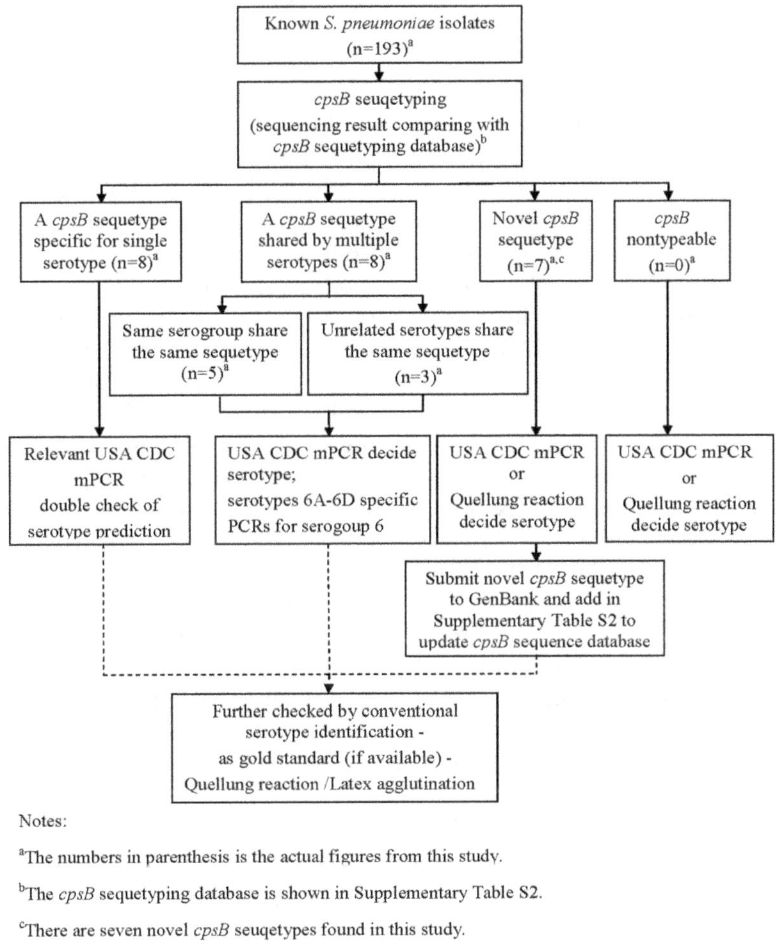

Fig. 1 The *Streptococcus pneumoniae* serotype prediction algorithm – a strategy based on *cpsB* sequetyping and selected mPCR. Step 1. The *cpsB* sequetyping was performed on all 193 *S. pneumoniae* isolates. Sequencing results compared with *cpsB* sequetyping database. 21 different sequetypes were identified; included serotype-specific sequetypes, sequetypes shared by multiple serotypes and novel *cpsB* sequetypes. Step 2. Modified and selected USA CDC sequential multiplex PCR to double check, or resolve discrepant results, or identify those that shared the same *cpsB* sequetype. Step 3. Serotypes 6A-6D specific PCRs were performed for serogroup 6 isolates. Step 4. Submit all novel *cpsB* sequetypes to GenBank and update *cpsB* sequetyping database

Serotypes 6A-6D specific PCRs

In a previous study, we developed serotype-specific PCR to identify serotypes 6A, 6B, 6C and 6D [4]. Using the same protocol and primers, sequential single PCRs were performed with three primer sets to distinguish these serotypes.

Antimicrobial susceptibility testing

In vitro susceptibility tests were performed using disk diffusion and the following antibiotics were used; erythromycin, clindamycin, levofloxacin, vancomycin, tetracycline, sulfamethoxazole-trimethoprim and chloramphenicol (Oxoid, UK). The minimum inhibitory concentrations for penicillin and ceftriaxone were determined by E-test (AB Biodisk, Solna, Sweden). All tests were performed following the United States Clinical and Laboratory Standards Institute (CLSI) recommendations, and CLSI M100-S25 version of the antibiotic susceptibility breakpoints for *S. pneumoniae* was adopted as criteria for determining drug resistance [20]. *S. pneumoniae* ATCC 49619 was used as the quality-control strain. Isolates not susceptible to three or more classes of antimicrobials were considered multidrug-resistant (MDR).

Statistical analysis

Data on serotype distribution of the isolates were analyzed using SPSS version 13.0 (SPSS Inc., Chicago, IL) statistical software. Association between serotypes and clinical presentation was tested using χ^2 test or Fisher's exact test. A two-tailed cutoff of $P < 0.05$ was considered statistically significant.

Results

Clinical data

During the study period, 193 non-duplicate *S. pneumoniae* isolates were collected from hospitalized children with pneumococcal infections. The patients included 121 boys and 72 girls; 126 (65.3 %) children were < 2 years old; 61 (31.6 %) were 2–5 years old; and 6 (3.1 %) were > 5 years old. The distribution of cases by clinical presentation was as follows: non-severe pneumonia (134, 69.4 %), severe and very severe pneumonia (38, 19.7 %), primary bacteremia (17, 8.8 %), meningitis (2, 1 %), urinary tract infections (1, 0.5 %) and cellulitis (1, 0.5 %) (Additional file 1: Table S1).

Development of reference *cpsB* sequence sequetyping database

We developed a comprehensive *S. pneumoniae* serotype *cpsB* sequence (732-bp) sequetyping reference database for all the 95 described serotypes, including all 390 available GenBank sequences with full length of the *cpsB* sequence name (see Additional file 3: Table S2, Additional file 2: Figure S1). When the same sequetype was shared by two or more serotypes, the sequetype name included all the different serotypes in ascending numerical order (e.g., 24 F-24B-33 F-33A-35A-1).

The *cpsB* sequetyping results for studied clinical isolates

All the 193 isolates included in the study could be amplified by *cpsB* PCR and yielded satisfactory sequencing results (Table 1, Additional file 4: Table S3). Based on *cpsB* sequence heterogeneity at one or more sites for all isolates, 21 different sequetypes were identified: eight serotype-specific sequetypes could predict isolates to serotype level (3, 9 V, 6B, 10B, 14, 19A, 23 F, 23A); five sequetypes shared by different serotypes but in the same serogroups (6C-6D-1, 6B-6E-6X-1, 15B-15C-1, 19 F-19A-1, and 28 F-28A-1) could predict isolates to the serogroup level; and three sequetypes shared by different serotypes - serotypes 13 and 20, 15A and 33B, 17A and 34, could not be differentiated from each other. Of the 193 isolates tested, 66 (34.2 %) were sequetyped to the serotype level and 107 (55.4 %) to the serogroup level.

When the Blastn result was not a 100 % match with any GenBank sequences, the sequences (if with good sequencing quality for both directions) potentially represented

Table 1 Serotype distribution among 193 *S. pneumoniae* isolates as determined by *cpsB* sequetyping and selected sequential mPCR

Serotype/ Serogroup	No. of isolates with serotypes determined by		Novel sequetypes
	mPCR/6A-6D specific PCR	*cpsB* sequetyping[a]	
3	3 ($n = 2$)	1 bp-3-2 ($n = 2$)	3-sz-1 (3–5)
6A	6/6A ($n = 12$)	2 bp-6C-6D-1 ($n = 12$)	6A-sz-1 (6A-5)
6B	6/6B ($n = 13$)	6B-1 ($n = 1$) 6B-6E-6X-1 ($n = 12$)	
6C	6/6C ($n = 2$)	6C-6D-1 ($n = 2$)	
9 V/9A	9 V/9A ($n = 3$)	9 V-1 ($n = 3$)	
10B	unknown ($n = 1$)[d]	10B-1 ($n = 1$)	
14	14 ($n = 14$)	14-1 ($n = 14$)	
15 F/15A	15 F/15A ($n = 2$)	3 bp-15A-33B-1 ($n = 2$)[b]	15 F/15A-sz-1(15 F-15A-1)
15B/15C	15B/15C ($n = 13$)	15B-15C-1 ($n = 13$)	
19 F	19 F ($n = 67$)	19 F-19A-1 ($n = 67$)	
19A	19A ($n = 23$)	19A-2 ($n = 23$)	
20	20 ($n = 2$)	13-20A-20B-1 ($n = 2$)[b]	
23 F	23 F ($n = 33$)	23 F-1 ($n = 20$) 11 bp-11 F-1 ($n = 9$)[c] 6A-6B-6 F ($n = 2$)[c] 2 bp-6A-6B-6 F-1 ($n = 1$)[c] 13-20A-20B ($n = 1$)[c]	23 F-sz-1 (23 F-2) 23 F-6A-6B-6 F-sz-1 23 F-sz-2 (23 F-2) 23 F-13-20A-20B-1
23A	23A ($n = 2$)	23A-1 ($n = 2$)	
28 F/28A	unknown ($n = 1$)[d]	28 F-28A-1 ($n = 1$)	
34	34 ($n = 1$)	17A-34-1 ($n = 1$) [b]	
unknown	unknown ($n = 2$)[d]	unknown ($n = 2$)	

[a]21 different sequetypes were identified
[b]Five isolates with ambiguous sequetype result, mPCR confirmed them
[c]Thirteen 23 F isolates were of new sequetypes after mPCR was performed
[d]Four isolates were untypeable by mPCR. Two isolates were identified by *cpsB* sequetyping. Two isolates were also unknown by sequencing

new *cpsB* sequetypes. For example, four new 23 F *cpsB* sequetypes, confirmed by 23 F specific PCR were found among thirteen 23 F isolates (Additional file 4: Table S3). Among the 27 serogroup 6 isolates, the distribution of sequetypes was as follows; 6B-1 (1/27, 3.7 %), 6C-6D-1 (14/27, 51.8 %), 6B-6E-6X-1 (12/27, 44.4 %). Two isolates (ID 250, 268) produced *cpsB* amplicons but they were non-typeable by both *cpsB* sequetyping and sequential multiplex PCR (Additional file 4: Table S3).

Sequential multiplex PCR results

After *cpsB* sequetyping results were known, isolates that presumptively belonged to relevant serotypes were further tested by multiplex PCR to confirm the results, resolve discrepant results, or identify those that shared the same *cpsB* sequetype (Table 1, Additional file 4: Table S3, and Fig. 1). Overall, 115 (59.5 %) of sequetyping results needed confirmation by selected mPCR to give a definite serotype. The level of agreement between *cpsB* sequetyping and multiplex PCR results was 92.2 %. Five isolates, for which sequencing gave ambiguous result as serotypes 15A-33B-1 (2 isolates), 13-20A-20B-1 (2 isolates), and 17A-34-1 (1 isolate), were confirmed by mPCR that they were serotypes 15 F/15A, 20 and 34, respectively. Thirteen serotype 23 F isolates belonging to four new *cpsB* sequetypes, were assigned new sequetype names after mPCR confirmed them as serotype 23 F. Four isolates identified by *cpsB* sequetyping as 10B, 28 F/28A, were non-typeable by mPCR because the serotype primer sets were not included in the USA CDC multiplex reaction scheme (Table 1, Additional file 4: Table S3). Two isolates (ID 250, 268 in Additional file 4: Table S3) showed unknown sequetype in *cpsB* sequetyping, and were also not amplified by any specific primer sets.

Serotypes 6A-6D specific PCRs results

The distribution of serotypes 6A-6D among the 27 serogroup 6 isolates were: 6A (12/27, 44.4 %), 6B (13/27, 48.1 %) and 6C (2/27, 7.4 %) and serotype 6D was not detected.

Serotype distribution

Using the sequence-based method selectively supplemented with sequential multiplex PCR and serotypes 6A-6D specific PCRs strategy, sixteen serotypes were identified from 193 *S. pneumoniae* isolates. They included 19 F (67, 34.7 %), 23 F (33, 17.1 %), 19A (23, 11.9 %), 14 (14, 7.3 %), 15B/15C (13, 6.7 %), 6B (13, 6.7 %), 6A (12, 6.2 %), 9 V/9A (3, 1.6 %); serotypes 6C, 3, 15 F/15A and 20 (2 each, 1.1 %); serotypes 10B, 28 F/28A and 34 (1 each, 0.5 %). The 10-valent PCV (PCV-10) vaccines cover 67.4 % of the serotypes identified, whilst the 13-valent PCV (PCV-13) covers 86.5 %. A total of 126 isolates were from patients less than 2 years of age, including 39 isolates of serotypes 19 F (30.9 %), 23 of 23 F (18.3 %), 16 of 19A (12.7 %), 10 of 15B/15C (7.9 %), 10 of 6A (7.9 %), 9 of 14 (7.1 %), 8 of 6B (6.3 %); 2 each of 20 and 15 F/15A (1.6 %); and 1 each of 9 V/9A, 3, 34, 10B and 23A (0.8 %). PCV-10 covers 70.6 % of these strains whilst PCV-13 covers 92 %. There was no significant difference between serotype distribution and clinical presentation (see Additional file 5: Table S4).

Antimicrobial susceptibility

Susceptibility results for the *S. pneumoniae* isolates are shown in Table 2. The resistance rates for erythromycin, clindamycin, sulfamethoxazole-trimethoprim and tetracycline, ranged from 87.6 to 97.4 %. According to the revised CLSI breakpoints for parenteral penicillin, the prevalence rates for penicillin resistance were 1.0 and 88.6 % in the non-meningitis and meningitis isolates, respectively. The proportion of isolates resistant to ceftriaxone was 5.2 % for non-meningitis, and 25.4 % for meningitis isolates. All the isolates were susceptible to vancomycin. The percentage of MDR isolates was 86.8 % (167/193), and the most common pattern was resistance to erythromycin + clindamycin + sulfamethoxazole-trimethoprim (167/193, 86.8 %), followed by resistance to erythromycin + clindamycin + sulfamethoxazole-trimethoprim + tetracycline (150/193, 77.9 %), and erythromycin + clindamycin + sulfamethoxazole-trimethoprim + tetracycline + chloramphenicol (22/193, 11.5 %). Antibiotic resistance was clustered mainly in serotype 19 F, with resistant rates to parenteral penicillin, ceftriaxone and erythromycin of 1.5, 14.9, and 97 % respectively. The other half of the penicillin resistant isolates was identified as serotype 23 F (3 %) (Additional file 6: Table S5). For the penicillin, ceftriaxone parenteral resistant non-meningitis isolates, the multidrug resistance patterns were; erythromycin + clindamycin + sulfamethoxazole-trimethoprim + tetracycline + chloramphenicol + penicillin + ceftriaxone ($n = 1$); erythromycin + clindamycin + sulfamethoxazole-trimethoprim + tetracycline + penicillin + ceftriaxone ($n = 1$); erythromycin + clindamycin + sulfamethoxazole-trimethoprim + tetracycline + ceftriaxone ($n = 6$); erythromycin + clindamycin + sulfamethoxazole-trimethoprim + ceftriaxone ($n = 2$).

Discussion

Most DNA-based methods allow the identification of a limited number of *S. pneumoniae* serotypes or serogroups. Since not all of the 95 described capsular types cause serious infections, it is important to develop a capsular typing scheme targeting serotypes most frequently associated with serious diseases [11]. In addition, after introduction of the pneumococcal conjugate vaccines, serotyping or serotype prediction assays are needed to

Table 2 Prevalence of antibiotic susceptibility to nine antimicrobials for 193 *S. pneumoniae* isolates from children

Antimicrobial	No. (%) of isolates			MIC (ug/mL)		
	Susceptible	Intermediate	Resistant	MIC_{50}	MIC_{90}	Range
Penicillin						0.016–8.0
Non-meningitis isolates						
Parenteral	176 (91.2)	15 (7.8)	2 (1.0)	1	2	
Oral	22 (11.4)	95 (49.2)	76 (39.4)	1	2	
Meningitis isolates	22 (11.4)	0 (0)	171 (88.6)	1	2	
Ceftriaxone						0.016–6.0
Non-meningitis isolates	144 (74.6)	39 (20.2)	10 (5.2)	0.75	2	
Meningitis isolates	83 (43.0)	61 (31.6)	49 (25.4)	0.75	2	
Erythromycin	2 (1.0)	3 (1.6)	188 (97.4)			
Vancomycin	193 (100)	0(0)	0(0)			
Levofloxacin	191 (99)	2 (1.0)	0 (0)			
Tetracycline	9 (4.7)	12 (6.2)	172 (89.1)			
Chloramphenicol	168 (87.0)	0 (0)	25 (13)			
Sulfamethoxazole-trimethoprim	14 (7.3)	10 (5.2)	169 (87.6)			
Clindamycin	5 (2.6)	1 (0.5)	187 (96.9)			

monitor serotype switch from vaccine serotypes to non-vaccine serotypes [21].

Because of the existence of 95 different *S. pneumoniae* capsular types, it is difficult to develop a simple practical molecular typing scheme based on genetic approaches. In the present study, we developed a strategy to address this challenge. To our knowledge, it is the most comprehensive *cpsB* sequetyping database to date. Having more serotype sequetypes and sequetypes with multiple identical *cpsB* sequences in the sequetyping database, leads to more accurate serotype prediction compared to Leung's study.

For most of our local isolates (except 2 non-serotypeable), *cpsB* sequetyping would be a more straightforward way to predict serotypes. Although molecular assays are generally considered unaffordable for most developing countries, PCR reagents are commonly available in most laboratories in China, and are relatively inexpensive. Furthermore, commercial sequencing is also affordable, convenient and cheap (~U$ 2.5/each reaction) for the majority of clinical labs. In our laboratory, *cpsB* sequencing is performed when a sufficient number of samples have been submitted for a run, which makes the cost very reasonable, and enables the lab to operate more efficiently. However, we found that many GenBank sequences share the same *cpsB* sequences (Additional file 3: Table S2), between both related serotypes (antigenic cross-reaction) and unrelated serotypes (no antigenic cross-reaction), probably due to recombination events [22]. In this study, sequetyping characterized 34.2 % isolates to serotype level and 55.4 % isolates to serogroup level. Multiplex PCR (mPCR) was needed to make a definite serotype prediction or increase the serotype prediction accuracy. But in most cases, *cpsB* sequetyping had already defined the test isolates to a smaller serotype group range, which made mPCR set selection much easier and saved from having to perform eight sequential mPCR. We only needed to resolve those *cpsB* sequetypes which were shared by different serotypes (e.g., 13-20A-20B, 15A-33B, 17A-34) or for isolates non-typeable by *cpsB* sequetyping (Fig. 1). In fact, only 115 (59.5 %) of sequetyping results needed to be confirmed by selected sets of mPCR in this study.

Furthermore, using the mPCR, most serotypes were identified in the first three sets of mPCR reactions, and only seven (3.6 %) isolates required further testing of up to eight sequential sets of multiplex reactions. After we update our new *cpsB* sequetyping database in the future, the number of isolates requiring mPCR confirmation would be much less than 59.5 % isolates, with most of them identified in the first three mPCR reactions. We also identified some new sequetypes within serotypes 23 F, 6A, 15 F/15A, 3 and rare serotype 20, which will improve the serotype prediction accuracy besides reducing the necessity of performing eight sequential multiplex reactions.

Although molecular methods are becoming increasingly utilized for pneumococcal typing, phenotypic methods including Quellung reaction and latex agglutination, remain the most reliable way to discover possible false-positive PCR results, which is fairly rare, but can occur (Fig. 1) [23]. However, some isolates are genotypeable by microarray or sequencing, but non-typeable by the Quellung reaction and latex agglutination [10, 24], suggesting caution must be exercised when interpreting controversial results

(Fig. 1). In reality, genotyping, no matter how accurate it is, is only a method for prediction of serotypes/serogroups, not a replacement method for conventional serotyping, because "serotype" is traditionally a phenotypic rather than a genotype based definition.

The distribution of *S. pneumoniae* serotypes differ by geographic region. Several studies conducted over the years in China demonstrated great diversity in the distribution of *S. pneumoniae* serotypes by region [25, 26]. Bao'an district, the biggest administrative region in Shenzhen City, has a population of 6 million, of which 90 % are floating (temporary) residents as this city shares a border with Hong Kong. In this region, the immunization level for PCV7 vaccine has been less than 1 % for the past 5 years. Our study identified 16 serotypes, seven (19 F, 23 F, 19A, 14, 15B/15C, 6B and 6A) of which accounted for 90.7 % of the isolates, which is in general agreement to another study in Shenzhen [3]. Furthermore, our study confirmed previous findings showing that serotype 19A is one of the most common serotypes in Shenzhen [3] and China [27], which is not related to the introduction of PCV-7 vaccine, but to widespread antimicrobial use, similar to the situation in Korea [28]. A further 15 (7.8 %) of the 193 isolates belonged to serogroup 15 (2 serotype 15 F/ 15A isolates; 13 serotype 15B/15C isolates), which is quite similar to the pre-PVC7 period proportion in Hong Kong for serogroup 15 (5.7 %) [29].

It has been reported that serotypes 1, 2, 7, 9, 14, and 16 are among the most invasive serotypes, whilst serotypes 3, 6, 15, 19, and 23 are considered least invasive serotypes [30, 31]. However, Picazo et al. reported that serotype 19A was linked to non-respiratory IPDs in children of <24 months [32], whilst Hausdorff et al. found that serotypes 1 and 14 were more often isolated from blood, and serogroups 3, 19, and 23, more often isolated from middle ear fluid [33]. In the present study, no significant differences were noted between serotype and clinical presentation, which could be due to limited number of isolates and/or disease categories studied.

Prevention of pneumococcal disease includes vaccination with pneumococcal polysaccharide conjugate vaccines especially in children. Based on the distribution of serotypes in all patients in our study population (age from 27 days to 6 years and 5 months), the PCV-10 vaccine would cover 67.4 % of the serotypes, whilst the PCV-13 vaccine would cover 86.5 % of the serotypes found in the area. The major target population for vaccination and prevention is children under 2 years of age. PCV-13 still showed higher coverage (92 %) in <2 year old patients in our study population compare to PCV-10 (70.6 %). Specifically, the significantly increased coverage by PCV13 in our study population is due to high prevalence of serotypes 19A (23, 11.9 %) and 6A (12, 6.2 %), which together with serotype 3, are contained in the PCV-13 vaccine but not in the PCV-10 [3]. These findings suggest that PCV-13 should be the major target for future development and applications in our community, since PCV-7 is no longer available, and PCV-10 has less coverage.

The low prevalence rate of parenteral penicillin resistance (1.0 %) among the non-meningitis isolates in our study is noted, and suggests that hospitalized children with non-meningitis pneumococcal infections can be treated with parenteral penicillin. It has been reported that seven (6A, 6B, 9 V, 14, 19A, 19 F, 23 F) out of 95 serotypes are associated with antibiotic resistance [34]. Interestingly, these seven serotypes accounted for 85.5 % of our 193 isolates, which could explain the high prevalence rate of multidrug resistance (86.8 %) in the present study (Additional file 6: Table S5).

This study has several limitations. First, the number of isolates from blood and cerebrospinal fluid was small, which limited statistical power. Furthermore, 87.6 % isolates were from sputum, some of which may be colonizing organisms since certain *S. pneumoniae* serotypes have a propensity for colonization without necessarily causing disease. However, it is believed that invasive disease originates from colonization and that serotype distribution among colonizing strains, is an indicator of the diversity of pneumococcal strains circulating in the community [35]. Furthermore, our sputum specimen sampling strategy, including using the quality criteria, would have minimized the level of contamination from colonizing strains. Secondly, all data presented here is from one of the biggest district hospitals, so we can't overplay the data to represent more rural regions though it would be representative of our Bao'an District hospitalized children.

Conclusions

This study provides a cost-effective alternative *S. pneumoniae* serotype prediction strategy to conventional serotyping. We showcased the utility of this new serotyping strategy by identifying serotypes of 193 *S. pneumoniae* isolates from children. This strategy enables most routine laboratories equipped with PCR to predict the majority of pneumococcal serotypes without the need for an expensive set of serological reagents in China. This study confirms that serotype 19A is common in China, and that PCV13 vaccine would be important for future vaccination in areas such as Shenzhen. Considering the low resistance rate in non-meningitis isolates to parenteral penicillin, clinicians should be encouraged to increase the use of penicillin to treat penicillin-susceptible non-meningitis pneumococcal infections, instead of using broader-spectrum antimicrobials. Continued surveillance of the serotype distribution and antimicrobial susceptibility of *S. pneumoniae* isolates in China is warranted.

Availability of data and materials

The datasets supporting the conclusions of this article are included within the article and its additional files. Patient age and gender were part of the original dataset used in our study. We have, however, removed this information from the clinical dataset provided in Additional file 1: Table S1 in order to protect the patients' identity. The GenBank/EMBL/DDBJ accession numbers for the new *cpsB* sequences from this study have been submitted to GenBank with accession numbers KT164777-KT164783 and are listed in Additional file 4: Table S3.

Additional files

Additional file 1: Table S1. Clinical information of our 193 isolates.

Additional file 2: Figure S1. The algorithm show how we build up the comprehensive GenBank *cpsB* seuquetyping database as Additional file 3: Table S2.

Additional file 3: Table S2. Comprehensive *cpsB* sequetyping database based on GenBank sequences (until Jan 1, 2015).

Additional file 4: Table S3. The *cpsB* sequetyping results of our 193 local isolates.

Additional file 5: Table S4. Serotype distribution by clinical presentation among our 193 *S. pneumonie* isolates from children.

Additional file 6: Table S5. Percentages of resistant to antibiotics for serotypes with 10 or more isolates.

Abbreviations

CDC: centers for disease control and prevention; CLSI: the Clinical and Laboratory Standards Institute; MDR: multidrug- resistance; mPCR: multiplex PCR; PCV-10: 10-valent PCV; PCV-13: 13-valent PCV; PCV7: 7-valent pneumococcal conjugate vaccine; *S. pneumoniae*: *Streptococcus pneumoniae*.

Competing interests

The authors declare that they have no competing interests.

Authors' contributions

PJ conceived the study, participated in its design, executed the studies and drafted the manuscript. LW cultured the isolates, performed drug sensitivity testing and assisted in preparation of the manuscript. FK participated in the design of the study, performed the sequencing results analysis, coordinated acquisition and interpretation of data, and helped to modify the manuscript. SH and TK helped to edit the manuscript. QZ coordinated the execution of the studies and corrected the manuscript. All authors read and approved the final manuscript.

Acknowledgements

The authors appreciate the assistance of Zehao Yan, who provided DNA preparation.

Funding

The research was supported by Shenzhen Science and Technology Research and Development funds (JCYJ20140416085544654) and Guangdong Provincial Science and Technology Department Funds (2014A020212382).

Author details

[1]Pediatric Center, Zhujiang Hospital, Southern Medical University, Guangzhou 510282, P. R. China. [2]Paediatric Intensive Care Unit, Bao'an Maternity & Child Health Hospital affiliated with Jinan University, Shenzhen, P. R. China. [3]Department of Clinical Laboratory, Bao'an Maternity & Child Health Hospital affiliated with Jinan University, Shenzhen, P. R. China. [4]Centre for Infectious Diseases and Microbiology Laboratory Services, ICPMR – Pathology West, University of Sydney, Westmead Hospital, Darcy Road, Westmead, NSW, Australia. [5]Charles Sturt University, Leeds Parade, Orange, NSW, Australia.

References

1. O'Brien KL, Wolfson LJ, Watt JP, Henkle E, Deloria-Knoll M, McCall N, et al. Burden of disease caused by *Streptococcus pneumoniae* in children younger than 5 years: global estimates. Lancet. 2009;374(9693):893–902.
2. Xue L, Yao KH, Yu SJ, Liu ZJ, Qian J, Shen XZ, et al. Molecular epidemiology of serotype 19A *Streptococcus pneumoniae* isolated from children in Beijing, 1997–2006. Chin Med J. 2011;124(12):1769–74.
3. Ma X, Zhao R, Ma Z, Yao K, Yu S, Zheng Y, et al. Serotype distribution and antimicrobial resistance of *streptococcus pneumoniae* isolates causing invasive diseases from Shenzhen Children's hospital. PLoS One. 2013;8(6):e67507.
4. Jin P, Kong F, Xiao M, Oftadeh S, Zhou F, Liu C, et al. First report of putative *Streptococcus pneumoniae* serotype 6D among nasopharyngeal isolates from Fijian children. J Infect Dis. 2009;200(9):1375–80.
5. Calix JJ, Nahm MH. A new pneumococcal serotype, 11E, has a variably inactivated wcjE gene. J Infect Dis. 2010;202(1):29–38.
6. Ko KS, Baek JY, Song JH. Capsular gene sequences and genotypes of "serotype 6E" *Streptococcus pneumoniae* isolates. J Clin Microbiol. 2013; 51(10):3395–99.
7. Turner P, Turner C, Jankhot A, Phakaudom K, Nosten F, Goldblatt D. Field evaluation of culture plus latex sweep serotyping for detection of multiple pneumococcal serotype colonisation in infants and young children. PLoS One. 2013;8(7):e67933.
8. Batt SL, Charalambous BM, McHugh TD, Martin S, Gillespie SH. Novel PCR-restriction fragment length polymorphism method for determining serotypes or serogroups of *Streptococcus pneumoniae* isolates. J Clin Microbiol. 2005;43(6):2656–61.
9. Kong F, Brown M, Sabananthan A, Zeng X, Gilbert GL. Multiplex PCR-based reverse line blot hybridization assay to identify 23 *Streptococcus pneumoniae* polysaccharide vaccine serotypes. J Clin Microbiol. 2006;44(5):1887–91.
10. Kong F, Wang W, Tao J, Wang L, Wang Q, Sabananthan A, et al. A molecular-capsular-type prediction system for 90 *Streptococcus pneumoniae* serotypes using partial cpsA-cpsB sequencing and wzy- or wzx-specific PCR. J Med Microbiol. 2005;54(Pt 4):351–56.
11. Pai R, Gertz RE, Beall B. Sequential multiplex PCR approach for determining capsular serotypes of *Streptococcus pneumoniae* isolates. J Clin Microbiol. 2006;44(1):124–31.
12. Tomita Y, Okamoto A, Yamada K, Yagi T, Hasegawa Y, Ohta M. A new microarray system to detect *Streptococcus pneumoniae* serotypes. J Biomed Biotechnol. 2011;2011:352736.
13. Leung MH, Bryson K, Freystatter K, Pichon B, Edwards G, Charalambous BM, et al. Sequetyping: serotyping *Streptococcus pneumoniae* by a single PCR sequencing strategy. J Clin Microbiol. 2012;50(7):2419–27.
14. Raymond F, Boucher N, Allary R, Robitaille L, Lefebvre B, Tremblay C, et al. Serotyping of *Streptococcus pneumoniae* based on capsular genes polymorphisms. PLoS One. 2013;8(9):e76197.
15. Selva L, del Amo E, Brotons P, Munoz-Almagro C. Rapid and easy identification of capsular serotypes of *Streptococcus pneumoniae* by use of fragment analysis by automated fluorescence-based capillary electrophoresis. J Clin Microbiol. 2012;50(11):3451–57.
16. Agweyu A, Kibore M, Digolo L, Kosgei C, Maina V, Mugane S, et al. Prevalence and correlates of treatment failure among Kenyan children hospitalised with severe community-acquired pneumonia: a prospective study of the clinical effectiveness of WHO pneumonia case management guidelines. Trop Med Int Health. 2014;19(11):1310–20.
17. Patrick R, Murray. Manual of Clinical microbiology 9th Edition: Specimen collection, Transport, and Processing: Bacteriology. Am Soc Microbiol. 2007; 1:319–320.
18. Kim SH, Song JH, Chung DR, Thamlikitkul V, Yang Y, Wang H, et al. Changing trends in antimicrobial resistance and serotypes of *streptococcus pneumoniae* isolates in Asian countries: an Asian network for surveillance of resistant pathogens (ANSORP) study. Antimicrob Agents Chemother. 2012; 56(3):1418–26.
19. Zhang YJ, Chen YS, Wang ZW, Li YQ, Wang DX, Shang Y, et al. Serological and molecular capsular typing, antibiotic susceptibility and multilocus sequence typing of *Streptococcus pneumoniae* isolates from invasive and non-invasive infections. Chin Med J (Engl). 2013;126(12):2296–303.

20. Clinical and Laboratory Standards Institute. Performance standards for antimicrobial susceptibility testing; 25st informational supplement, vol. 31. Wayne: Clinical and Laboratory Standards Institute; 2015. p. 90–5. M100-S25.
21. Tocheva AS, Jefferies JM, Rubery H, Bennett J, Afimeke G, Garland J, et al. Declining serotype coverage of new pneumococcal conjugate vaccines relating to the carriage of *Streptococcus pneumoniae* in young children. Vaccine. 2011;29(26):4400–04.
22. Coffey TJ, Daniels M, Enright MC, Spratt BG. Serotype 14 variants of the Spanish penicillin-resistant serotype 9V clone of *Streptococcus pneumoniae* arose by large recombinational replacements of the cpsA-pbp1a region. Microbiology. 1999;145(Pt 8):2023–31.
23. Siira L, Kaijalainen T, Lambertsen L, Nahm MH, Toropainen M, Virolainen A. From Quellung to multiplex PCR, and back when needed, in pneumococcal serotyping. J Clin Microbiol. 2012;50(8):2727–31.
24. Scott JR, Hinds J, Gould KA, Millar EV, Reid R, Santosham M, et al. Nontypeable pneumococcal isolates among navajo and white mountain apache communities: are these really a cause of invasive disease? J Infect Dis. 2012;206(1):73–80.
25. Liu Y, Wang H, Chen M, Sun Z, Zhao R, Zhang L, et al. Serotype distribution and antimicrobial resistance patterns of *Streptococcus pneumoniae* isolated from children in China younger than 5 years. Diagn Microbiol Infect Dis. 2008;61(3):256–63.
26. Yao KH, Wang LB, Zhao GM, Zheng YJ, Deng L, Huang JF, et al. Pneumococcal serotype distribution and antimicrobial resistance in Chinese children hospitalized for pneumonia. Vaccine. 2011;29(12):2296–301.
27. Xue L, Yao K, Xie G, Zheng Y, Wang C, Shang Y, et al. Serotype distribution and antimicrobial resistance of *Streptococcus pneumoniae* isolates that cause invasive disease among Chinese children. Clin Infect Dis. 2010;50(5):741–44.
28. Choi EH, Kim SH, Eun BW, Kim SJ, Kim NH, Lee J, et al. Streptococcus pneumoniae serotype 19A in children. South Korea Emerg Infect Dis. 2008; 14(2):275–81.
29. Liyanapathirana V, Nelson EA, Ang I, Subramanian R, Ma H, Ip M. Emergence of serogroup 15 *Streptococcus pneumoniae* of diverse genetic backgrounds following the introduction of pneumococcal conjugate vaccines in Hong Kong. Diagn Microbiol Infect Dis. 2015;81(1):66–70.
30. Brueggemann AB, Griffiths DT, Meats E, Peto T, Crook DW, Spratt BG. Clonal relationships between invasive and carriage *Streptococcus pneumoniae* and serotype- and clone-specific differences in invasive disease potential. J Infect Dis. 2003;187(9):1424–32.
31. Smith T, Lehmann D, Montgomery J, Gratten M, Riley ID, Alpers MP. Acquisition and invasiveness of different serotypes of *Streptococcus pneumoniae* in young children. Epidemiol Infect. 1993;111(1):27–39.
32. Picazo J, Ruiz-Contreras J, Casado-Flores J, Giangaspro E, Del Castillo F, Hernandez-Sampelayo T, et al. Relationship between serotypes, age, and clinical presentation of invasive pneumococcal disease in Madrid, Spain, after introduction of the 7-valent pneumococcal conjugate vaccine into the vaccination calendar. Clin Vaccine Immunol. 2011;18(1):89–94.
33. Hausdorff WP, Bryant J, Kloek C, Paradiso PR, Siber GR. The contribution of specific pneumococcal serogroups to different disease manifestations: implications for conjugate vaccine formulation and use, part II. Clin Infect Dis. 2000;30(1):122–40.
34. Dagan R, Klugman KP. Impact of conjugate pneumococcal vaccines on antibiotic resistance. Lancet Infect Dis. 2008;8(12):785–95.
35. Chen Y, Deng W, Wang SM, Mo QM, Jia H, Wang Q, et al. Burden of pneumonia and meningitis caused by *Streptococcus pneumoniae* in China among children under 5 years of age: a systematic literature review. PLoS One. 2011;6(11):e27333.

Permissions

All chapters in this book were first published in PEDIATRICS, by BioMed Central; hereby published with permission under the Creative Commons Attribution License or equivalent. Every chapter published in this book has been scrutinized by our experts. Their significance has been extensively debated. The topics covered herein carry significant findings which will fuel the growth of the discipline. They may even be implemented as practical applications or may be referred to as a beginning point for another development.

The contributors of this book come from diverse backgrounds, making this book a truly international effort. This book will bring forth new frontiers with its revolutionizing research information and detailed analysis of the nascent developments around the world.

We would like to thank all the contributing authors for lending their expertise to make the book truly unique. They have played a crucial role in the development of this book. Without their invaluable contributions this book wouldn't have been possible. They have made vital efforts to compile up to date information on the varied aspects of this subject to make this book a valuable addition to the collection of many professionals and students.

This book was conceptualized with the vision of imparting up-to-date information and advanced data in this field. To ensure the same, a matchless editorial board was set up. Every individual on the board went through rigorous rounds of assessment to prove their worth. After which they invested a large part of their time researching and compiling the most relevant data for our readers.

The editorial board has been involved in producing this book since its inception. They have spent rigorous hours researching and exploring the diverse topics which have resulted in the successful publishing of this book. They have passed on their knowledge of decades through this book. To expedite this challenging task, the publisher supported the team at every step. A small team of assistant editors was also appointed to further simplify the editing procedure and attain best results for the readers.

Apart from the editorial board, the designing team has also invested a significant amount of their time in understanding the subject and creating the most relevant covers. They scrutinized every image to scout for the most suitable representation of the subject and create an appropriate cover for the book.

The publishing team has been an ardent support to the editorial, designing and production team. Their endless efforts to recruit the best for this project, has resulted in the accomplishment of this book. They are a veteran in the field of academics and their pool of knowledge is as vast as their experience in printing. Their expertise and guidance has proved useful at every step. Their uncompromising quality standards have made this book an exceptional effort. Their encouragement from time to time has been an inspiration for everyone.

The publisher and the editorial board hope that this book will prove to be a valuable piece of knowledge for researchers, students, practitioners and scholars across the globe.

List of Contributors

Qian Peng and Hanmin Liu
Department of Pediatric Cardiology, West China Second University Hospital/West China Women's and Children's Hospital, West China School of Medicine, Sichuan University, Chengdu 610041, China
Key Laboratory of Birth Defects and Related Diseases of Women and Children (Sichuan University), Ministry of Education, Chengdu 610041, China

Qian Peng
Department of Pediatrics, Sichuan Academy of Medical Sciences and Sichuan Provincial People's Hospital, Chengdu 610072, China

Yan Deng
Department of Cardiovascular Ultrasound and Non-invasive Cardiology, Sichuan Academy of Medical Sciences and Sichuan Provincial People's Hospital, Chengdu 610072, China

Yuan Yang
Department of Medical Genetics, West China Hospital, West China School of Medicine, Sichuan University, Chengdu 610041, China

Khansoudaphone Phakhounthong, Podjanee Jittamala and Pan-ngum
Department of Tropical Hygiene (Biomedical and Health Informatics), Faculty of Tropical Medicine, Mahidol University, Bangkok, Thailand

Pimwadee Chaovalit
National Electronics and Computer Technology Center (NECTEC), Bangkok, Thailand

Podjanee Jittamala, Stuart D. Blacksell, Nicholas P. J. Day, Lisa J. White and Wirichada Pan-ngum
Mahidol-Oxford Tropical Medicine Research Unit, Faculty of Tropical Medicine, Mahidol University, Bangkok, Thailand

Stuart D. Blacksell, Paul Turner, Nicholas P. J. Day and Lisa J. White
Centre for Tropical Medicine and Global Health, Nuffield Department of Medicine, University of Oxford, Oxford, UK

Michael J. Carter
Institute of Child Health, University College London, London, UK

Paul Turner, Kheng Chheng, Soeung Sona, Varun Kumar and Nicholas P. J. Day
Angkor Hospital for Children, Siem Reap, Cambodia

Gunta Laizane, Marita Cikovska, Ilze Grope and Dace Gardovska
Department of Paediatrics, Riga Stradins University, Vienibas gatve 45, Riga LV-1004, Latvias

Anda Kivite and Inese Stars
Department of Public Health and Epidemiology, Riga Stradins University, Kronvalda boulevard 9, Riga LV-1010, Latvia

Min Li, Jia Liu, Huan Yi, Li Xu and Fuhua Peng
Multiple Sclerosis Center, Department of Neurology, the Third Affiliated Hospital of Sun Yat-Sen University, Guangzhou, Guangdong 510630, China

Xiufeng Zhong
State Key Laboratory of Ophthalmology, Zhongshan Ophthalmic Center, Sun Yat-sen Univeristy, Guangzhou, Guangdong 510060, China

Marina Kreitschmann
Private Practice Dr. Thomas Hinz, Dr. Uta Neumann, Stoeckstraße 106, 44649 Herne, Germany

Lea C. Epping
Private Practice, Weststraße 1, 49176 Hilter, Germany

Ariane Hohoff and Thomas Stamm
Department of Orthodontics, University of Münster, Albert-Schweitzer-Campus 1, 48149 Münster, Germany

Cristina Sauerland
Institute of Biostatistics and Clinical Research, University of Münster, Schmeddingstraße 56, 48149 Münster, Germany

Molla Taye
Department of Anatomy, School of Medicine, College of Medicine and Health Sciences, the University of Gondar, Gondar, Ethiopia

Mekbeb Afework
Department of Anatomy, School of Medicine, College of Health Sciences, Addis Ababa University, Addis Ababa, Ethiopia

Wondwossen Fantaye
School of Dentistry, College of Health Sciences, Addis Ababa University, Addis Ababa, Ethiopia

Ermias Diro
School of Medicine, College of Medicine and Health Sciences, the University of Gondar, Gondar, Ethiopia

Alemayehu Worku
School of Public Health, College of Health Sciences, Addis Ababa University, Addis Ababa, Ethiopia

Yu-lin Kang, Ying Wu, Shen Hao, Xin-yu Kuang, Wen-yan Huang and Guang-hua Zhu
Department of Nephrology and Rheumatology, Shanghai Children's Hospital, Shanghai Jiao Tong University, Shanghai, China

Yu-cai Zhang and Yun Cui
Pediatric Intensive Care Unit, Shanghai Children's Hospital, Shanghai Jiao Tong University, Shanghai, China

Karin Zimmermann, Eva Cignacco and Katri Eskola
Department Public Health (DPH), Nursing Science, University of Basel, Bernoullistrasse 28, 4056 Basel, Switzerland

Karin Zimmermann
Paediatric Palliative Care, University Children's Hospital Zurich, Children's Research Center CRC, Steinwiesstrasse 75, 8032 Zurich, Switzerland

Karin Zimmermann
Department of Pediatrics, Inselspital Bern University Hospital, Bern, Switzerland

Eva Cignacco
Health Division, University of Applied Sciences Bern, Bern, Switzerland

Sandra Engberg
School of Nursing, University of Pittsburgh, 3500 Victoria Street, Pittsburgh, PA 15261, USA

Anne-Sylvie Ramelet
Institute of Higher Education and Research in Healthcare – IUFRS, University of Lausanne, Route de la Corniche 10, 1010 Lausanne, Switzerland
Nurse Research Consultant, Department of Woman-Mother-Child, Lausanne University Hospital CHUV, Lausanne, Switzerland

Nicolas von der Weid
Paediatric Haematology-Oncology, University Children's Hospital UKBB, Spitalstrasse 33, 4056 Basel, Switzerland

Katri Eskola and Eva Bergstraesser
Triemli Hospital Zurich, Zurich, Switzerland

Bobby P. Smyth and Khalifa Elmusharafs
Department of Public Health and Primary Care, Trinity College Dublin, Dublin Ireland
Graduate Entry Medical School, University of Limerick, Limerick, Ireland

Bobby P. Smyth
National Drug Treatment Centre, 30/31 Pearse St, Dublin 2, Ireland

Walter Cullen
Academic General Practice, School of Medicine, University College Dublin, Belfield, Dublin 4, Ireland

Bobby P. Smyth
HSE Addiction Service, Bridge House, Cherry Orchard Hospital, Dublin 10, Ireland

Joana Kist-van Holthe, Tirza Blom, Laura Melchers, Teatske Altenburg, Remy HiraSing and Mai Chinapaw
Department of Public and Occupational Health, Amsterdam Public Health Research Institute, VU Medical Center, Amsterdam, the Netherlands

Alcira Janga-Jansen, Tahirih van Kanten and Marian Luinstra-Passchier
Department of Public Health, Openbaar Lichaam Bonaire, Bonaire, the Netherlands

Elena Chiappini, Antonina Marta Cangelosi, Luisa Galli and Maurizio de Martino
Department of Health Sciences, Anna Meyer Children's University Hospital, University of Florence, Viale Pieraccini, 24, 50100 Florence, Italy

Paolo Becherucci and Monica Pierattelli
Primary Care Paediatrician, Florence, Italy

Vidit Bhargava and Daniel Tawfik
Department of Pediatrics, Division of Pediatric Critical Care, Lucile Salter Packard Children's Hospital, 770 Welch Road, Suite 435, Palo Alto, CA 94304, USA

Bruce Niebuhr
Department of Pediatrics, University of Texas Medical Branch, Galveston, TX, USA

Sunil K. Jain
Department of Pediatrics, Division of Neonatology, University of Texas Medical Branch, Galveston, TX, USA

Jie Li, Rong Zhu, Yuxiang Yan, Yanxia Luo and Yan He
Department of Epidemiology and Biostatistics, School of Public Health, Capital Medical University, No. 10 Xitoutiao, You'anmen Wai, Fengtai District, Beijing 100069, People's Republic of China

Jie Li, Da Huo, Yiwei Du, Zhichao Liang, Yang Yang, Lei Jia, Lijuan Chen and Quanyi Wang
Institute for Infectious Disease and Endemic Disease Control, Beijing Center for Disease Prevention and Control, No.16, Hepingli Middle Street, Beijing 100013, People's Republic of China

Nehla Ghedira, Karim Ben Ameur, Rania Sakka, Emna Kerkeni, Fatma-Zohra Chioukh and Kamel Monastiri
Research Unit 01/UR/08-14, Faculty of Medicine of Monastir, University of Monastir, Avenue Avicenne, 5019 Monastir, Tunisia

Nehla Ghedira, Arnaud Lagarde, Sahar Elouej, Sylviane Olschwang, Jean-Pierre Desvignes, Valerie Delague, Nicolas Lévy and Annachiara De Sandre-Giovannoli
Aix Marseille University, INSERM, GMGF, Marseille, France

Karim Ben Ameur, Rania Sakka, Fatma-Zohra Chioukh and Kamel Monastiri
Department of Intensive Care and Neonatal Medicine, Fattouma Bourguiba University Hospital, Monastir,Tunisia

Arnaud Lagarde, Sylviane Olschwang, Nicolas Lévy and Annachiara De Sandre-Giovannoli
Departement of Medical Genetics, Childrens' Hospital La Timone, 264 Rue Saint Pierre, Marseille, France

Sylviane Olschwang
Groupe Ramsay Générale de Santé, Hôpital Clairval, Marseille, France

Sahar Elouej and Sonia Abdelhak
Institut Pasteur de Tunis, Laboratoire de Genomique Biomedicale et Oncogenetique LR11IPT05, Tunis, Tunisia

S. Haithar and M. Kumar
Department of Psychiatry, College of Health Sciences, University of Nairobi, Nairobi 00101, Kenya

M. W. Kuria and M. Kumar
Research Department of Clinical, Health and Educational Psychology, University College London, London WC1E 7HB, UK

A. Sheikh
Department of Clinical Medicine and Therapeutics, College of Health Sciences, University of Nairobi, Nairobi 00202, Kenya

A. Vander Stoep
Psychiatry and Behavioral Sciences and Epidemiology, 6200 NE 74th Street, Suite 210, Seattle, WA 88115-1538, USA

Ayana Chimdessa
School of Nursing and Midwifery, College of Health Sciences, Wollega University, Nekemte, Ethiopia

Amsale Cheire
College of Health Science, Addis Ababa University, Addis Ababa, Ethiopia

Randall W. Grout, Rachel Thompson-Fleming and Stephen M. Downs
Children's Health Services Research, Department of Pediatrics, Indiana University School of Medicine, 410 W. 10th Street, HS 2000, Indianapolis, IN 46202, USA

Aaron E. Carroll
Pediatric and Adolescent Comparative Effectiveness Research, Department of Pediatrics, Indiana University School of Medicine, 410 W. 10th Street, HS 2000A, Indianapolis, IN 46202, USA

Aaron E. Carroll and Stephen M. Downs
Regenstrief Institute, Inc, 1101 W. 10th Street, Indianapolis, IN 46202, USA

Rachel Thompson-Fleming
Children's Hospital of Wisconsin, 8915 W Connell Ct, Milwaukee, WI 53326, USA

Qinghong Meng, Lijun Li, Wei Shi, Qing Wang and Kaihu Yao
Beijing Key Laboratory of Pediatric Respiratory Infection Diseases, Key Laboratory of Major Diseases in Children, Ministry of Education, National Clinical Research Center for Respiratory Diseases, National Key Discipline of Pediatrics (Capital Medical University), Beijing Pediatric Research Institute, Beijing Children's Hospital, Capital Medical University, National Center for Children's Health, Beijing 100045, China

Mingjie Ding, Yanqin Liu and Xiang Ma
Respiratory department, Qilu Children's Hospital, Shandong University, Ji'nan 250022, China

Jingyi Shi, Chunxia Wang, Yun Cui and Yucai Zhang
Department of Critical Care Medicine, Shanghai Children's Hospital, Shanghai Jiao Tong University, No.355 Luding Road, Putuo District, Shanghai 200062, China

Chunxia Wang and Yucai Zhang
Institute of Pediatric Critical Care, Shanghai Jiao Tong University, No.355 Luding Road, Putuo District, Shanghai 200062, China

Anna E. Epperson
Stanford Prevention Research Center, Department of Medicine, Stanford University, 1265 Welch Road, Suite 300, Palo Alto, CA 94305, USA

Jan L. Wallander
Psychological Sciences and Health Sciences Research Institute, University of California, Merced, 5200 Lake Rd, Merced, CA 95340, USA

Marc N. Elliott
RAND Corporation, 1776 Main Street, Santa Monica, CA 90401, USA

Mark A. Schuster
Division of General Pediatrics, Boston Children's Hospital, 300 Longwood Ave, Boston, MA 02115, USA
Department of Pediatrics, Harvard Medical School, 25 Shattuck St, Boston, MA 02115, USA
Kaiser Permanente School of Medicine, 100 S. Los Robles Avenue, Pasadena, CA 91101, USA

Johanna M. Uitti, Paula A. Tähtinen and Aino Ruohola
Department of Paediatrics and Adolescent Medicine, Turku University Hospital, Turku, Finland
Department of Paediatrics and Adolescent Medicine, University of Turku, Turku, Finland

Sanna Salanterä
Department of Nursing Science, University of Turku, Turku, Finland
Hospital District of Southwest Finland, Turku, Finland

Miia K. Laine
Department of Clinical Microbiology, Turku University Hospital, Turku, Finland

Degnet Teferi Asres, Amanuel Nana and Girma Nega
Department of Applied Human Nutrition, Biotechnology Research Institute, Bahir Dar Institute of Technology, Bahir Dar University, Bahir Dar, Ethiopia

Gereltuya Dorj, Tsetsegmaa Sanjjav and Byambatsogt Gendenragchaa
School of Pharmacy and Biomedicine, Mongolian National University of Medical Sciences, S.Zorig Street, Ulaanbaatar 14210, Mongolia

Bruce Sunderland
School of Pharmacy, Bentley, Curtin University, GPO Bentley, WA 6845, Australia

Gantuya Dorj
School of Public Health, Mongolian National University of Medical Sciences, S. Zorig Street, Ulaanbaatar 14210, Mongolia

Idrissa Diawara, Khalid Zerouali and Naima Elmdaghri
Laboratoire de Microbiologie, Faculté de Médecine et de Pharmacie, Hassan II University of Casablanca, B.P 5696 Casablanca, Morocco
Service de Microbiologie, CHU Ibn Rochd, B.P 2698 Casablanca, Morocco

Naima Elmdaghri
Institut Pasteur du Maroc, 1 Louis Pasteur place, Casablanca, Morocco

Lucretia M. Hoffman
Forsyth County Department of Public Health, 201 N Chestnut St, Winston-Salem, NC, USA

Abderrahman Abid
Service des Maladies Infectieuses Pédiatriques, Hôpital d'Enfants Abderrahim Harouchi, CHU Ibn Rochd, Casablanca, Morocco

Molly A Martin
University of Illinois at Chicago, 840 South Wood Street, M/C 856, Chicago, IL 60612, USA

Steven K. Rothschild, Elizabeth Lynch and Kelly Karavolos
Rush University Medical Center, 1700 W Van Buren, Suite 470, Chicago, IL 60612, USA

Katherine Kaufer Christoffel and Anna Barnes
Lurie Children's Hospital, 225 E Chicago Ave, Chicago, IL 60611, USA

Militza M. Pagán
Puerto Rican Cultural Center, 2700 W Haddon Ave, Chicago, IL 60622, USA

Jose Luis Rodriguez
Greater Humboldt Park Community of Wellness, 1116 N. Kedzie, Chicago, IL 60651, USA

Antonieta Diaz
University of Illinois at Chicago, Jane Addams College of Social Work, 1040 West Harrison Street, Chicago, IL 60607, USA

Diana Plata
Rush University Medical Center, College of Medicine, 600 S Paulina St, Chicago, IL 60612, USA

Sandra Villalpando
University of Illinois at Chicago, College of Medicine, 808 S Wood St, Chicago, IL 60612, USA

Ping Jin and Qiyi Zeng
Pediatric Center, Zhujiang Hospital, Southern Medical University, Guangzhou 510282, P. R. China

Ping Jin
Paediatric Intensive Care Unit, Bao'an Maternity and Child Health Hospital affiliated with Jinan University, Shenzhen, P. R. China

Lijuan Wu
Department of Clinical Laboratory, Bao'an Maternity and Child Health Hospital affiliated with Jinan University, Shenzhen, P. R. China

Shahin Oftadeh, Timothy Kudinha and Fanrong Kong
Centre for Infectious Diseases and Microbiology Laboratory Services, ICPMR - Pathology West University of Sydney, Westmead Hospital, Darcy Road, Westmead, NSW, Australia

Timothy Kudinha
Charles Sturt University, Leeds Parade, Orange, NSW, Australia

Index

www.ingramcontent.com/pod-product-compliance
Lightning Source LLC
LaVergne TN
LVHW080703210926
848485LV00003B/413